Understanding Clinical Papers

Third Edition

David Bowers
Leeds Institute of Health Sciences, School of Medicine, University of Leeds, UK

Allan House
Leeds Institute of Health Sciences, School of Medicine, University of Leeds, UK

David Owens
Leeds Institute of Health Sciences, School of Medicine, University of Leeds, UK

Bridgette Bewick
Leeds Institute of Health Sciences, School of Medicine, University of Leeds, UK

WILEY Blackwell

This edition first published 2014 © 2014 by John Wiley and Sons, Ltd.

Second edition published 2006 © 2006 by John Wiley and Sons Ltd
First edition published 2001 © 2001 by John Wiley and Sons Ltd.

Registered office: John Wiley & Sons, Ltd, The Atrium, Southern Gate, Chichester, West Sussex, PO19 8SQ, UK

Editorial offices: 9600 Garsington Road, Oxford, OX4 2DQ, UK
The Atrium, Southern Gate, Chichester, West Sussex, PO19 8SQ, UK
111 River Street, Hoboken, NJ 07030-5774, USA

For details of our global editorial offices, for customer services and for information about how to apply for permission to reuse the copyright material in this book please see our website at www.wiley.com/wiley-blackwell

Library of Congress Cataloging-in-Publication Data

Bowers, David, 1938- author.
    Understanding clinical papers / David Bowers, Allan House, David Owens, Bridgette Bewick. – Third edition.
        p. ; cm.
    Includes bibliographical references and index.
    ISBN 978-1-118-23282-8 (pbk.)
    I. House, Allan, author. II. Owens, David, 1954- author. III. Bewick, Bridgette, author. IV. Title.
    [DNLM: 1. Journalism, Medical. 2. Reading. 3. Writing. WZ 345]
    R853.S7
    610.72′4–dc23
                                                                                                        2013019471

A catalogue record for this book is available from the British Library.

Wiley also publishes its books in a variety of electronic formats. Some content that appears in print may not be available in electronic books.

Cover image: iStock, #4724283 © jmbatt
Cover design by Andy Meaden

Set in 10/12pt Times by Thomson Digital Noida, India
Printed and bound in Malaysia by Vivar Printing Sdn Bhd

2   2014

Understanding
Clinical Papers

>re

Contents

Preface to the First Edition

Buy this book if you are a health-care professional and you want some guidance in understanding the clinical research literature. It is designed to help you with reading research papers, by explaining their structure and the vocabulary they use. These essential first steps will make interpretation of clinical research that much easier for you. For example, the book will help with questions like:

- "Who were the authors, what is their standing, and can they be trusted?"
- "What question or questions did they want to answer, and what was the clinical importance of doing so?"
- "Who were the subjects in the study, how were they chosen, and were the methods used the most suitable?"
- "How were the data collected? Was this the best approach?"
- "What methods did the authors use to analyse the data, and were the methods employed appropriate?"
- "What did they find? Were their conclusions consistent with their results"
- "Were there any shortcomings in the study? Do the authors acknowledge them?"
- "What are the clinical implications of their results?"
- "Does it all make sense?"

This book is *not* an introduction to medical statistics, study design, epidemiology, systematic reviews, evidence-based medicine, or critical appraisal, although we inevitably touch on all of these things (and more). Even so, if you are not already well versed in some of these fields, you should know a lot more by the time you get to the end.

We have concentrated on improving our readers understanding of *quantitative* research papers, and while qualitative papers contain several important elements which we have not been able to cover here, there are many other areas, particularly at the beginning and ends of papers, which readers of qualitative papers will find relevant to their needs.

Primarily, this book should be of interest to the following individuals:

- Clinicians currently practising. This would include GPs, doctors in hospitals, in the community and in public health, nurses, midwives, health visitors, health educators and promoters, physiotherapists, dietitians, chiropodists, speech therapists, radiographers, pharmacists, and other clinically-related specialists.
- Clinicians of all types engaged in research activities: as part of their training; as a condition of their clinical duties; for postgraduate studies and courses; or for professional qualifications.
- Those involved with the education and training of health professionals in colleges of health, in universities, and in in-house training and research departments.
- College, undergraduate, and postgraduate students in all medical and clinical disciplines which involve any element of research methods, medical statistics, epidemiology, critical appraisal, clinical effectiveness, evidence-based medicine, and the like.

In addition, this book should appeal to individuals who although are not themselves clinicians none-the-less find themselves in a clinical setting, and need some understanding of what the published clinical research in their area means. These people would include

- Clinical auditors and quality assessors.
- Clinical managers.
- Service managers, administrators and planners.
- Those working in health authorities and in local government social and health departments.
- Purchasers of health provision.
- People not actually employed in a clinical arena but who none-the-less have a professional or personal interest in the medical literature. For example, members of self-help and support groups (e.g. migraine, stroke, diabetes, Alzheimer's, etc.); medical journalists; research-fund-providers; the educated, interested, lay public.

We have structured the contents of the book into a series of units whose sequence mirrors that of papers in most of the better-quality journals. Thus we start with the preliminaries (title, authors, institution, journal type and status, and so on) and end with the epilogue (discussion, conclusions and clinical implications). Throughout the book we have used a wide variety of extracts from recently published papers to illuminate our textual comments. In these we have focussed largely, but not solely, on examples of *good* practice in the hope that this will provide readers with some "how it should be done" benchmarks. Any errors remain of course our own.

David Bowers, Allan House, David Owens
Leeds, 2001

Preface to the Third Edition

It seems to us quite a long time since the second edition of *Understanding Clinical Papers* was published (in 2005). In the intervening years we have again (as we did for the previous editions) received from readers many favourable comments, as well as some useful suggestions. One suggestion that struck us as being eminently sensible, coinciding with our own thoughts, was that we should introduce material into the book which would help readers understand clinical papers with a *qualitative* design. Such papers are increasingly seen in the mainstream clinical journals (in addition of course to the specialist qualitative journals) and we feel that we should be providing readers with some help in making sense of this content.

The inclusion of five new chapters containing this qualitative material is the most important change in our book from the second edition. We are very pleased to have been able to welcome an experienced qualitative researcher as a co-author, who has contributed this new material.

In addition, we have, not surprisingly, taken the opportunity to update many of the examples of clinical papers with which we illustrate the ideas contained throughout the book. At the same time, we have sharpened and clarified the text where we felt it was needed. We have added small amounts of new material here and there – where we felt that these additions, drawn from our familiarity with the evolving health research literature, would improve the book.

The book should appeal, as before, to doctors, nurses, health visitors, physiotherapists, radiographers, dietitians, speech therapists, health educators and promoters, podiatrists, and all of those other allied professionals (and students in each of these disciplines) – and to all of those involved in health research.

David Bowers, Allan House, David Owens, Bridgette Bewick
Leeds, 2013

I

Setting the Scene:
Who Did What, and Why

1

Some Preliminaries

Before you start reading a paper, you could usefully ask one or two questions which help set the work in context:

- Who wrote the paper?
- In what sort of journal does the paper appear?
- Who (and what) is acknowledged?

WHO WROTE THE PAPER?

Often, one person writes an article such as a review or an editorial. This is less common for papers describing the results of a research study. Because most research is a joint enterprise, papers describing research studies are usually published under the names of a number of people – the research team. From the list of authors, you can tell:

- *The range of expertise of the research team.* Professional backgrounds of the authors (and sometimes their level of seniority) are often included, with the address of each.
- *The research centre or centres involved in the study.* This is useful when you've been reading for a while and you know whose work to look out for – for whatever reason!
- *The principal researcher.* He or she is often named first, or sometimes identifiable as the only author whose full address and contact details are listed (called the corresponding author).

Figure 1.1 shows a typical example of a research project which required a collaborative effort.

The list of authors may be quite long. The more people involved with a study, the less likely it is that one of them has a pre-eminent position, so there may be no principal author. The authors may simply be listed in alphabetical order.

When a large study involving many sites is published, it may be that the work is written up by a small team, on behalf of the larger group. You may then find that there are no named authors, or only one or two, and the rest of the team is listed elsewhere – as in Figure 1.2. This type of multiple authorship is unavoidable if everybody is to get credit for participating in large studies.

An undesirable form of multiple authorship arises if members of an academic department attach their names to a paper when they had nothing to do with the study. This is sometimes called 'gift authorship', although it isn't always given very freely. To try to stop this practice, many journals now expect each author to explain exactly what part he or she has played in the study. For this, and other useful information, you should turn to the Acknowledgements at the end of the paper.

Understanding Clinical Papers, Third Edition. David Bowers, Allan House, David Owens and Bridgette Bewick.
© 2014 John Wiley & Sons, Ltd. Published 2014 by John Wiley & Sons, Ltd.

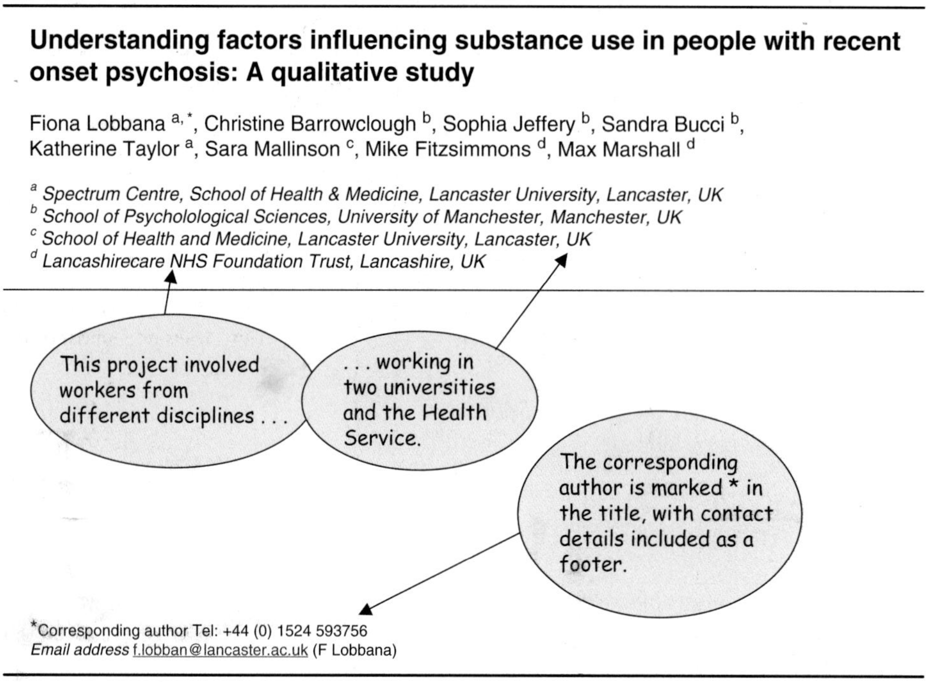

Understanding factors influencing substance use in people with recent onset psychosis: A qualitative study

Fiona Lobbana [a,*], Christine Barrowclough [b], Sophia Jeffery [b], Sandra Bucci [b], Katherine Taylor [a], Sara Mallinson [c], Mike Fitzsimmons [d], Max Marshall [d]

[a] Spectrum Centre, School of Health & Medicine, Lancaster University, Lancaster, UK
[b] School of Psycholological Sciences, University of Manchester, Manchester, UK
[c] School of Health and Medicine, Lancaster University, Lancaster, UK
[d] Lancashirecare NHS Foundation Trust, Lancashire, UK

This project involved workers from different disciplines . . .

. . . working in two universities and the Health Service.

The corresponding author is marked * in the title, with contact details included as a footer.

*Corresponding author Tel: +44 (0) 1524 593756
Email address f.lobban@lancaster.ac.uk (F Lobbana)

FIGURE 1.1   Authors and research centres listed at the start of a research article. Reprinted from Lobbana F, Barrowclough C, Jeffery S, Bucci S, Taylor K, Mallinson S, *et al.* Understanding factors influencing substance use in people with recent onset psychosis: a qualitative study. *Social Science & Medicine* 2010, 70 (8): 1141–7, © 2010, with permission from Elsevier.

IN WHAT SORT OF JOURNAL DOES THE PAPER APPEAR?

Not all journals are the same. Some are mainly aimed at members of a particular professional group, and therefore include political news, commentaries, and personal opinions. Others publish only research articles which have not appeared elsewhere, while some aim to mix these functions.

In some journals, the letters pages are designed to allow readers to express their opinions about articles which have appeared in previous issues. In others, the letters pages contain only descriptions of original studies.

What appears in a journal is decided by the Editor, nearly always with the help and advice of an Editorial Committee. The best journals also seek opinions from external referees who comment on papers sent to them and advise on suitability for publication. Because these referees are usually experts in the same field as the authors of the paper, this process is called 'peer reviewing'. It isn't always easy to tell whether papers for a journal are peer-reviewed, which is unfortunate because the peer-reviewing process is the best means of establishing the quality of a journal's contents. You shouldn't trust the results of any data-containing study if it appears in a journal which does *not* use the peer-reviewing system.

Some journals produce *supplements*, which are published in addition to the usual regular issues of the main journal. They may be whole issues given over to a single theme or to describing presentations from a conference or symposium. Often they are produced (unlike the main journals) with the help of sponsorship from pharmaceutical companies. Papers in these supplements may not have been reviewed by the same process as papers in main journals and for that reason they tend not to be of as high quality.

Angiographically Defined Collateral Circulation and Risk of Stroke in Patients with Severe Carotid Artery Stenosis

Robert D. Henderson, FRACP; Michael Wliasziw, PhD; Allan J. Fox, MD;
Peter M. Rothwell, MD; Henry J. M. Barnett, MD;
For the North American Symptomatic Carotid Endarterectomy Trial (NASCET) Group

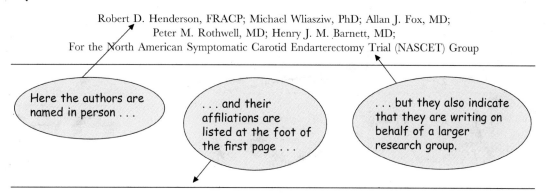

Received August 27, 1999; final revision received October 1, 1999; accepted October 1, 1999.
From the John P. Robarts Research Institute (R.D.H., M.E., H.J.M.B.) and Departments of Epidemiology and Biostatistics (M.E.), Clinical Neurological Sciences (M.E., A.J.F., H.J.M.B.), and Diagnostic Radiology (A.J.F.), University of Western Ontario, London, Ontario, Canada; and Department of Clinical Neurology, Radcliffe Infirmary, Oxford, UK (P.M.R.).
Correspondence to H.J.M. Barnett MD, John P. Robarts Research Institute, 100 Perth Dr, PO Box 5015, London, Ontario N6A5K8, Canada, E-mail barnett@rri.on.ca

FIGURE 1.2   Authorship on behalf of a large research group. Reproduced from Henderson RD, Wliasziw M, Fox AJ, Rothwell PM, Barnett HJM, for the North American Symptomatic Carotid Endarterectomy Trial Group. Angiographically defined collateral circulation and risk of stroke in patients with severe carotid artery stenosis. Stroke 2000, 31: 128–32, with permission from Wolters Kluwer Health publising.

One way to judge the quality of a journal is to check its *impact factor* – a measure of the frequency with which papers in the journal are quoted by other researchers.* The impact factor is only a rough guide because high-quality journals that cover very specialised topics will inevitably have lower ratings than journals with a wider readership.

WHO (AND WHAT) IS ACKNOWLEDGED?

It is tempting to treat the Acknowledgements at the end of a paper as being a bit like the credits after a film – only of interest to insiders. But they contain interesting information. For example, who is credited with work, but does not feature as an author? This is often the fate of medical statisticians and others who offer specialist skills for the completion of one task in the study. If the study required special expertise – such as advanced statistics, economic analysis, supervision of therapists – then the necessary 'expert' should be a member of the research team and acknowledged. If not, then either the expert was not a member of the team or somebody isn't getting credit where it is due. To ensure that co-authorship is earned, and to guard against research fraud, the Acknowledgements in many journals now also contain a statement from each author about his or her individual contribution.

---

* You can check the impact factor of a journal at a number of websites, including (for example) the Thomson Reuters (formerly ISI) *Journal Citation Reports*. These are available through many Health Science libraries and websites (e.g. http://isiknowledge.com/jcr).

Gender differences in HIV-1 diversity at time of infection

E. Michelle Long, Harold L. Martin, Jr, Joan K. Kriess,
Stephanie M. J. Rainwater, Ludo Lavreys, Denis J. Jackson, Joel Rakwar,
Kishorchandra Mandaliya & Julie Overbaugh

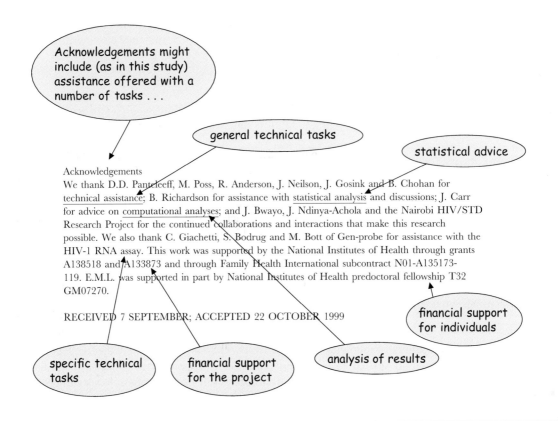

Acknowledgements
We thank D.D. Panteleeff, M. Poss, R. Anderson, J. Neilson, J. Gosink and B. Chohan for technical assistance; B. Richardson for assistance with statistical analysis and discussions; J. Carr for advice on computational analyses; and J. Bwayo, J. Ndinya-Achola and the Nairobi HIV/STD Research Project for the continued collaborations and interactions that make this research possible. We also thank C. Giachetti, S. Bodrug and M. Bott of Gen-probe for assistance with the HIV-1 RNA assay. This work was supported by the National Institutes of Health through grants A138518 and A133873 and through Family Health International subcontract N01-A135173-119. E.M.L. was supported in part by National Institutes of Health predoctoral fellowship T32 GM07270.

RECEIVED 7 SEPTEMBER; ACCEPTED 22 OCTOBER 1999

FIGURE 1.3 Acknowledgement of statistical, financial, and other support at the end of a paper. Reprinted by permission from Macmillan Publishers Ltd: Long EM, Martin HL, Kriess JK, Rainwater SMJ, Lavreys L, Jackson DJ, *et al.* Gender differences in HIV-1 diversity at time of infection. *Nature Medicine* 2000, 6: 71–5, © 2000.

The Acknowledgements section from the first paper we looked at showed what additional help the research team received (Figure 1.3). It also contains an indication of the *source of funding* that supported the research. This is of interest because external funding *may* bring with it extra safeguards as to the rigour with which work was conducted. On the other hand, it may lead to a *conflict of interest* (for example if a pharmaceutical or other commercial company has funded research into one of its own products).

Declaring a conflict of interest is *not* the same as admitting to a guilty secret. Its aim is to ensure that readers, when they are making their judgements about the study, are informed that there may be non-scientific influences on the conduct or interpretation of a study.

2

The Abstract and Introduction

At or near the beginning of most quantitative papers you will find an Abstract and an Introduction.

THE ABSTRACT

If the title of an article doesn't give you a clear enough idea of what it's about, then most papers reporting primary research data start with an Abstract – a brief summary of the whole paper that appears immediately below the title.

The purpose of this brief summary is to help the reader decide if they want to go on to read the paper in detail, by outlining the content of the research and its main findings. A good Abstract should help the reader decide – if this study has been well conducted, then is it one about which I would be interested enough to read further?

Some journals require authors to provide structured Abstracts – using headings equivalent to those that appear in the main text. A typical example is shown in Figure 2.1, from a study of a day treatment programme for patients with eating disorders. Some Abstracts are unstructured and simply give a brief narrative account of the accompanying paper as in Figure 2.2, from a qualitative study on the attitudes of young male offenders to fatherhood. The decision about which style of Abstract to use is determined not by the author, but by the journal.

A list of Keywords may accompany the Abstract, if the journal requires it. Their purpose is to assist readers who are searching for articles on particular topics. For such a list the words may come from a standard source decided by the journal or they may be chosen by the authors themselves.

THE INTRODUCTION

After the abstract comes an introductory section. Its aim is to provide some background information that makes it clear why the study described in the paper has been undertaken. The general topic area of the paper may be very familiar, but even so (perhaps especially so) the authors will probably give some summary of its importance, possibly along the lines of:

- *Is it clinically important?* Is it about a symptom that affects quality of life or causes major treatment difficulties?
- *Is there a public health importance?* Is it about an illness that represents a big burden for the community – in terms of chronic handicap, or costs to health or social services?
- *Is the interest theoretical?* Will further study help us to understand the causes of a condition or its consequences?

Understanding Clinical Papers, Third Edition. David Bowers, Allan House, David Owens and Bridgette Bewick.
© 2014 John Wiley & Sons, Ltd. Published 2014 by John Wiley & Sons, Ltd.

Day treatment programme for patients with eating disorders: randomized controlled trial

Seongsook Kong

Aim This paper reports a randomized controlled trial to compare the effects of day-treatment programmes for patients with eating disorders with those of traditional outpatient treatment.

Background Eating disorders are common, especially in adolescents, and their worldwide prevalence is increasing. Treatment interventions for patients with eating disorders have traditionally been offered on an outpatient or inpatient basis, but the recent introduction of day-hospital programmes offers the possibility of greater cost-effectiveness and relapse-prevention for this population.

Methods Volunteers from an outpatient clinic for eating disorders were randomly assigned either to a treatment group ($n=21$), participating in a modified day treatment programme based on the Toronto Day Hospital Program, or to a control group ($n=22$) receiving a traditional outpatient programme of interpersonal psychotherapy, cognitive behaviour therapy and pharmacotherapy. Data were collected from January to December 2002 using the Eating Disorder Examination, Eating Disorder Inventory-2, Beck Depression Inventory, and Rosenberg Self-Esteem Scale.

Results Participants in the day treatment programme showed significantly greater improvements on most psychological symptoms of the Eating Disorder Inventory-2, frequency of binging and purging, body mass index, depression and self-esteem scores than the control group. They also showed significant improvement in perfectionism, but the group difference was not significant.

Conclusion Nurses in day treatment programmes can play various and important roles establishing a therapeutic alliance between patient and carer in the initial period of treatment. In addition, the cognitive and behavioural work that is vital to a patient's recovery, that is, dealing with food issues, weight issues and self-esteem, is most effectively provided by a nurse therapist who maintains an empathic involvement with the patient.

Keywords Day treatment, depression, eating disorders, nursing, outcome, self-esteem

A structured Abstract uses headings also found in a full paper.

Some Abstracts give actual results, others summarise the main findings.

FIGURE 2.1   An example of a structured Abstract – this one from a trial of two treatment programmes for patients with eating disorders. Reproduced from Kong (2005) with permission from John Wiley & Sons.

Figure 2.3 shows the Introduction to a study which examined the effect of two ways of presenting information to women who were making decisions about antenatal testing.

These questions will normally be discussed by *reference to existing evidence*. The Introduction to a paper is not the place to look for a comprehensive literature review, and introductory sections in most papers are brief, but there are one or two pointers to help you decide if the evidence is being presented in a fair and unbiased way:

Experiences of, and attitudes towards, pregnancy and fatherhood amongst incarcerated young male offenders: Findings from a qualitative study

Katie Margaret Buston*
*Medical Research Council Social and Public Health Sciences Unit,
4 Lilybank Gardens, Glasgow G12 8RZ, UK*

ARTICLE INFO

It is not a hard-and-fast rule, but qualitative research is more often accompanied by an unstructured Abstract.

Article history:
Available on line 21 October 2010

Keywords:

Teenage parenthood

Fatherhood

Pregnancy

Young offenders

Sex and relationships education

Parenting interventions

Scotland

Some journals ask authors to include a list of Keywords to accompany their Abstract.

Abstract

Teenage parenthood is problematised in the UK. Attention is increasingly falling on the potential or actual father yet we still know relatively little about young men's experiences and attitudes in this area. This paper focuses on the experiences of, and attitudes towards, pregnancy and fatherhood amongst a sample of men incarcerated in a Scottish Young Offenders Institute. In-depth interviews were conducted with 40 inmates, aged 16-20, purposively sampled using answers from a questionnaire administered to 67 inmates. Twelve men reported eighteen pregnancies for which they were, definitely or possibly, responsible. All but one of the pregnancies were unplanned. Five of the men were fathers: two were still in a relationship with the mother of their child and were in close contact with her and the child while incarcerated, three, all of whom had separated from their partner before the birth, had patchy contact with the mother and child before and/or during their sentence. All five of the men expressed a strong desire to be 'a good father'. Amongst the interview sample as a whole, most said they did not feel ready to become fathers. The main reason given was being unable to fulfil what they regarded as the key role of financial provider. Most of the men had given little or no thought to the possibility of a sexual partner becoming pregnant. Contraceptive use was high, however, amongst the minority who reported thinking about this possibility. The paper concludes by considering the cultural context of the men's attitudes and the potential for intervention development for incarcerated male young offenders in the areas of Sex and Relationships Education and parenting.

FIGURE 2.2   An unstructured Abstract accompanied by a list of Keywords indicating the article's content. Reprinted from Buston, 2010. Experiences of, and attitudes towards, pregnancy and fatherhood amongst incarcerated young male offenders: findings from a qualitative study. *Social Science & Medicine* 2010, 71 (12): 2212–8, © 2010, with permission from Elsevier.

- Is there reference to a systematic review (see Chapter 33)? Or if not, to a search strategy which the authors used to identify relevant evidence? For an example, see Figure 2.4, taken from a study of the association between birthweight and adult blood pressure.
- Is the evidence mainly from the authors' own group or do the authors quote a range of evidence, even if it is not in support of their own views?

Randomised controlled trial comparing effectiveness of touch screen with leaflet for providing women with information on prenatal tests

Wendy Graham, Pat Smith, A Kamal, A Fitzmaurice, N Smith, N Hamilton

Introduction

Informed choice has been an important component of health care in the United Kingdom for almost a decade. One area in which this principle has long been applied is prenatal testing. Specific initiatives have been launched to promote women's awareness of best evidence on the effectiveness of specific tests and active participation in decisions about their care. The number of conditions for which screening is offered continues to grow rapidly, and women consequently face increasingly complex decisions. Studies have illuminated many dimensions to this complexity, including the professional and organisational barriers to informed choice, the huge variations in the scope and accuracy of information given, and the problem of receiving unsolicited and unanticipated information from screening. What is also clear is that informed choice depends on an effective partnership between the user, the provider and the communication medium.

Throughout the NHS, efforts are being made to evaluate traditional methods of conveying information, such as leaflets, and to develop and assess new approaches. This paper reports the results of a recent trial to evaluate a touch screen information system for providing information on prenatal tests to women.

> The authors start by emphasising the difficulty for women in exercising informed choice in a complex area.

> They go on to indicate the role of communication in making that choice easier . . .

> . . . and they point to the increased interest in evaluating new ways of helping people make choices.

FIGURE 2.3 Explaining the background to a research study. Reproduced from Graham W, Smith P, Kamal A, Fitzmaurice A, Smith N, Hamilton N. Randomised controlled trial comparing effectiveness of touch screen with leaflet for providing women with information on prenatal tests. *BMJ* 2000, 320: 155–60, © 2000, with permission from BMJ Publishing Group Ltd.

- Many clinical studies are carried out because the evidence is ambiguous or contradictory. Is there a dilemma which is posed by the evidence and is it clearly spelled out in the Introduction?

Generally speaking, the justification for a new study is that the existing evidence is unsatisfactory and a typical Introduction summarizes why, as in Figure 2.4. The commonest justifications for new research are that:

- Different studies have come to different conclusions about the topic and it isn't possible to come to an answer without new work.
- The evidence cannot be applied in the setting being considered by the authors. For example, good evidence may cease to be of value simply because it is old – trials showing the benefit of treatment may no longer be useful if a disorder changes so that its sensitivity to treatment changes. Similarly, evidence from one part of the world cannot always be applied freely elsewhere.

Association between birth weight and adult blood pressure in twins: historical cohort study

N R Poulter, C L Chang, A J MacGregor, H Snieder, T D Spector

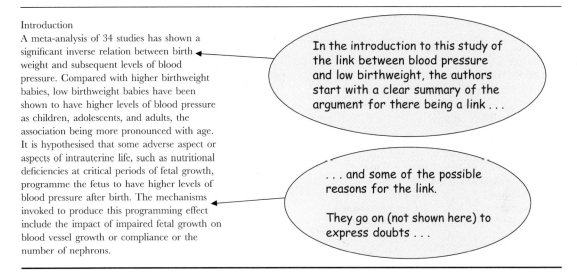

Introduction
A meta-analysis of 34 studies has shown a significant inverse relation between birth weight and subsequent levels of blood pressure. Compared with higher birthweight babies, low birthweight babies have been shown to have higher levels of blood pressure as children, adolescents, and adults, the association being more pronounced with age. It is hypothesised that some adverse aspect or aspects of intrauterine life, such as nutritional deficiencies at critical periods of fetal growth, programme the fetus to have higher levels of blood pressure after birth. The mechanisms invoked to produce this programming effect include the impact of impaired fetal growth on blood vessel growth or compliance or the number of nephrons.

In the introduction to this study of the link between blood pressure and low birthweight, the authors start with a clear summary of the argument for there being a link . . .

. . . and some of the possible reasons for the link.

They go on (not shown here) to express doubts . . .

FIGURE 2.4   Meta-analytic review quoted in a paper's Introduction. Reproduced from Poulter NR, Chang CL, MacGregor AJ, Snieder H, Spector TD. Association between birth weight and adult blood pressure in twins: historical cohort study. *BMJ* 1999, 319: 1330–3, © 1999, with permission from BMJ Publishing Group Ltd.

- The evidence may be incomplete. For example, we may know that rates of smoking are increasing among young women but we don't know why.
- The evidence may be of poor quality, so that no conclusion can be drawn from it. See, for example, Figure 2.5 from a study on the detection of depression in primary care.

If these elements of the Introduction are well presented, then it should be clear what the paper is about and why the authors have chosen to conduct the work that they have. Armed with this background briefing, you can now move on to check the *specific objectives* of the authors' work.

ETHICAL CONSIDERATIONS

Nearly all studies in health-care that involve contact with people will require ethical approval. What that means is that the researchers will have had to submit their proposals to a panel of experts, such as a local research ethics committee, who decide whether the project is ethical or not. For example, the risks of any research should be outweighed by its benefits and participants should have been given the opportunity to participate or not as they wished, without their decision influencing their medical care.

Most authors will indicate that their study has been approved by the appropriate body governing research ethics – usually either in the Methods section or the Acknowledgements. Increasingly, authors

Effects of a clinical-practice guideline and practice-based education on detection and outcome of depression in primary care: Hampshire Depression Project randomised controlled trial

C Thompson, A L Kinmonth, L Stevens, R C Peveler, A Stevens, K J Ostler, R M Pickering, N G Baker, A Henson, J Preece, D Cooper, M J Campbell

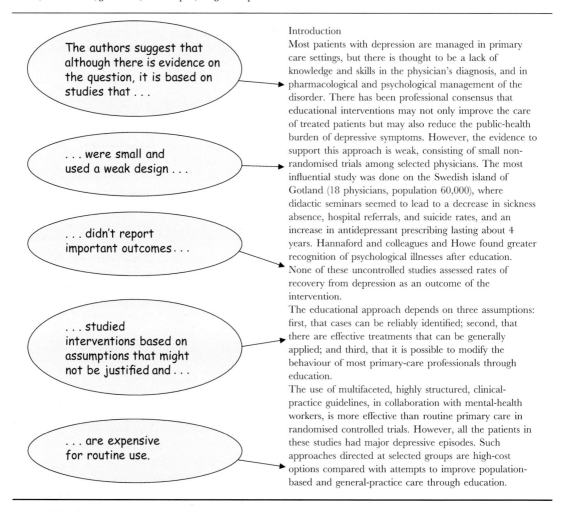

Introduction

Most patients with depression are managed in primary care settings, but there is thought to be a lack of knowledge and skills in the physician's diagnosis, and in pharmacological and psychological management of the disorder. There has been professional consensus that educational interventions may not only improve the care of treated patients but may also reduce the public-health burden of depressive symptoms. However, the evidence to support this approach is weak, consisting of small non-randomised trials among selected physicians. The most influential study was done on the Swedish island of Gotland (18 physicians, population 60,000), where didactic seminars seemed to lead to a decrease in sickness absence, hospital referrals, and suicide rates, and an increase in antidepressant prescribing lasting about 4 years. Hannaford and colleagues and Howe found greater recognition of psychological illnesses after education. None of these uncontrolled studies assessed rates of recovery from depression as an outcome of the intervention.

The educational approach depends on three assumptions: first, that cases can be reliably identified; second, that there are effective treatments that can be generally applied; and third, that it is possible to modify the behaviour of most primary-care professionals through education.

The use of multifaceted, highly structured, clinical-practice guidelines, in collaboration with mental-health workers, is more effective than routine primary care in randomised controlled trials. However, all the patients in these studies had major depressive episodes. Such approaches directed at selected groups are high-cost options compared with attempts to improve population-based and general-practice care through education.

The bubble callouts in the figure read:

- The authors suggest that although there is evidence on the question, it is based on studies that . . .
- . . . were small and used a weak design . . .
- . . . didn't report important outcomes . . .
- . . . studied interventions based on assumptions that might not be justified and . . .
- . . . are expensive for routine use.

FIGURE 2.5 Some reasons why previous research may be inadequate for current needs. Reprinted from *The Lancet* 355: Thompson C, Kinmonth AL, Stevens L, Peveler RC, Stevens A, Ostler KJ, *et al*. Effects of a clinical-practice guideline and practice-based education on detection and outcome of depression in primary care: Hampshire Depression Project randomised controlled trial. 2000; 185–9, © 2000, with permission from Elsevier.

will mention any particular ethical dilemmas raised by their research either in the Introduction or the Discussion of their paper. Where there are particular questions raised by a study, the authors may expand upon them (including, for example, details of the information given to participants and the way in which consent was obtained).

Does HIV status influence the outcome of patients admitted to a surgical intensive care Unit? A prospective double blind study

Satish Bhagwanjee, David JJ Muckart, Prakash M Jeena, Prushini Moodley

Introduction

Limited resources and the high cost of intensive care have compelled clinicians to rationalise the allocation of resources. For example, in our unit it is policy not to admit patients with incurable malignant disease, and end-stage liver disease, and patients with multiple organ failure who are deemed non-salvageable. The lack of objective data made it unclear whether patients with HIV infection should be treated similarly. To allow rationalisation of the admissions policy with respect to these patients we conducted a prospective study to determine the prevalence of HIV infection among patients admitted to the unit and assess the impact of HIV status (HIV positive, HIV negative, AIDS) on outcome. The study embraced a major ethical dilemma. On the one hand, the clinician has an obligation of non-maleficence – that is, patients must not be harmed by the actions of the doctor. On the other hand, the doctor has an obligation to society to ensure that available resources are appropriated fairly, based on objective evidence. Though the basic ethical tenets of patient autonomy, justice, beneficence, and non-maleficence are useful, they are only the starting points for ethical decision making.

Subjects and methods The study was conducted in the 16 bed surgical intensive care unit at King Edward VIII Hospital, a large teaching hospital in Durban. All patients admitted to the unit over six months (September 1993 to February 1994) were included. There were no exclusions. Informed consent was not sought. The study protocol was approved by the ethics committee of the University of Natal.

This research studied a topic identified by the authors as being of great ethical importance ...

... implicitly, the ethical importance of the work was taken to justify the inclusion of non-consenting (unconscious) patients.

FIGURE 2.6   Discussion of ethical considerations from a study into the outcomes of surgical patients and their HIV status. Reproduced from Bhagwanjee S, Muckart DJJ, Jeena PM, Moodley P. Does HIV status influence the outcome of patients admitted to a surgical intensive care unit? A prospective double blind study. *BMJ* 1997, 314: 1077, © 1997, with permission from BMJ Publishing Group Ltd.

Certain types of research cause particular ethical concerns. For example, young children, or those with cognitive impairment or learning disability, or patients who are unconscious, cannot give consent to participate in research that nonetheless asks extremely important questions about clinical care. In these situations, researchers may undertake research with ethical approval, provided certain criteria are met (see Figure 2.6 from a study of HIV status and surgical outcomes).

3

The Aims and Objectives

Following the Introduction, you should look for a clear statement of the *purposes* of the current work. This statement can come in two forms: the aims of the study and the objectives.

- *Aims* are general statements about purpose. For example, the authors might wish to examine the attitudes of hospital nurses to colleagues with mental health problems.
- *Objectives* are specific questions, suggested by previous research or theory. For example, 'Does taking the oral contraceptive pill increase the risk of stroke among women of childbearing age?'. One particular sort of objective is to *test an hypothesis*.

Because the terminology of hypothesis testing is so widely used, we will start there.

HYPOTHESES

Often, studies will ask more than one question, so they will have several hypotheses. In these circumstances, you should look for a *main hypothesis* (Figures 3.1 and 3.2) and the other questions will form *subsidiary or secondary hypotheses*.

There are important reasons why a study should have only one main question:

- If a study tests many hypotheses, then just by chance it is likely to produce positive results for some of them. (See Chapter 27 on hypothesis testing and the possibility of false-positive results from *multiple testing*.)
- We can trust a negative result only if we know that a study was large enough; otherwise, there is a possibility of false-negative results. Many researchers therefore make an *estimate of sample size* to help them decide how big to make their study so that they can avoid this sort of error (see Chapter 10). To do that calculation they need to know what the main outcome of interest is, and the *main outcome* will be chosen to test the main hypothesis.

There used to be a conventional way of stating a study's hypothesis, which involved the use of a *null hypothesis* and the description of a study set up to *disprove or refute an hypothesis*. Although this approach is still sometimes taught, you will almost never come across examples in papers. The null hypothesis was a way of stating a question in the form 'situation A is no different from situation B'. It arose because certain statistical tests operate by testing whether an assumption of similarity is likely to be true.

The need to refute rather than prove an hypothesis is similarly based on a technical point – about the nature of scientific evidence. In fact, nearly everybody now states their hypotheses in a straightforward way. The English doesn't have to be difficult to follow for the science to be right!

Understanding Clinical Papers, Third Edition. David Bowers, Allan House, David Owens and Bridgette Bewick.
© 2014 John Wiley & Sons, Ltd. Published 2014 by John Wiley & Sons, Ltd.

Effects of a clinical-practice guideline and practice-based education on detection and outcome of depression in primary care: Hampshire Depression Project randomised controlled trial

C Thompson, A L Kinmonth, L Stevens, R C Peveler, A Stevens, K J Ostler, R M Pickering, N G Baker, A Henson, J Preece, D Cooper, M J Campbell

The Hampshire Depression Project was designed as a randomised controlled trial of an educational programme that could be generalised across primary-care settings. Our main hypotheses were that an education group of primary-care physicians would show greater sensitivity and specificity for recognition of depressive symptoms than a control group of physicians, and that an educated group of practice teams would achieve greater recovery rates in their patients than a control group of practices.

> In the final paragraph of the Introduction to the report from the Hampshire Depression Project (see Chapter 2), the authors state their hypotheses.

FIGURE 3.1 Statement of a study's main hypothesis. Reprinted from *The Lancet* 355: Thompson C, Kinmonth AL, Stevens L, Peveler RC, Stevens A, Ostler KJ, *et al.* Effects of a clinical-practice guideline and practice-based education on detection and outcome of depression in primary care: Hampshire Depression Project randomised controlled trial. 2000; 185–9, © 2000, with permission from Elsevier.

Affective aggression in patients with temporal lobe epilepsy: A quantitative MRI study of the amygdala

L. Tebartz van Elst, F.G. Woermann, L. Lemieux, P.J. Thompson and M.R. Trimble

Rationale for this study
The aim of our study was to investigate amygdala pathology in patients suffering from temporal lobe epilepsy and additional affective aggression, specifically IED. In particular, we hypothesized that, in patients with temporal lobe epilepsy and intermittent affective aggression, amygdala sclerosis in the context of hippocampal sclerosis would be more common than in control patients. Further more, we wanted to test if there is an association between aggression, on the one hand, and hippocampal sclerosis, low IQ and poor social adjustment, on the other hand, in patients with temporal lobe epilepsy.

> It is (unfortunately) rare to see the questions stated clearly in a separate section of a paper's introduction.

> In this study there were two hypotheses.

FIGURE 3.2 A study with two hypotheses. Reproduced from Tebartz van Elst L, Woermann FG, Lemieux L, Thompson PJ, Trimble MR. Affective aggression in patients with temporal lobe epilepsy: a quantitative MRI study of the amygdala. *Brain* 2000, 123: 234–43, with permission from Oxford University Press.

OBJECTIVES THAT ARE NOT HYPOTHESIS TESTING

Not all questions are framed as hypotheses, even in quantitative research. For example, in a study examining the rate of antibiotic resistance among post-operative wound infections the authors might have no definite rate in mind.

And many studies are not designed to test hypotheses at all – for example some are designed to generate new ideas and questions for future research. This is especially true of qualitative research, which is generally speaking more exploratory – asking a question when we might not know what answers to expect and where we don't want to measure something but to understand its nature. In other words, although qualitative studies do not usually test hypotheses, they are still designed to answer a question. For example, in the study illustrated in Figure 3.3 the researchers were asking the question: 'What do people with progressive life-limiting illness want to know about their condition – for example about its consequences and its treatment?'.

Meeting information needs of patients with incurable progressive disease and their families in South Africa and Uganda: multicentre qualitative study

Lucy Selman, Irene J Higginson, Godfrey Agupio, Natalya Dinat, Julia Downing, Liz Gwyther, Thandi Mashao, Keletso Mmoledi, Anthony P Moll, Lydia Mpanga Sebuyira, Barbara Panajatovic Richard Harding

ABSTRACT

Objectives To explore the information needs of patients with progressive, life limiting disease and their family caregivers in South Africa and Uganda and to inform clinical practice and policy in this emerging field.

Design Semistructured qualitative interview study.

Setting Four palliative care services in South Africa and one in Uganda, covering rural, urban, and peri-urban locations.

Participants 90 patients and 38 family caregivers enrolled in palliative care services; 28 patients had cancer, 61 had HIV infection (including 6 dual HIV/cancer diagnoses), and 1 had motor neurone disease.

Results Five themes emerged from the data. (1) Information sources: a lack of information from general healthcare providers meant that patients and caregivers had to draw on alternative sources of information. (2) Information needs: patients and caregivers reported needing more information in the key areas of the causes and progression of the disease, its symptoms and treatment, and financial/social support. (3) Impact of unmet needs: poor provision of information had a detrimental effect on patients' and caregivers' ability to cope. (4) Communication: negative experiences of communication with general healthcare staff . . .

The question in this qualitative study was expressed as an objective.

FIGURE 3.3   The (structured) Abstract of a qualitative study, starting with an implicitly stated question. Reproduced from Selman L, Higginson IJ, Godfrey A, Dinat N, Downing J, Gwyther L, *et al*. Meeting information needs of patients with incurable progressive disease and their families in South Africa and Uganda: multicentre qualitative study. *BMJ* 2009, 338: b1326, © 2009, with permission from BMJ Publishing Group Ltd.

Illness careers and continuity of care in mental health services: A qualitative study of service users and carers

Ian Rees Jones, Nilufar Ahmed, Jocelyn Catty, Susan McLaren, Diana Rose, Til Wykes,Tom Burns, for the Echo group

Available online 3rd July 2009

Abstract

Continuity of care is considered by patients and clinicians as an essential feature of good quality care in long-term disorders, yet there is general agreement that it is a complex concept and the lack of clarity in its conceptualisation and operationalisation has been linked to a deficit of user involvement. In this paper we utilize the concept of the 'patient career' to frame patient accounts of their experiences of the mental health care system. We aimed to capture the experiences and views of users and carers focusing on the meanings associated with particular (dis)continuities and transitional episodes that occurred over their illness career.

As part of a large longitudinal study of continuity of care in mental health a sub-sample of 31 users was selected together with 14 of their carers. Qualitative interviews framed around the service user's illness career explored general experiences of relationship with services, care, continuity and transition from both user and carer perspectives.

Five key themes emerged: relational (dis)continuity; depersonalized transitions; invisibility and crisis; communicative gaps; and social vulnerability. One of the important findings was the fragility of continuity and its relationship to levels of satisfaction. Supportive, long-term relationships could be quickly undermined by a range of factors and satisfaction levels were often closely related to moments of transition where these relationships were vulnerable.

Examples of continuity and well managed transitions highlighted the importance of professionals personalizing transitions and situating them in the context of the daily life of service users. Further research is required to identify how best to negotiate these key points of transition in the future.

> The aim of a qualitative study is rarely if ever to test an hypothesis.

FIGURE 3.4   The aim of the qualitative study. Reprinted from Jones IR, Ahmed N, Catty J, McLaren S, Rose D, Wykes T, *et al.* Illness careers and continuity of care in mental health services: a qualitative study of users and carers. *Social Science & Medicine* 2009, 69: 632–9, © 2009, with permission from Elsevier.

In other cases it can be harder to see exactly what the question is. For example, the study illustrated in Figure 3.4 talks about capturing experiences and views of service users and carers, which doesn't sound like an objective, but perhaps a general aim. However, if you read the rest of the paragraph in this Abstract it becomes clearer that there is a more specific question, if quite a complex one: 'Is the idea of a patient career useful in helping us to organize our thoughts about how service users describe their experiences of mental health services?'.

A particular type of objective is to develop new hypotheses for testing in future research, so-called hypothesis-generating. Sometimes hypotheses are generated by subgroup analysis and *post hoc* examinations of the data produced by quantitative research (Figure 3.5). Hypothesis generation of this sort

Crisis telephone consultation for deliberate self-harm patients: effects on repetition

M. O. Evans, H. G. Morgan, A. Hayward and D. J. Gunnell

In this study, the question concerns the impact of a 'crisis card' (which gives details of how to seek help in future crises) on patients seen after an episode of deliberate self-harm.

In the last section of the Introduction, the authors spell out the reasons why they decided to undertake subgroup analysis.

Sub-group analyses
In the light of the findings from the earlier study, we were interested in determining whether the effect of the intervention differed in those with and without a past history of DSH. We also investigated whether men and women responded differently. The size of the study was, however, insufficient to detect small but nevertheless potentially important differences. In order to investigate whether the effects of the crisis card differed in these groups, the statistical significance of an interaction term between treatment group and each of these two variables was determined in logistic regression models using the likelihood ratio statistic. No other sub-group analyses were undertaken.

FIGURE 3.5 Subgroup analysis used to explore possible associations which were not sought as part of the study's original hypotheses. Reproduced from Evans MO, Morgan HG, Hayward A, Gunnell DJ. Crisis telephone consultation for deliberate self-harm patients: effects on repetition. *British Journal of Psychiatry* 1999, 175: 23–7, with permission from The Royal College of Psychiatrists, Copyright RCP © 1999.

should be regarded as unreliable, but for all that it may produce interesting ideas. Be careful to look out for it, because some authors present these as established results rather than ideas for future work.

STUDIES WITH UNCLEAR OBJECTIVES

If you cannot find a mention of the study's objectives expressed as aims or specific questions, you may yet be able to find them expressed in less clear-cut ways. Examples include 'exploring associations' or (worse) 'examining issues'. You will need to be particularly careful about studies with such vague objectives: because they are not asking a specific question, it is not easy to tell whether the results are meaningful. Quantitative studies with unclear prior questions can produce results that are due to chance – especially as a result of *post hoc* or multiple testing. Qualitative studies, when they start without a clear question, do not tend to produce misleading results as much as uninteresting ones.

As a final note, we want to say something about why we think it's worth so much effort to clarify the exact aims and objectives of a study. To do so, we will outline a small thought experiment. Suppose you are working as a general medical practitioner and a mother brings a child to you, saying she is worried that he is not growing and is shorter than all his peers. The appropriate initial response would be a piece of quantitative research to answer the question: 'Is this boy short for his age?'. You would measure his height, checking it against suitable norms.

Suppose now you see another child whose mother is worried that he seems unhappy and withdrawn, but she does not understand why that should be. You are likely to want to undertake some qualitative research – asking him in a relaxed and unstructured but purposeful way whether he does indeed feel unhappy, and if so why? In other words you *match the design of your inquiry to the question you are asking*. Now, it would be possible to have a chat with the first boy and ask him his experiences of growing up and being (perhaps) on the short side, and you could give the second child an age-appropriate standardised mood rating scale. You will have produced results but not answers because in neither case would your method of inquiry be appropriate to your (or the mother's) specific prior questions.

We hope that when you read research reports you will therefore have in mind your own queries: are the aims and objectives clear, and is the researchers' chosen method the best one to meet their aims and objectives?

II

Design Matters:
What Type of Study is It?

4

Descriptive Studies: Qualitative

Once you are clear about the aims and objectives of a study, and any hypotheses that have been posed, the next important question to ask is: 'What sort of study did the authors undertake?'. The various kinds of study design that are commonly found in clinical journals form the subject of this chapter and Chapters 5–8 – starting here with *qualitative* studies. *Quantitative* research, and its subcategories of design, is described across Chapters 5–7. The last chapter of this section (Chapter 8) goes on to describe so-called *mixed methods* studies, where the qualitative and quantitative approaches are combined in various ways.

QUALITATIVE RESEARCH

Qualitative research has proliferated greatly since the 1990s as a method for investigating illness and health-care, becoming a regular feature in most good clinical journals. In general, the method involves observation of people's experience of illness and of health-care, or examines how they are managing ill health or diagnostic investigation, without attempts to manipulate or alter either health or its care – an approach sometimes called *naturalistic* research. The data collected, analysed, and described in the report of a qualitative study will be based on words rather than numbers. These data are usually collected by way of carefully arranged conversations with the people concerned, or, less often, from diaries or other accounts, or through direct observation of their experiences.

Typically, qualitative research sets out aims but not hypotheses, tending to explain experiences or events but not to predict what may happen to other people. The pursuit of hypotheses in research (see Chapter 3) tends to be a feature of investigations that involve some kind of comparison: does some action (e.g. smoking) make certain illnesses more likely or is one treatment (e.g. an antibiotic) more effective than another? These kinds of hypothesis-driven studies form the *quantitative* analytic and intervention studies of the kind that are introduced in Chapters 6 and 7. Qualitative research, on the other hand, offers invaluable insights when little is known about a topic, in particular where it is important to know about people's attitude towards health-care. For example, common topics for qualitative enquiry concern people's views about whether to undergo tests or procedures and the effects of treatments on people's lives. An example is shown in Figure 4.1, where women who had a strong family history of breast cancer were asked about gene testing, whether they might consider prophylactic mastectomy in order to avoid cancer, and, for some of the women, their experience of mastectomy and reconstruction. The research pointed to a need for improved information and support for women in this predicament – at multiple stages of a complex pathway of decisions, procedures, care, and resumption of lifestyle.

Understanding Clinical Papers, Third Edition. David Bowers, Allan House, David Owens and Bridgette Bewick.
© 2014 John Wiley & Sons, Ltd. Published 2014 by John Wiley & Sons, Ltd.

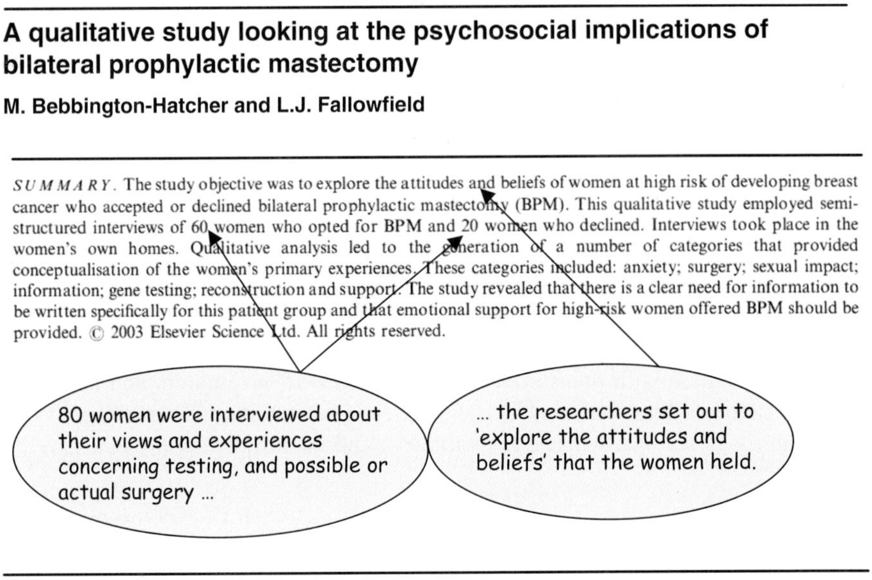

A qualitative study looking at the psychosocial implications of bilateral prophylactic mastectomy

M. Bebbington-Hatcher and L.J. Fallowfield

SUMMARY. The study objective was to explore the attitudes and beliefs of women at high risk of developing breast cancer who accepted or declined bilateral prophylactic mastectomy (BPM). This qualitative study employed semi-structured interviews of 60 women who opted for BPM and 20 women who declined. Interviews took place in the women's own homes. Qualitative analysis led to the generation of a number of categories that provided conceptualisation of the women's primary experiences. These categories included: anxiety; surgery; sexual impact; information; gene testing; reconstruction and support. The study revealed that there is a clear need for information to be written specifically for this patient group and that emotional support for high-risk women offered BPM should be provided. © 2003 Elsevier Science Ltd. All rights reserved.

(80 women were interviewed about their views and experiences concerning testing, and possible or actual surgery ...)

(... the researchers set out to 'explore the attitudes and beliefs' that the women held.)

FIGURE 4.1 A qualitative study examining views and experience of tests and interventions. Reproduced from Bebbington-Hatcher M, Fallowfield LJ. A qualitative study looking at the psychosocial implications of bilateral prophylactic mastectomy. *The Breast*, 2003, 12: 1–9, © 2003, with permission from Elsevier.

TYPES OF QUALITATIVE STUDY

Although there is no widely accepted classification of qualitative research that mirrors the useful classification of quantitative research (Chapter 5), there are a variety of ways of carrying out qualitative studies. There are several commonly encountered theoretical approaches, a variety of sampling techniques, and a number of methods of data gathering. These three components of the research process are by no means separate from one another; two are dealt with below as if individual topics, while sampling techniques are dealt with in Chapter 11.

Theoretical Approaches

Perhaps the most frequently encountered qualitative approach in health-care research is known as *grounded theory*, in which the researcher generates theory from the data – in contrast to the typical quantitative device of holding a hypothesis and then gathering data to support or refute it. In studies undertaken according to the precepts of grounded theory, it is usual practice to move between fieldwork and analysis – analysing early data before collecting later data, and using the interim analysis to adjust the later data collection – a procedure sometimes termed *continuous comparison*.

This framework for the research process is particularly suited to situations where the researcher has little prior understanding or knowledge of the data; where the researcher already has detailed knowledge, grounded theory might not represent the best approach. Figure 4.2 displays an extract from a study that used grounded theory as the basis for an examination of patients' views and experiences of what is widely called an *enhanced recovery programme* (ERP) for the treatment of colorectal cancer; there is already evidence from trials of its effectiveness. The complex ERP pathway includes: provision of extensive preoperative counselling to prepare patients for early rehabilitation, tailored anaesthesia and surgery to reduce operative stress, and early post-operative feeding and activity to improve gut function and mobility.

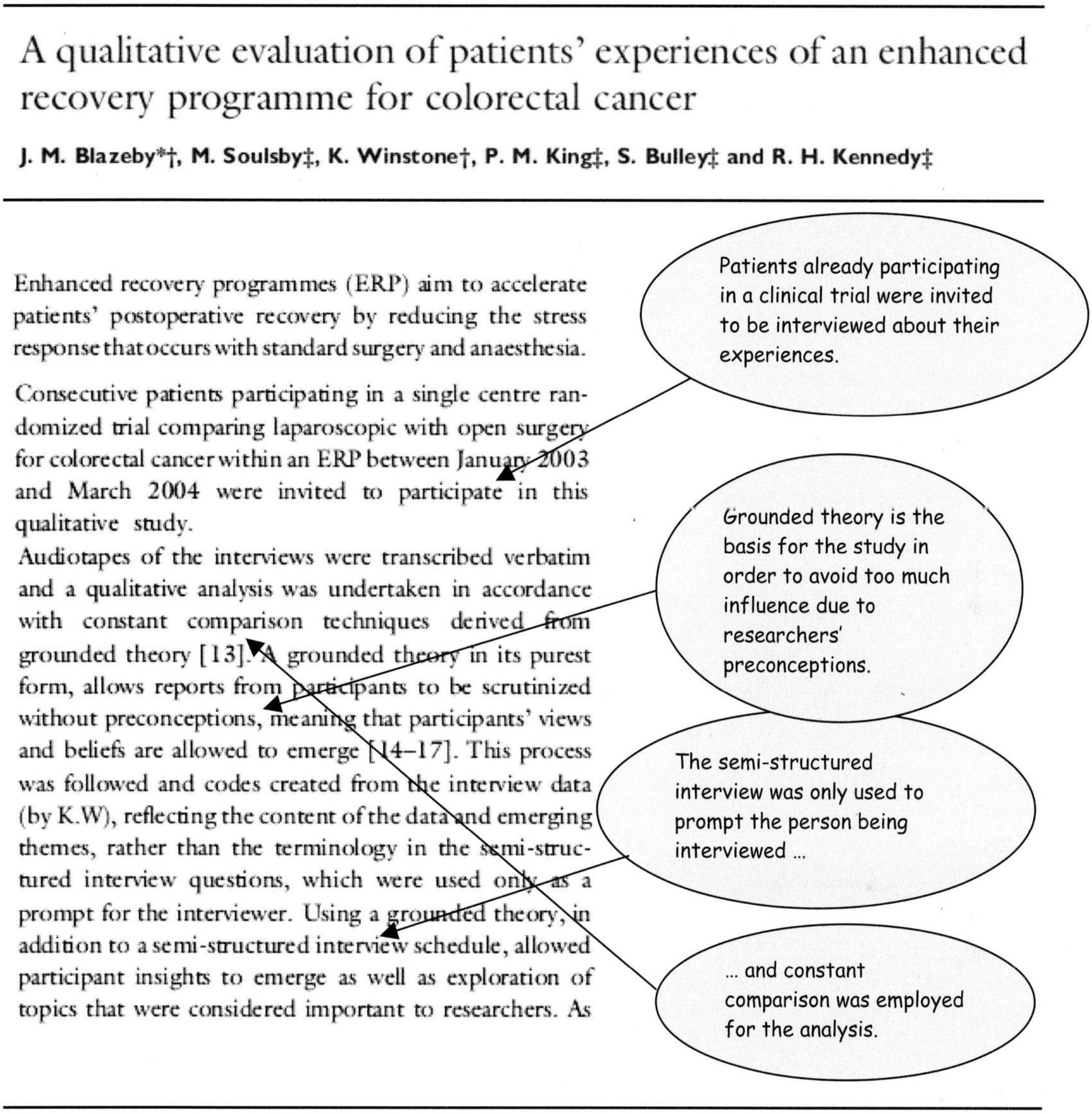

A qualitative evaluation of patients' experiences of an enhanced recovery programme for colorectal cancer

J. M. Blazeby*†, M. Soulsby‡, K. Winstone†, P. M. King‡, S. Bulley‡ and R. H. Kennedy‡

Enhanced recovery programmes (ERP) aim to accelerate patients' postoperative recovery by reducing the stress response that occurs with standard surgery and anaesthesia.

Consecutive patients participating in a single centre randomized trial comparing laparoscopic with open surgery for colorectal cancer within an ERP between January 2003 and March 2004 were invited to participate in this qualitative study.

Audiotapes of the interviews were transcribed verbatim and a qualitative analysis was undertaken in accordance with constant comparison techniques derived from grounded theory [13]. A grounded theory in its purest form, allows reports from participants to be scrutinized without preconceptions, meaning that participants' views and beliefs are allowed to emerge [14–17]. This process was followed and codes created from the interview data (by K.W), reflecting the content of the data and emerging themes, rather than the terminology in the semi-structured interview questions, which were used only as a prompt for the interviewer. Using a grounded theory, in addition to a semi-structured interview schedule, allowed participant insights to emerge as well as exploration of topics that were considered important to researchers. As

> Patients already participating in a clinical trial were invited to be interviewed about their experiences.

> Grounded theory is the basis for the study in order to avoid too much influence due to researchers' preconceptions.

> The semi-structured interview was only used to prompt the person being interviewed …

> … and constant comparison was employed for the analysis.

FIGURE 4.2 Grounded theory as the theoretical basis for a study examining patients' experience of care. Reproduced from Blazeby JM, Soulsby M, Winstone K, King PM, Bulley S, Kennedy RH (2010) with permission from John Wiley & Sons.

The findings, in a way that is typical of a grounded study, are set out to portray the setting of the research – using lots of examples of the participants' own words. In the research illustrated by Figure 4.2, here is one example of a patient's views concerning how the hospital should carry out its procedures: 'I'm a firm believer of being at home rather than in the hospital purely because of the ability to do what I want rather than to be part of a routine'.

Other theoretical approaches are available, including some that pay more attention to the meaning rather than the description of events or experiences in health-care; *interpretative phenomenological analysis* (IPA) is a popular form of such research. The interviews bear similarities with those carried out in a grounded theory study – with a topic guide (see below and Chapter 21) providing a loose structure for the

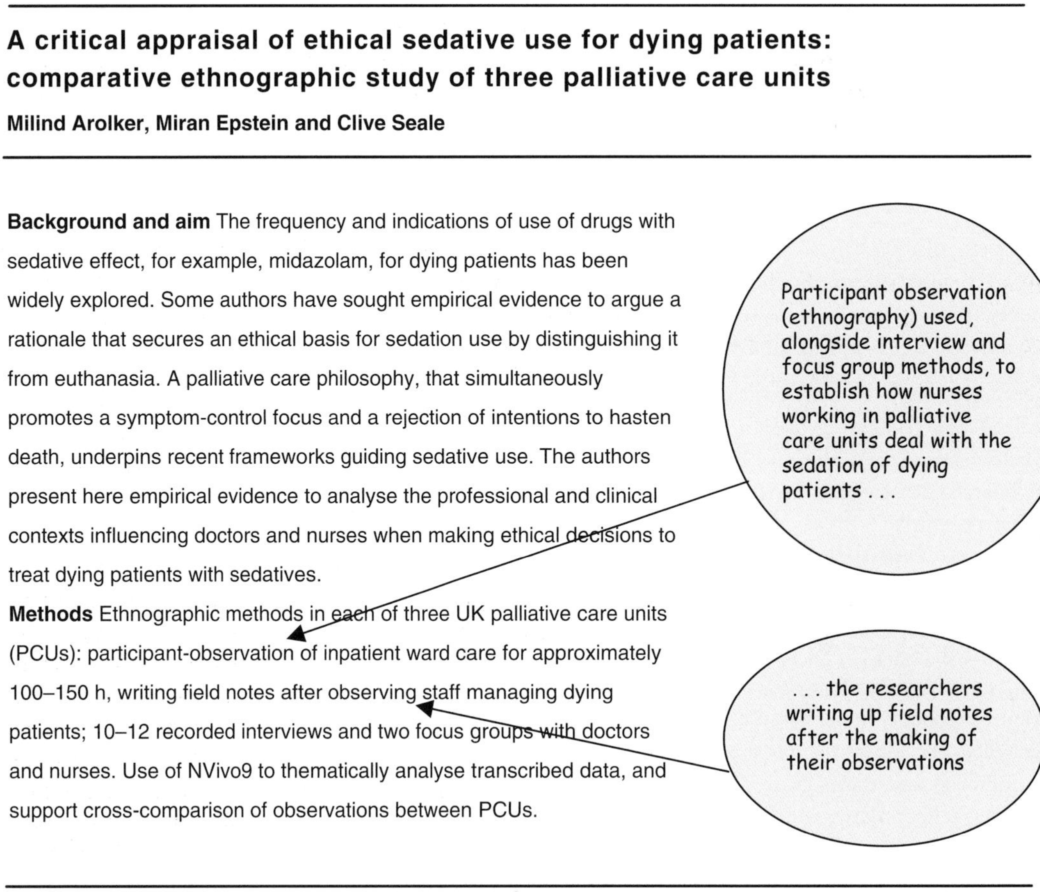

A critical appraisal of ethical sedative use for dying patients: comparative ethnographic study of three palliative care units

Milind Arolker, Miran Epstein and Clive Seale

Background and aim The frequency and indications of use of drugs with sedative effect, for example, midazolam, for dying patients has been widely explored. Some authors have sought empirical evidence to argue a rationale that secures an ethical basis for sedation use by distinguishing it from euthanasia. A palliative care philosophy, that simultaneously promotes a symptom-control focus and a rejection of intentions to hasten death, underpins recent frameworks guiding sedative use. The authors present here empirical evidence to analyse the professional and clinical contexts influencing doctors and nurses when making ethical decisions to treat dying patients with sedatives.

Methods Ethnographic methods in each of three UK palliative care units (PCUs): participant-observation of inpatient ward care for approximately 100–150 h, writing field notes after observing staff managing dying patients; 10–12 recorded interviews and two focus groups with doctors and nurses. Use of NVivo9 to thematically analyse transcribed data, and support cross-comparison of observations between PCUs.

Participant observation (ethnography) used, alongside interview and focus group methods, to establish how nurses working in palliative care units deal with the sedation of dying patients . . .

. . . the researchers writing up field notes after the making of their observations

FIGURE 4.3 A qualitative study employing ethnographic (participant observation) techniques. Reproduced from Arolker M, Epstein M, Seale C. A critical appraisal of ethical sedative use for dying patients: comparative ethnographic study of three palliative care units. *Supportive & Palliative Care* 2012, 2: A34, © 2012, with permission from BMJ Publishing Group Ltd.

interview. The difference will often lie in trying to get rather closer to the participants' accounts of events and background – getting to know the person and his or her context quite well. Often the sample is small and the data from each person very detailed. Interviews are sometimes supplemented by other material such as diaries, personal written accounts, and letters. Some IPA researchers deliberately target participants who are articulate and likely to be particularly forthcoming. The research questions tend to concentrate on meaning: 'What is it like to receive a diagnosis of pre-senile dementia?', 'Why don't some people with insulin-dependent diabetes attend specialist clinic for advice and treatment?'.

Another, less frequently encountered, qualitative method is that of *ethnography* or *participant observation*. The researcher directly observes the matter being studied, interpreting the behaviour and activities observed. The technique, although possible in many settings, such as the provision of health or social care, or in health workers' training, has been especially useful in studies of marginal or high-risk health behaviour such as with commercial sex workers or injecting drug users. In an attempt to understand the target group's daily lives, the researcher might live with them or work alongside them, becoming one of them for a time (Figure 4.3). Most especially, the idea is of seeing the world as they do, seeing the same meanings in what takes place.

This section has described the above three approaches to show something of the spread of lines of attack; qualitative researchers use numerous other named and unnamed techniques and devices, and there are many good books that describe and explain them. The next section says a little more about the collection of data from individuals and from groups.

Practical Data Gathering

Most frequently, qualitative health researchers interview individuals. They do not try to draw their samples, as quantitative researchers do, in a way that provides a subset of the population that represents the population in a probabilistic kind of way. Rather, they frequently use what is termed a *purposive* procedure: they use predetermined criteria to select people to invite for the study. For example, patients attending hospital because of self-harm (usually overdose or self-cutting) were invited for an interview to discover their views about the care and attention that they received at the hospital Emergency Department; the researchers purposively attempted to recruit approximately equal numbers of people who had taken an overdose or cut themselves, equal numbers of males and females, and equal numbers of people attending for the first time or at a repeat attendance. Sampling in qualitative research is described in some detail in Chapter 11.

Reports of qualitative research usually describe the way in which the data were collected. Often the data are gathered through the interview of a series of individuals, although groups of people (generally termed *focus groups*) are also widely used. Whether it is a study with individual interviews or one engaged with groups, the researchers will generally have set out for themselves an organised way of posing questions. The structure of the questioning can be extremely loose, perhaps little more than an occasional prompt on a broadly drawn subject, through to detailed and in-depth enquiry in an organised order of questioning.

Most often the questioning, in individual interviews or focus groups, lies somewhere between these two poles and the researcher constructs a *topic guide* in which there are a number of open-ended questions arranged in an order that is not necessarily adhered to should the conversation pursue its own direction. Sometimes, the topic guide is rather more structured and the qualitative researcher may refer to it as a *semi-structured interview*. The content of questions varies widely, but will usually pay attention to the participants' attitudes and experiences (Figure 4.4). Topic guides are referred to in more detail in Chapter 21. Where the method is participant observation, the data are recorded in rather different ways, often using field notes – written as the observations are being made or soon afterwards (Figure 4.3).

It is normal practice to make audio recordings of all of the interviews and to transcribe them: the researcher, or someone paid by the researcher, listens to the recording and types out what has been said by both parties, or by everyone in the group, verbatim. Focus groups ought to provide an extra ingredient that should enrich the data: the group process itself ought to help the participants to explore, consider, clarify, and reflect on their views and their reports of experience – with the participants each assisting the researcher in eliciting one another's responses. Whether derived from individual interviews or from focus groups, the transcribed written material becomes the basis for the analysis – discussed in Chapter 34.

Patients, prisoners, or people? Women prisoners' experiences of primary care in prison: a qualitative study

Emma Plugge, Nicola Douglas and Ray Fitzpatrick

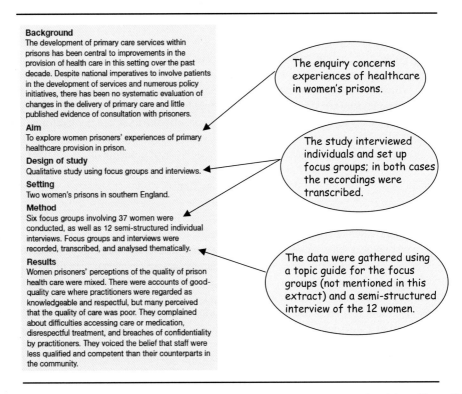

Background
The development of primary care services within prisons has been central to improvements in the provision of health care in this setting over the past decade. Despite national imperatives to involve patients in the development of services and numerous policy initiatives, there has been no systematic evaluation of changes in the delivery of primary care and little published evidence of consultation with prisoners.

Aim
To explore women prisoners' experiences of primary healthcare provision in prison.

Design of study
Qualitative study using focus groups and interviews.

Setting
Two women's prisons in southern England.

Method
Six focus groups involving 37 women were conducted, as well as 12 semi-structured individual interviews. Focus groups and interviews were recorded, transcribed, and analysed thematically.

Results
Women prisoners' perceptions of the quality of prison health care were mixed. There were accounts of good-quality care where practitioners were regarded as knowledgeable and respectful, but many perceived that the quality of care was poor. They complained about difficulties accessing care or medication, disrespectful treatment, and breaches of confidentiality by practitioners. They voiced the belief that staff were less qualified and competent than their counterparts in the community.

The enquiry concerns experiences of healthcare in women's prisons.

The study interviewed individuals and set up focus groups; in both cases the recordings were transcribed.

The data were gathered using a topic guide for the focus groups (not mentioned in this extract) and a semi-structured interview of the 12 women.

FIGURE 4.4   A qualitative study involving focus groups and individual interviews. Reprinted from Plugge E, Douglas N, Fitzpatrick R. Patients, prisoners, or people? Women prisoners' experiences of primary care in prison: a qualitative study. *British Journal of General Practice* 2008, 58 (554): e1–8, with permission from the Royal College of General Practitioners.

5

Descriptive Studies: Quantitative

Broadly speaking, quantitative research may be either *observational* or *experimental*. In the first, the researcher actively observes patients by doing things like asking questions and taking samples, but does not experiment with the patient's treatment or care. In a typical *experimental* study, in contrast, the researcher *intervenes* to ensure that some or all of a group of people receive a treatment, service, or experience.

It can be helpful to divide observational studies into two groups according to their complexity (Figure 5.1). On the one hand, *descriptive* observational studies ask questions like: 'What are the clinical or biochemical characteristics of people who have rheumatoid arthritis?', 'How common a condition is asthma?', 'How disabled do people become over a decade of follow-up after a diagnosis of multiple sclerosis?'. On the other hand, some observational studies *compare* groups to try to answer more complex questions: 'Do people who smoke get more heart disease than those who don't smoke?', 'Are women who experienced venous thrombosis more likely to have been taking the oral contraceptive pill than women who didn't sustain a thrombosis?'. Studies that ask these kinds of non-experimental (observational) questions, but which involve comparisons, are often described as *analytic*.

Analytic observational studies are dealt with in Chapter 6 and *experimental (intervention) studies* in Chapter 7. The remainder of this chapter tackles the simplest forms of quantitative observation – *descriptive studies*. We find it useful to subdivide descriptive studies into four types:

- Case reports
- Case series
- Cross-sectional studies (simple cross-sectional studies determining, for example, how common (prevalent) a condition is; more complex cross-sectional studies involving comparisons are dealt with under analytic research in Chapter 6)
- Longitudinal studies

CASE REPORTS

Some would say that case reports are scarcely research at all. They usually take the form of an unusual clinical case that illustrates something about the cause or the outcome of the person described that the author hopes will intrigue you. Perhaps the author's care over detail – eliciting symptoms, possible precipitants, and treatments offered – takes the case report out of the ordinary clinical arena and justifies the title of research. Research journal editors vary in their views – some publish such reports and others do not.

Understanding Clinical Papers, Third Edition. David Bowers, Allan House, David Owens and Bridgette Bewick.
© 2014 John Wiley & Sons, Ltd. Published 2014 by John Wiley & Sons, Ltd.

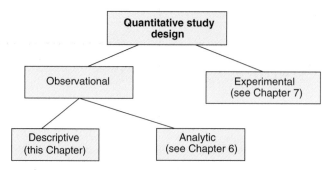

FIGURE 5.1   Types of research study design.

CASE SERIES

A respectable form of research is a description of clinical findings seen in a succession of patients who seem to display a similar condition: the *case series*. Something unexpected has turned up – more cases than usual of a rare disorder perhaps, or an apparent excess of some clinical sign – hence the motive for writing-up the series of cases. For example, Figure 5.2 shows how clinicians used a case series to point to dangers of playing around on bouncy castles.

Sometimes the author of a case series notices some common feature that the cases share and speculates that this factor might help to explain the condition. A famous example of such studies includes the early descriptions of the birth abnormalities that became linked with the drug thalidomide.

Injuries sustained on "bouncy castles"

Gian Singer, Lawrence S Freedman

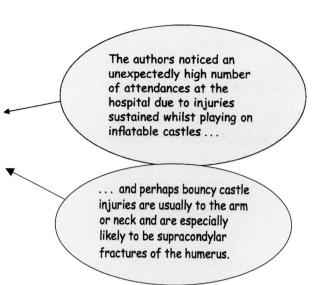

SIR,—We wish to report the dangers of playing on "bouncy castles." A bouncy castle is an inflatable children's playground, consisting essentially of a rubber mattress inflated with air. Three walls generally surround the castle, with the fourth side open to allow entry and exit, but some castles are open on all four sides. They are popular in fairgrounds and recreational halls. During last summer five children and one adult were treated at Northwick Park Hospital for injuries sustained while they were playing on bouncy castles. All injuries were to the arm or neck.

Three supracondylar fractures of the humerus occurred. Two of these required open reduction and internal fixation with Kirschner wires. The third was managed with a collar and cuff support. A girl aged 6 sustained a fracture of the mid-shaft of the humerus, which was managed with a hanging cast support. The neck injuries occurred in a 52 year old man and a 12 year old boy. These were both soft tissue injuries caused by flexion and were managed conservatively.

FIGURE 5.2   Extract from case series of bouncy castle injuries. Reproduced from Singer G, Freedman LS. Injuries sustained on "bouncy castles". *BMJ* 1992, 304: 912, © 1992, with permission from BMJ Publishing Group Ltd.

CROSS-SECTIONAL STUDIES

Unlike the case series, which usually reports an unexpected clinical encounter, the researchers of a cross-sectional study deliberately set out to assemble a group of study subjects – often patients in current or recent contact with part of the health service – and describe the presence and absence of various clinical features. For example, responding to the case series of bouncy castle injuries (Figure 5.2), another researcher extracted from a national survey of leisure accidents the clinical and circumstantial details of 105 bouncy castle injuries (Figure 5.3) – providing us with a more representative picture. This new, premeditated study of 105 cases is a fairly typical cross-sectional study. It seems to show that, when the matter is examined using a suitably selected sample, there is no convincing evidence that bouncy castle

More injuries from "bouncy castles"

S Levene

SIR,—In response to Gian Singer and Lawrence S Freedman's letter[1] I have analysed national figures for accidents involving "bouncy castles." The Department of Trade and Industry's leisure accidents surveillance system records all people injured in accidents other than home, industrial, or road traffic accidents who present to a sample of 11 hospitals throughout the United Kingdom, with 24 hour accident and emergency departments receiving at least 10 000 cases a year. One hundred and five such people were recorded, suggesting a national estimate of roughly 4000 people injured severely enough for them to present to hospital.

Thirty people were injured by falling off the castle (17 male, 13 female; five aged 0–4, 12 aged 5–9, 12 aged 10–14, and one aged 22). Parts of the body commonly injured were the foot, ankle, or toe (10 cases) and the arm, elbow, wrist, or hand (eight cases). Most injuries were minor bruising, cuts, or swelling (20 cases), but there were six fractures and three sprains or strains. Two children required admission for fractures to the arm or elbow. The locations of the bouncy castles varied: six were at fairgrounds and five at indoor sports centres.

Seventy five people were injured on the castle itself (31 male, 44 female; eight aged 0–4, 33 aged 5–9, 27 aged 10–14, and seven adults). Thirty two fell over and 14 were struck by another child, usually after the patient had fallen over. The arm, elbow, wrist, or hand (27 cases), the face and neck (nine cases), and the ankle or foot (15 cases) were commonly injured. Fifty injuries were minor, with nine fractures, 10 sprains and strains, and two dislocations. Fairgrounds (10 cases) were the most common site for the castle.

This author responded to publication of the case series by extracting (from data collected for a large leisure accident surveillance system) information about 105 cases of bouncy castle injury—presenting us with a cross-sectional study

Because of their larger number and their systematic collection, these patients are likely to be more representative than the six people who happened to attend the hospital where the case series was based . . .

. . . and it is plain that the injuries are not only to the head and neck; there is, after all, no specific bouncy castle enjury.

FIGURE 5.3   Extract from cross-sectional study about bouncy castle injuries. Reproduced from Levene S. More injuries from "bouncy castles". *BMJ* 1992, 304: 1311–2, © 1992, with permission from BMJ Publishing Group Ltd.

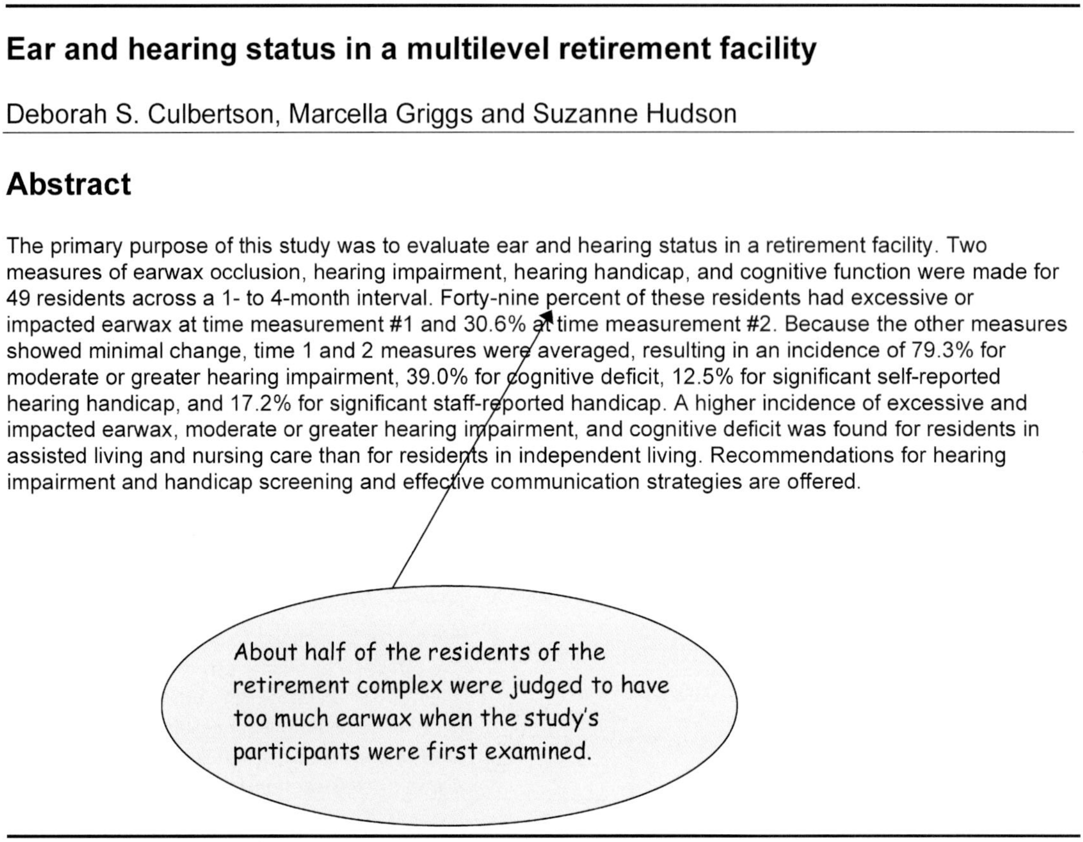

Ear and hearing status in a multilevel retirement facility

Deborah S. Culbertson, Marcella Griggs and Suzanne Hudson

Abstract

The primary purpose of this study was to evaluate ear and hearing status in a retirement facility. Two measures of earwax occlusion, hearing impairment, hearing handicap, and cognitive function were made for 49 residents across a 1- to 4-month interval. Forty-nine percent of these residents had excessive or impacted earwax at time measurement #1 and 30.6% at time measurement #2. Because the other measures showed minimal change, time 1 and 2 measures were averaged, resulting in an incidence of 79.3% for moderate or greater hearing impairment, 39.0% for cognitive deficit, 12.5% for significant self-reported hearing handicap, and 17.2% for significant staff-reported handicap. A higher incidence of excessive and impacted earwax, moderate or greater hearing impairment, and cognitive deficit was found for residents in assisted living and nursing care than for residents in independent living. Recommendations for hearing impairment and handicap screening and effective communication strategies are offered.

About half of the residents of the retirement complex were judged to have too much earwax when the study's participants were first examined.

FIGURE 5.4 Prevalence of a clinical feature, determined in a cross-sectional study. Reprinted from Culbertson DS, Griggs M, Hudson S. Ear and hearing status in multilevel retirement facility. *Geriatric Nursing* 2004, 25: 93–6, © 2004, with permission from Elsevier.

injuries cause a specific fracture of the elbow region but, instead, lead to all manner of soft tissue, joint, and bony injuries – anywhere on the body.

A particular type of cross-sectional, single-group study is one in which incidence or prevalence of a condition is determined. A *prevalence* study determines how many cases of a condition or disease there are in a given population or it might establish the frequency of a clinical finding in a study sample. For example, researchers might use hospital and pharmacy records to establish how many people have insulin-receiving diabetes in a defined hospital catchment area. Then again, another study might estimate the proportion of older people in residential facilities whose ears are occluded by earwax (Figure 5.4).

Incidence studies are rather similar but refine the above kind of study in two ways: the incidence of a condition is the number of *new* cases arising in a defined population over a defined *time*. Figure 5.5 describes such a study – to determine in a defined area of 22 adjoining electoral wards in South London, the number of first-in-a-lifetime strokes, according to ethnic origin. The researchers established the incidence (sometimes called *inception rate*) of stroke in each of the ethnic groups under scrutiny – per 1000 population per year. Strictly speaking it is this incorporation of time, as well as the proportion of cases, that makes incidence a rate, while prevalence is merely a proportion.

Incidence and case fatality rates of stroke subtypes in a multiethnic population: the South London Stroke Register

C D A Wolfe, A G Rudd, R Howard, C Coshall, J Stewart, E Lawrence, C Hajat, T Hillen.

The South London Stroke Register (SLSR) was established to investigate ethnic differences in the natural history of stroke. Initial findings reported that the overall incidence rate ratio for stroke was 2.2 in the black population compared with the white population. This paper considers for the first time the incidence of first in a lifetime stroke by clinical subtype … in a multiethnic community.

The authors investigated stroke incidence from a case register.

Data were collected prospectively by the registry team comprising a medical researcher and nurse trained research associates. Using 12 referral sources in hospital, the local community and neighbouring hospitals, stroke cases were identified as resident in a defined area corresponding to 22 wards of Lambeth, Southwark, and Lewisham Health Commission.

The total population (234 533) is 72% white, 21% black (11% black Caribbean, 7.5% West African, and 2.5% black mixed), and 3% Asian, Bangladeshi, and Pakistani with 4% "other". Hospital surveillance of stroke admissions included two teaching hospitals within and three outside the study area. Community surveillance of stroke included patients under the care of all general practitioners within and on the borders of the study area (n=147). The notification sources were accident and emergency departmental records, hospital wards, brain imaging requests, death certificates, coroners' records, general practitioners, hospital medical staff, community therapists, bereavement officers, hospital based stroke registries, general practice, computer records, and "miscellaneous", including notification by patients or relatives of patients.

In a defined area the data were collected from a wide range of sources of potential cases in hospitals and the community.

FIGURE 5.5 Extract from a cross-sectional (incidence) study about frequency of stroke. Reproduced from Wolfe CDA, Rudd AG, Howard R, Coshall C, Stewart J, Lawrence E, *et al*. Incidence and case fatality rates of stroke subtypes in a multiethnic population: the South London Stroke Register. *Journal of Neurology, Neurosurgery & Psychiatry* 2002, 72: 211–6, © 2002, with permission from BMJ Publishing Group Ltd.

Figure 5.5 shows how the data were collected from hospitals and the community. Some incidence research data, as in this case, are derived from *case-registers* – many of which have been set up with research and clinical service in mind, routinely recording data useful for both purposes. In other cross-sectional studies the researchers undertake a survey of the study sample, where this survey – whether by interview, or by electronic or paper self-report – has been set up specifically for the research project. For example, researchers might ask nurses who visit patients in their homes to describe, by filling in a paper questionnaire, how their patients are using prescribed medicines (Figure 5.6).

Nurses' observations and experiences of problems and adverse effects of medication management in home care

Carol Hall Ellenbecker, Susan C. Frazier and Sharon Verney

Abstract

The purpose of this nonexperimental, descriptive study was to explore and describe the current state of medication management for patients receiving services from certified home health care agencies (CHHAs). Data were collected by self-report from a convenience sample of 101 home health care nurses from 12 agencies in six states. Nurses reported on a total of 1467 patients. Results of this study support the findings from previous research on medication management of older people living in the community. The majority of older home care patients were taking more than five prescription drugs. Many patients were taking medications in ways that deviated from the prescribed medication regimen. The results also suggest that patients are experiencing many adverse effects from medication errors. The reasons for these errors were reported to be a result of individual patient characteristics and, most frequently, communication problems in the system. Results of this study support recommendations for technology application, regulatory and policy changes, further research, and nursing practice.

Community-based nurses were given a paper survey asking them, among other things, about their patients' receipt and use of prescribed medication, for example, whether the patients were taking multiple drugs and whether they skipped doses or took the wrong amounts.

FIGURE 5.6   Use of a survey method in a cross-sectional study. Reproduced from Ellenbecker CH, Frazier SC, Verney S. Nurses' observations and experiences of problems and adverse effects of medication management in home care. *Geriatric Nursing* 2004, 26: 164–70, © 2004, with permission from Elsevier.

LONGITUDINAL STUDIES

When researchers study a group of subjects over time in a *longitudinal study*, there is more research work to be done than in a cross-sectional study; subjects must be followed up one or more times to determine their *prognosis* or *outcome*.

The kinds of observational studies we've seen above are among the simplest form of clinical research. In the next chapter, more complex observational studies are described – *quantitative analytic* studies. What they have in common (and in this way they differ from the above study types) is that they generally involve *comparison* of two or more groups of people and often attempt to infer something about cause of symptoms or conditions.

6

Analytic Studies

Remember from the previous chapter that, compared with descriptive studies of a single group, analytic studies are more complex (and often more interesting). Analytic studies will usually involve some comparison, and frequently aim to elucidate cause and effect in some way. Four kinds of observational analytic study will be described here:

- Ecological studies
- Cross-sectional, two-group studies
- Case-control studies
- Cohort analytic studies

ECOLOGICAL STUDIES

A neat way of tackling questions about the cause of disease or other health events is to sit in a library (or, more likely, at a computer), locate routinely collected data, and put population data about disease frequency (e.g. regional deaths from lung cancer) together with data about exposure to a risk (e.g. regional data on tobacco consumption). By so doing, you might find that regions with high lung cancer death rates were also the ones with high tobacco consumption. Suppose also that you found the opposite – that low mortality areas were associated with low tobacco consumption – then your findings would support a link between the supposed risk (smoking) and the target disorder (lung cancer).

The real study used as an example in Figure 6.1 concerns whether smoking might be an important risk factor for the loss of life arising from fires in people's homes. Researchers from Atlanta, Georgia looked into this observation by assembling data for the year 2004 from two separate databases – one that holds death certificate data by state and another that provides smoking data by state. The graph set out in Figure 6.1 shows how the researchers use the data to shed more light on whether smoking is associated with death in domestic fires.

But you may by now have spotted a flaw in this type of study: we don't know whether the individual people who died in house fires were smokers. Put another way, it is possible for a study of this design to come up with these findings even if every person who died in a house fire was a non-smoker. This flaw is sometimes called the *ecological fallacy* and is a consequence of the use of aggregated data rather than the more usual research method of collecting data for each individual study participant. The other three types of analytic study set out below are more satisfactory approaches to cause-and-effect questions because they are able to relate the supposed risk factor directly to the outcome in each study participant.

Understanding Clinical Papers, Third Edition. David Bowers, Allan House, David Owens and Bridgette Bewick.
© 2014 John Wiley & Sons, Ltd. Published 2014 by John Wiley & Sons, Ltd.

Ecological level analysis of the relationship between smoking and residential-fire mortality

S T Diekman, M F Ballesteros, L R Berger, R S Caraballo, S R Kegler

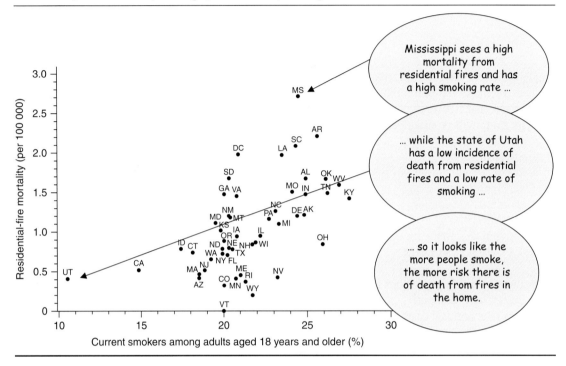

FIGURE 6.1 Findings from an ecological study about smoking and domestic fires. Reproduced from Diekman ST, Ballesteros MF, Berger LR, Carabello RS, Kegler SR. Ecological level analysis of the relationship between smoking and residential-fire mortality. *Injury Prevention* 2008, 14: 228–31, © 2008, with permission from BMJ Publishing Group Ltd.

CROSS-SECTIONAL, TWO-GROUP STUDIES

Some cross-sectional studies aim to shed light on cause and effect by recording whether people with a disease were more likely than people without the same disease to experience exposure to a risk factor. For example, for more than half a century researchers have recognised that patients with schizophrenia, when compared with the general population, are more likely to come from lower socio-economic classes. What is a lot less clear is whether lower socio-economic status is a risk factor for schizophrenia or, conversely, whether schizophrenia causes a slide down the socio-economic scale. The cross-sectional study design – in which the researcher measures in each subject a supposed risk factor at the same time as recording the presence of a condition – will nearly always have this *chicken or egg* problem (which comes first?).

In a study of bullying (Figure 6.2), the researchers persuaded 904 co-educational secondary school pupils aged 12–17 years to declare whether they were bullied or not and to self-report their feelings – including a scale that measured their level of anxiety. They found that those who reported being bullied also reported more anxiety. Notice that the study design does not preclude either possibility: that bullying exacerbates anxiety or that anxious children are more likely to be targets for bullies.

Bullying in schools: self reported anxiety, depression, and self esteem in secondary school children

G Salmon, A James, D M Smith

Variable	Being bullied or bullying	
	No	Yes
Bullied children (mean score for being bullied) ≥ 2)		
School:		
A	377	24
B	489	14
School year:		
8	224	16
9	237	8
10	194	9
11	211	5
Sex:		
Male	439	23
Female	427	15
Mean (SD) score:		
Anxiety	9.71 (6.00)	17.71 (6.75)
Esteem	29.27 (4.75)	24.97 (6.38)
Lying	2.52 (2.10)	3.37 (2.33)
Depression	5.88 (5.13)	12.92 (7.95)

Notice that bullied children have higher anxiety and depression and lower self-esteem. But is it because they are bullied or do these characteristics lead to the bullying?

This cross-sectional study doesn't have a design that can determine the direction of any effect.

FIGURE 6.2 Extract from table of summary statistics from cross-sectional study of bullying and self-reported anxiety (values are numbers of schoolchildren unless stated otherwise). Reproduced from Salmon G, James A, Smith DM. Bullying in schools: self reported anxiety, depression, and self esteem in secondary school children. *BMJ* 1998, 317: 924–5, © 1998, with permission from BMJ Publishing Group Ltd.

It is a limitation of cross-sectional designs that the direction of any effect cannot be determined because the supposed risk factor and the outcome are identified at the same time. The next two analytic study designs tackle this weakness and are able to identify the direction of any effect.

CASE-CONTROL STUDIES

A more satisfactory way of investigating cause and effect is to concentrate on a clinical scenario in which the characteristic that you suspect might be a risk factor and the outcome can only have arisen in that order. Consider for a moment smoking and lung cancer: it is plain that contracting lung cancer cannot have led someone to become a long-standing heavy smoker.

Notice though that it is the pre-existence of heavy smoking that defines the difference between this example and the cross-sectional example above. If a researcher wanted to know whether high blood pressure made stroke more likely, and chose to measure blood pressure in two groups of patients who were and were not victims of stroke, then any finding that hypertension was more prevalent in stroke patients might be a consequence of the stroke rather than a contributory cause. If, on the other hand, each set of patients had previously had their blood pressure recorded some years before, then the finding that stroke patients had a past excess of hypertension might very well point to high blood pressure being a risk factor for stroke.

Case-control study is the label applied to a study such as the one just mentioned, about high blood pressure and stroke. The group of people with the condition are called the *cases* and they are compared with another group who are free of the disease and are called the *controls*. The comparison to be drawn is the exposure of each of the two groups to a supposed risk factor: were the cases more often exposed to the risk than were the controls? For further discussion of cases and controls, see Chapters 12 and 13.

In the study in Figure 6.3, researchers in Dorset and York undertook a case-control study to help to settle controversy over measles vaccination in childhood and whether it predisposes to development in

---

A case-control study of measles vaccination and inflammatory bowel disease

Mark Feeney, Andrew Clegg, Paul Winwood, Jonathon Snook, for the East Dorset Gastroenterology Group

---

Summary

Background The cause of inflammatory bowel disease (IBD) remains to be established. Evidence has linked measles infection in early childhood with the subsequent risk of developing IBD, particularly Crohn's disease. A cohort study raised the possibility that immunisation with live attenuated measles vaccine, which induces active immunity to measles infection, might also predispose to the later development of IBD, provoking concerns about the safety of the vaccine.

Method We report a case-control study of 140 patients with IBD (including 83 with Crohn's disease) born in or after 1968, and 280 controls matched for age, sex and general practitioner (GP) area, designated to assess the influence of measles vaccination on later development of IBD. Documentary evidence of childhood vaccination history was sought from GP and community health records.

Findings Crude measles vaccination rates were 56.4% in patients with IBD and 57.1% among controls. Matched odds ratios for measles vaccination were 1.08 (95% CI 0.62–1.88) in patients with Crohn's disease, 0.84 (0.44–1.58) in patients with ulcerative colitis, and 0.97 (0.64–1.47) in all patients with IBD.

Interpretation These findings provide no support for the hypothesis that measles vaccination in childhood predisposes to the later development of either IBD overall or Crohn's disease in particular.

In a case-control study subjects get into their study group according to whether they have the disease or not.

For an explanation of what the odds ratios tell us, see Chapter 24; and see Chapter 26 for how to interpret the confidence intervals.

FIGURE **6.3** Summary of a case-control study. Reprinted from *The Lancet* 350: Feeney M, Clegg A, Winwood P, Snook J, for the East Dorset Gastroenterology Group. A case-control study of measles vaccination and inflammatory bowel disease. 1997, 764–6, © 1997, with permission from Elsevier.

adulthood of inflammatory bowel disease – ulcerative colitis and Crohn's disease. They ascertained the vaccination history, from general practice records, of 140 patients with definite inflammatory bowel disease (the cases). For each of these patients they randomly selected from the same general practitioner's list two people of the same age and sex (the controls); they then ascertained the vaccination history of these control patients. They found that 79 of the 140 cases (56%) had received measles vaccine compared with 160 of the 280 (57%) controls – almost exactly the same proportions. The authors conclude that their findings provide no support for the notion that measles vaccination in childhood predisposes to later development of inflammatory bowel disease.

COHORT ANALYTIC STUDIES

Another way of identifying any relation between measles vaccine and inflammatory bowel disease would have been to compare the eventual outcome for people who were or were not vaccinated – a *cohort study* – sometimes termed a *cohort analytic study*, thereby emphasising the comparative (or analytic) objective of the investigation. In this hypothetical example, the subjects of the research would have been divided by the researcher according to whether they were vaccinated or not. In the earlier, real, case-control study the study participants were divided by whether they had the disease or not; the designs are quite different.

In a real example of a cohort study shown in Figure 6.4, researchers in Canada looked into whether having received epidural anaesthesia during labour is a risk factor for post-partum back pain. The study participants were a consecutive series of 329 women who had a child delivered at the hospital. As it happened, about half of the women had opted for epidural anaesthesia – allowing their comparison with those who had alternative forms of pain relief. A research nurse interviewed all the patients and rated on a scale their degree of self-reported pain at three follow-up points during the 6 weeks following delivery.

COMPARING AND CONTRASTING CASE-CONTROL AND COHORT STUDIES

Compared with cohort studies, case-control studies are cheap and cheerful. First, they can be completed without waiting for the outcome to develop. Second, there is no need for enormous numbers of study subjects who do not develop the outcome; because in a case-control study it is already clear who has the outcome, only a convenient number (needed for reasonable statistical precision) of these 'controls' is needed. In a cohort study, however, there is no way of knowing who will get and not get the outcome – so everyone has to be included until the study end-point reveals who has developed the condition so far. For a great many relatively uncommon outcomes the case-control study is favoured for just these reasons. Examples of case-control studies include investigating whether deep venous thrombosis is related to taking the oral contraceptive pill, and whether depressive illness is related to adverse life events and difficulties.

On the other hand, there are serious shortcomings with case-control studies. They are prone to extra biases – in particular those concerned with recollection of past events. Suppose, for example, that a study hypothesis is that an adult condition such as motor neurone disease is predisposed to by certain kinds of childhood infections. It is likely that in an effort to understand why one has such an illness, sufferers with motor neurone disease may recall more such illnesses than controls who have no pressure to make such an effort. It is very difficult to avoid such bias.

Second, it is usually difficult to select a wholly suitable control group for a case-control study. In a case-control study concerned with smoking and lung cancer, for example, should those without lung cancer be people with other cancers, or patients with other respiratory conditions, or other patients at the hospital without chest disorder, or general practice cases (and should they exclude those with chest problems), or members of the general public who are not drawn from health-care contacts at all? None of these possible

Epidural anaesthesia and low back pain after delivery: a prospective cohort study

Alison Macarthur, Colin Macarthur, Sally Weeks

Abstract

Objective—To determine whether epidural anaesthesia during labour and delivery is a risk factor for postpartum back pain.

Design—Prospective cohort study with follow up at one day, seven days, and six weeks after delivery.

Setting—Teaching hospital in Montreal.

Subjects—329 women who delivered a live infant(s) during the study period. Exclusion criteria were back pain before pregnancy and delivery by elective caesarean section.

Intervention—Epidural anaesthesia during labour and delivery.

Main outcome measures and results—The primary outcome variable was development of postpartum low back pain. Back pain was quantified with self reports (yes/no), a pain score (numeric rating scale), and degree of interference with daily activities. Of the 329 women, 164 received epidural anaesthesia during labour and 165 did not. The incidence of low back pain in epidural *v* non-epidural group was 53% *v* 43% on day one; 21% *v* 23% on day seven; and 14% *v* 7% at six weeks. The relative risk for low back pain (epidural *v* non-epidural) adjusted for parity, delivery, ethnicity, and weight was 1.76 (95% confidence interval 1.06 to 2.92) on day one; 1.00 (0.54 to 1.86) on day seven; and 2.22 (0.89 to 5.53) at six weeks. There were no differences between the two groups in pain scores or the frequency of interference with daily activities. Similar results were

In a cohort analytic study subjects get into their study group according to whether they were exposed to the supposed risk or not.

For an explanation of what the relative risks tell us, see Chapter 24; and see Chapter 26 for how to interpret the confidence intervals.

FIGURE 6.4 Cohort analytic study examining the relation between post-partum back pain and epidural anaesthesia during labour. Reproduced from Macarthur A, Macarthur C, Weeks S. Epidural anaesthesia and low back pain after delivery: a prospective cohort study. *BMJ* 1995, 311: 1336–9, © 1995, with permission from BMJ Publishing Group Ltd.

groups is wholly suited or unsuited; in the end, the findings will often be hard to interpret whichever control group is selected (sometimes case-control studies use more than one control group for just such reasons). Put another way, the control group in a case-control study is intended by the researcher to represent, as if it were a small random sample, the great many people in the population who have not developed the outcome. Unfortunately, in practice, they are instead a specifically targeted group – easily identified and included in the research – but not actually providing the representation of the non-cases in the population that the researcher ideally wants.

Cohort analytic studies avoid the worst aspects of the above two problems. First, because exposure is assessed at the start of the study, it is not subject to false remembering later. Second, assessment of exposure to risk provides sensible exposed and unexposed groups, and avoids uncertainty over which comparison group to choose.

Both these kinds of analytic observational study are greatly prone to *confounding*. This matter is discussed in Chapters 13 and 30.

7

Intervention Studies

There is evidence to suggest that dietary supplementation before surgery can reduce post-operative complications. A clinical team in the UK wanted to find out whether it would be beneficial, in the treatment of colorectal cancer, to use oral supplementary drinks before the major operation to treat the cancer. They introduced 400 mL of high-energy and protein containing supplements daily in the days running up to the operation. In the study, about half of the 125 people who agreed to take part received the intervention; the other half did not. The patients were randomly allocated to one or other of these groups using a procedure governed by random numbers. As it turned out, the main outcome of interest was not significantly affected by the dietary supplements: those who had the supplements, and those who didn't, had about the same post-operative complication rate.

TRIALS

The study depicted in Figure 7.1 has three defining features. First, it is called a *trial* because the researchers have introduced experimentation; they have arranged for some subjects but not others to receive the intervention. Second, they fix it so that their two groups of subjects will differ only according to whether or not they had the intervention. We would therefore expect to see, for instance, as many underweight patients, as many patients with cancers at an advanced stage, and as many cigarette smokers in each of the two treatment groups. If so, none of these factors can have accounted for the difference found in outcomes; researchers often assert that these factors have been *controlled* for. But how can the groups be made similar in every way? This can happen only when allocation to one or other group is by a *randomised* procedure.

This kind of study, the *randomised controlled trial*, has become almost the only acceptable way of judging the benefit of a treatment (whether it be a drug, procedure, operation, psychological therapy, or other intervention). Although it would be a lot more convenient only to investigate what happens to the treated group, the problem is that if the treated patients were to get better it might have been for reasons unconnected with the treatment-for example, the condition might simply have resolved with time. But if, in a comparison of two similar patient groups, those who got the treatment improved more than those who did not get it, then we have compelling evidence in favour of the treatment; improvement due to the passage of time, or due to any other factor unrelated to the treatment, could not explain why the treated patients had the better outcome.

In a study from Sri Lanka (extract shown in Figure 7.2), where there are many species of poisonous snakes, and venomous bites are consequently a serious health hazard, researchers used the principle of the randomised controlled trial to answer an important treatment question: 'Can the dangerous side-effects of life-saving antivenom serum be counteracted?'.

Understanding Clinical Papers, Third Edition. David Bowers, Allan House, David Owens and Bridgette Bewick.
© 2014 John Wiley & Sons, Ltd. Published 2014 by John Wiley & Sons, Ltd.

An unblinded randomised controlled trial of preoperative oral supplements in colorectal cancer patients

S. T. Burden, J. Hill, J. L. Shaffer, M. Campbell & C. Todd.

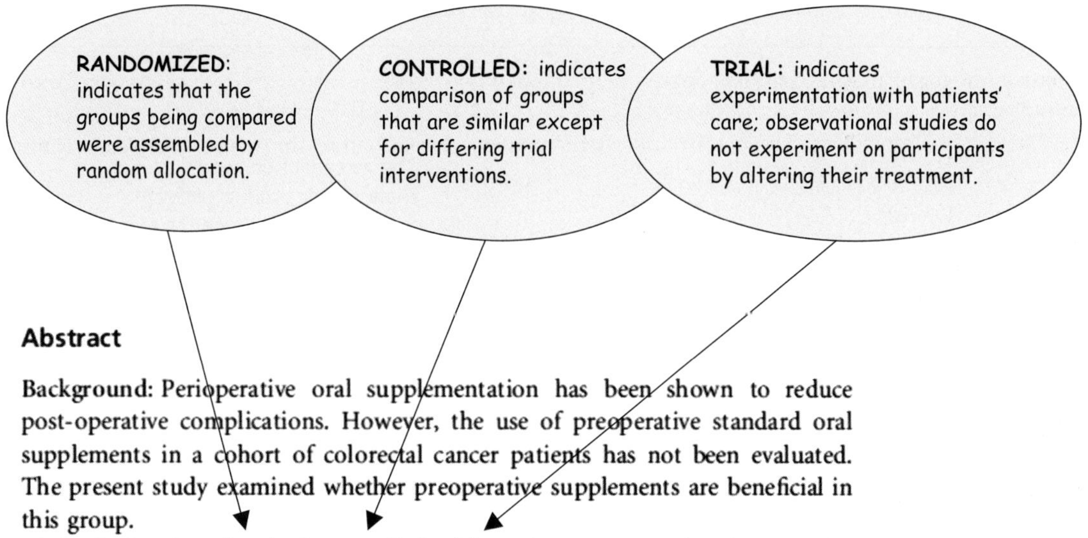

RANDOMIZED: indicates that the groups being compared were assembled by random allocation.

CONTROLLED: indicates comparison of groups that are similar except for differing trial interventions.

TRIAL: indicates experimentation with patients' care; observational studies do not experiment on participants by altering their treatment.

Abstract

Background: Perioperative oral supplementation has been shown to reduce post-operative complications. However, the use of preoperative standard oral supplements in a cohort of colorectal cancer patients has not been evaluated. The present study examined whether preoperative supplements are beneficial in this group.

Methods: In a randomised controlled trial, patients were assigned to receive 400 mL of oral supplement and dietary advice or dietary advice alone. Primary outcome was the number of post-operative complications. One hundred and twenty-five patients were recruited (59 randomised to the intervention group and 66 to the control group) and nine were excluded.

Results: In the intervention group, 24 (44%) patients had a complication compared to 26 (42%) in the control group ($P = 0.780$). In the intervention and control groups, there were eight (15%) and 16 (25%) surgical site infections, respectively ($P = 0.140$) and seven (13%) and 11 (17%) chest infections, respectively ($P = 0.470$). Subgroup analysis for hypothesis generation included 83 (71%) weight-losing patients, where there was a significant reduction in surgical site infections using the Buzby definition ($P = 0.034$), although this was not the case for the Centre for Disease Control definition ($P = 0.052$).

Conclusions: There was no evidence that preoperative supplements were beneficial in reducing the number of complications, although there may be some benefit for surgical site infections in selected weight-losing preoperative patients.

FIGURE 7.1   Summary of a randomised controlled trial investigating an intervention aimed at reducing post-operative complications in patients with colorectal cancer. Reproduced from Burden SR, Hill J, Shaffer JL, Campbell M, Todd C (2011) with permission from John Wiley & Sons.

Low dose subcutaneous adrenaline to prevent acute adverse reactions to antivenom serum in people bitten by snakes: randomised, placebo controlled trial

A P Premawardhena, C E de Silva, M M D Fonseka, S B Gunatilake, H J de Silva

Objective To assess the efficacy and safety of low dose adrenaline injected subcutaneously to prevent acute adverse reactions to polyspecific antivenom serum in patients admitted to hospital after snake bite.
Design Prospective, double blind, randomised, placebo controlled trial.
Setting District general hospital in Sri Lanka.
Subjects 105 patients with signs of envenomation after snake bite, randomised to receive either adrenaline (cases) or placebo (controls) immediately before infusion of antivenom serum.
Interventions Adrenaline 0.25 ml (1:1000).
Main outcome measures Development of acute adverse reactions to serum and side effects attributable to adrenaline.
Results 56 patients (cases) received adrenaline and 49 (controls) received placebo as pretreatment. Six (11%) adrenaline patients and 21 (43%) control patients developed acute adverse reactions to antivenom serum (P=0.0002). Significant reductions in acute adverse reactions to serum were also seen in the adrenaline patients for each category of mild, moderate, and severe reactions. There were no significant adverse effects attributable to adrenaline.
Conclusions Use of 0.25 ml of 1:1000 adrenaline given subcutaneously immediately before administration of antivenom serum to patients with envenomation after snake bite reduces the incidence of acute adverse reactions to serum.

The researchers want to know if adrenaline prevents dangerous side-effects caused by the life-saving antivenom serum . . .

. . . so they administered adrenaline to the half of the patients who were randomly selected to receive it.

Only 1 in 9 of those given adrenaline had a severe reaction to the antivenom serum, compared with nearly half of those not given adrenaline.

FIGURE 7.2   Summary of a randomised controlled trial seeking to identify improvement in care for snake-bite victims. Reproduced from Premawardhena AP, de Silva CE, Fonseka MMD, Gunatilake SB, de Silva HJ. Low dose subcutaneous adrenaline to prevent acute adverse reactions to antivenom serum in people bitten by snakes: randomised, placebo controlled trial. *BMJ* 1999, 318: 1041–3, © 1999, with permission from BMJ Publishing Group Ltd.

RANDOM ALLOCATION AND ITS CONCEALMENT

Clinical trials such as the examples above often declare that treatment was allocated randomly. In recent times though, there has been particular attention given to whether this process of randomisation was scrupulously adhered to at the point of treatment allocation – by concealing the imminent allocation from the person who first administers one or other treatment.

There are several ways of determining treatment randomly. Computers can generate random numbers or printed tables of random numbers can be referred to. Either way, the process can be carried out in advance, and the results put into sealed, opaque, and tamper-proof envelopes. The person who obtains the patient's consent to take part in the trial can then simply open the next envelope and proceed with the randomly allocated decision therein. Unfortunately, this admirable procedure is not beyond subversion; clinical researchers have been known to shine bright lights through envelopes to reveal the allocation, and to open several envelopes in advance of seeing potential subjects and then allocate treatment according to their non-random judgement. A better (more tamper-proof) system is distant randomisation, for example, by telephone or by the Internet. The researcher, after obtaining consent, calls up the randomisation service, registers the index patient's entry to the study, and only then is given the answer to the random allocation.

The advantage of these procedures is that the researcher's knowledge of the patient cannot influence the selection procedure. These methods have been proven to reduce selection biases, which otherwise seriously slant the trial results (usually appearing to favour markedly the new or active treatment). Trials that do not adequately report how they concealed allocation of treatment should be treated with suspicion.

This so-called *concealment of allocation* overlaps with 'blinding' (or 'masking') procedures. Blinding techniques (dealt with in Chapter 17) also involve hiding information about the treatment allocation, but are introduced at a later stage in the research investigation where efforts are made to avoid bias in the measurement or experience of outcomes of the treatment under scrutiny.

CONSENT AND RANDOMISATION IN TRIALS

Under most circumstances, patients cannot ethically be included in a randomised controlled trial without their informed consent. The information given to patients will usually include a description of the randomised allocation of treatment in a trial. It is, however, appropriate in some circumstances to randomise people without their consent, which is sought after the allocation has been made – but before the treatments are undertaken. This procedure (shown in Figure 7.3) is sometimes called post-randomisation consent or *Zelen's procedure*. Trial participants consent to any treatment and follow-up assessment they receive, but without being aware that they have been allocated that treatment by randomisation.

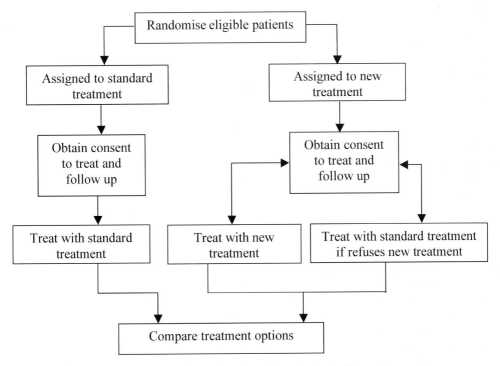

FIGURE 7.3 A flow-chart to illustrate Zelen's procedure for post-randomization consent.

The big advantage of randomisation is that it deals with confounding (see Chapter 13) so that, provided the trial is big enough to make chance unlikely to affect the result, any differences between patient groups will be due to the treatment offered.

Despite the merits of random allocation, for a variety of reasons many eligible patients do not end up in randomised trials. It may be that clinicians don't like asking their patients or that patients, when asked, refuse to be randomised. The upshot is that most trials do not study treatments in a fully representative sample of those patients who might be suitable for treatment in the real world.

To put it more technically – randomised controlled trials have high *internal validity* if they are well conducted. That is, their results tell you something real about the effects of treatments because confounding has been dealt with. But they have low *external validity* if only a small proportion of patients agree to participate. That is, you may not be able to generalise the results to the whole group of patients in which you are interested. For this reason it is important to know how many people who were eligible did not participate. Flow diagrams like those recommended in the guidelines of the CONSORT (Consolidated Standards of Reporting Trials) Statement (http://www.consort-statement.org) can be very useful in identifying the likely impact of non-participation on generalisability.

PLACEBOS OR TREATMENT-AS-USUAL

We know that when health-care professionals recommend some course of action, like giving a tablet or encouraging an exercise, it frequently has some beneficial effect – even if the tablet is chalk or the exercise quite unproved in benefit. In a randomised controlled trial in which the people who get the treatment under scrutiny improve more than those who don't get it, it is plausible that the benefit arises only because of this *placebo effect*. To get around such a problem, researchers frequently compare two apparently similar treatments, but where only one contains the supposedly active ingredient. Exactly that technique was used by the researchers in the snake-bite study referred to above (Figure 7.4).

Often, it would be unethical to withhold treatment and give placebo, when effective treatments are already available, so a new treatment is tested not against placebo, but against one of the standard

---

Low dose subcutaneous adrenaline to prevent acute adverse reactions to antivenom serum in people bitten by snakes: randomised, placebo controlled trial

A P Premawardhena, C E de Silva, M M D Fonseka, S B Gunatilake, H J de Silva

---

Subjects 105 patients with signs of envenomation after snake bite, randomised to receive either adrenaline (cases) or placebo (controls) immediately before infusion of antivenom serum.

In the snake venom trial, half the patients were given saline, identical in appearance to the adrenaline solution.

FIGURE 7.4   Extract from summary of snake-bite trial (Figure 7.2) describing the placebo treatment. Reproduced from Premawardhena AP, de Silva CE, Fonseka MMD, Gunatilake SB, de Silva HJ. Low dose subcutaneous adrenaline to prevent acute adverse reactions to antivenom serum in people bitten by snakes: randomised, placebo controlled trial. *BMJ* 1999, 318: 1041–3, © 1999, with permission from BMJ Publishing Group Ltd.

Comparison of microwave endometrial ablation and transcervical resection of the endometrium for treatment of heavy menstrual loss: a randomised trial

Kevin G Cooper, Christine Bain, David E Parkin

Background Various new endometrial ablation techniques have emerged for the treatment of menorrhagia. We undertook a randomised controlled trial comparing one new technique, microwave endometrial ablation (MEA), with a proven procedure, transcervical resection of the endometrium (TCRE), for women with heavy menstrual loss.
Methods 263 eligible and consenting women, referred for endometrial ablative surgery, were randomly assigned MEA (Microsulis plc, Waterlooville, Hampshire, UK; n=129) or TCRE (n=134). 230 participants were needed to give 80% power of demonstrating a 15% difference in satisfaction with treatment. All procedures were done under general anaesthesia 5 weeks after endometrial thinning with goserelin 3.6 mg. Questionnaires were completed at recruitment and at 12 months' follow-up. The primary outcome measures were patients' satisfaction with and the acceptability of treatment. Analysis was by intention to treat among women followed up to 12 months (n=116 MEA, n=124 TCRE).

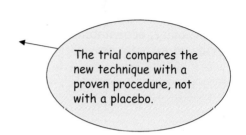

The trial compares the new technique with a proven procedure, not with a placebo.

FIGURE 7.5   Extract from the summary of a randomised controlled trial comparing two procedures to tackle heavy menstrual loss. Reprinted from *The Lancet* 354: Cooper KG, Bain C, Parkin DE. Comparison of microwave endometrial ablation and transcervical resection of the endometrium for treatment of heavy menstrual loss: a randomised trial. 1999; 1859–63, © 1999, with permission from Elsevier.

current treatments. An obvious example arises when comparing two surgical procedures. For example (Figure 7.5), when they evaluated surgical treatments of heavy menstrual loss, gynaecologists in Aberdeen compared operating time, length of stay in hospital, and patient satisfaction in a randomised controlled trial of resection (cutting away) of the uterus lining versus a technique using ablation (destruction) of the lining with microwaves. Plainly, a placebo could not have been an acceptable alternative to the microwave technique. In another case, a new treatment for lowering high blood pressure would usually need to be judged against an existing blood-pressure-lowering agent; in most circumstances ethics would preclude using placebo when there are available effective treatments.

PRAGMATIC AND EXPLANATORY TRIALS

If a new intervention is to be used in clinical practice then, ideally, its benefits will have been determined in randomised controlled trials. But if these trials have been carried out in narrowly defined ways with carefully selected groups of participants, is it credible that the findings will apply to routine care? Researchers who undertake clinical trials sometimes tackle this challenge – the application of science to the real world – by referring to *explanatory trials* and *pragmatic trials*. An explanatory trial attempts to advance scientific understanding by employing techniques that are like experimental procedures in a laboratory: study subjects are tightly defined with strict inclusion and exclusion criteria, and interventions are similarly narrow – perhaps delivering the same number of milligrams of a drug per kilogram of body weight for every participant who has been randomly allocated to the active treatment. A pragmatic trial, on the other hand, is designed with attention to the variability of patients and of their treatments in the routine clinical setting where the treatment is expected to be used.

Put another way, explanatory trials establish benefits that arise in rather idealised conditions, where these benefits are sometimes termed the *efficacy* of the intervention. Pragmatic trials, conversely, offer potentially greater opportunity to generalise the findings, because a range of patients are offered a range of treatments, just as they are in day-to-day practice; this kind of evaluation is sometimes termed the *effectiveness* of the intervention. Figure 7.6 sets out an extract from a pragmatic trial, in which patients

---

Accessibility, acceptability, and effectiveness in primary care of routine telephone review of asthma: pragmatic, randomised controlled trial

Pinnock H, Bawden R, Proctor S, Wolfe S, Scullion J, Price D, Sheikh A

Methods
Recruitment – All four general practices that took part in the study had nurses who were trained and experienced in providing proactive asthma care (table 1). From their computerised asthma registers the practices identified adults (≥ 18 years) who had asked for a bronchodilator inhaler prescription in the previous six months but who had not had a routine asthma review in the preceding 11 months. Patients were excluded if the diagnosis of asthma had been made within the previous year, if they had chronic obstructive pulmonary disease, if communication difficulties made a telephone consultation impossible, or (at the general practitioner's request) for major social or medical reasons. We wrote to all eligible patients inviting them to take part in the study.

There are a few reasonable exclusions but as many patients as possible are included.

Randomisation – Patients were centrally randomised in blocks of 10 to ensure that approximately equal numbers of patients were allocated to each arm of the study.

Intervention – Patients randomised to the telephone review group were sent a letter from their practice informing them that they had been allocated to receive a telephone review and that they should expect a call from the asthma nurse within a month. Nurses were told to make up to four attempts to contact the patient by phone. The nurses were given no instructions about the content of the review except that it should reflect their normal practice and be appropriate to each patient's clinical need. Details about the consultation, including failed attempts at phone calls and the duration of the consultation, were recorded immediately after the review on a piloted consultation record. Nurses arranged any follow up consultations (whether in the surgery or by telephone) they deemed clinically necessary. Patients were free to arrange any consultations they wished.

Patients allocated to the telephone review group received variable interventions, depending on their circumstances and the nurse's assessment of need.

Control group – Patients randomised to the face to face consultation arm were sent a written invitation to make an appointment to see the asthma nurse within a month. Clinical care and follow up were the same as for the intervention group but without a telephone option.

FIGURE 7.6   Extract from a pragmatic trial comparing face-to-face consultation for asthma sufferers with a telephone review by a nurse. Reproduced from Pinnock H, Bawden R, Proctor S, Wolfe S, Scullion J, Price D, *et al.* Accessibility, acceptability, and effectiveness in primary care of routine telephone review of asthma: pragmatic, randomised controlled trial. *BMJ* 2003, 326: 477–9, © 2003, with permission from BMJ Publishing Group Ltd.

with asthma who got a telephone review (the treatment-as-usual control group got a face-to-face consultation with the doctor instead) received a variety of interventions, depending on their responses and what the nurses thought they required. This example demonstrates that, in a pragmatic trial, it is the treatment or management protocol that is under scrutiny, whereas an explanatory trial usually examines the benefit of a single, highly specific treatment.

INTENTION-TO-TREAT ANALYSIS

The advantages of random allocation to treatments are easily destroyed if some trial subjects are not included in the analysis of the data at the end of the study. For example, some patients do not or cannot take the treatment to which they were allocated. If they are excluded from the analysis, the biases removed by the randomisation process creep back in. Instead, it is recommended practice for all subjects to be analysed within the group they were allocated to – even if they did not (for whatever reason) experience the treatment. This, at first sight rather odd, principle is known as *intention-to-treat analysis*. The researchers tell us that they used this form of analysis in the gynaecological trial described in Figure 7.5.

To understand the logic of this approach, imagine a trial in which 50 people are randomly allocated to receive Treatment A and 50 people are randomly allocated to receive Treatment B. All 50 people complete their course of Treatment A and at follow-up half of them are recovered from the condition being treated. In the Treatment B group only one person completes treatment and at follow-up she has recovered. We wouldn't want to argue that Treatment B was better than Treatment A because recovery was 100% for B and only 50% for A; we would want to know what happened to the 49 people who didn't complete Treatment B. Perhaps all of them stopped treatment after a day because of unacceptable side-effects, so only one in 50 (2%) of patients who took Treatment B actually recovered!

It follows, then, that the intention-to-treat approach can only be fully applied when complete data on the main outcome are available for all participants who were randomly allocated, even if they did not complete the course of treatment. In practice, these outcome data are incomplete in a high proportion of trials. In Chapter 17 we discuss how researchers attempt to deal with the challenge of undertaking an intention-to-treat analysis when they have not been able to collect follow-up data on all the people who have agreed to participate in a trial.

It is especially important that pragmatic trials, which aim to assess the real-world effectiveness of a treatment, take proper account of everyone who agreed to participate. Sadly though, all the methods proposed (Chapter 17) for dealing with missing data in trials are less than satisfactory. Consequently, although the assertion of 'intention-to-treat' by a trial's authors is intended to signal a robust analysis, it may simply mask unresolved bias. It is fair to say, however, that a flawed attempt at intention-to-treat is likely to be better than an analysis that pays no attention to the participants who underwent random allocation but dropped out somewhere along the way.

To make matters worse, because intention-to-treat analysis has become the customary expectation of those who fund or monitor or publish trials, researchers sometimes use the term loosely – presumably in the hope of impressing those reading their plans or their findings. Surveys of the analyses that are passed off as intention-to-treat show that many of the research studies are poorly described or insufficiently scrupulous in their execution.

8

Mixed Methods Research

Conventionally, descriptions of research methods have delineated two main types – the *qualitative* and the *quantitative*. It was not always so, but increasingly researchers have come to understand that there may be benefits from employing both approaches in the same project. When the two approaches are genuinely integrated, researchers refer to *mixed-methods* research.

Sometimes quantitative and qualitative approaches to data collection are employed simultaneously or *concurrently* (Figure 8.1). In this example, the researcher concurrently applied two methods of data collection and then analysed the qualitative results in the light of those from the standardised questionnaire.

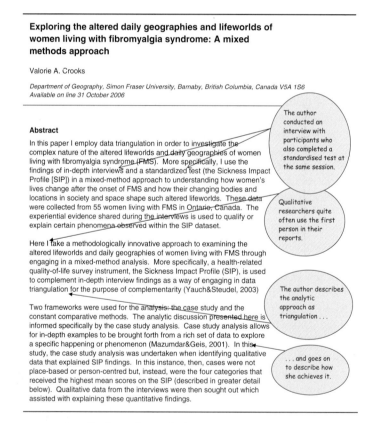

Exploring the altered daily geographies and lifeworlds of women living with fibromyalgia syndrome: A mixed methods approach

Valorie A. Crooks

Department of Geography, Simon Fraser University, Barnaby, British Columbia, Canada V5A 1S6
Available on line 31 October 2006

Abstract

In this paper I employ data triangulation in order to investigate the complex nature of the altered lifeworlds and daily geographies of women living with fibromyalgia syndrome (FMS). More specifically, I use the findings of in-depth interviews and a standardized test (the Sickness Impact Profile [SIP]) in a mixed-method approach to understanding how women's lives change after the onset of FMS and how their changing bodies and locations in society and space shape such altered lifeworlds. These data were collected from 55 women living with FMS in Ontario, Canada. The experiential evidence shared during the interviews is used to qualify or explain certain phenomena observed within the SIP dataset.

Here I take a methodologically innovative approach to examining the altered lifeworlds and daily geographies of women living with FMS through engaging in a mixed-method analysis. More specifically, a health-related quality-of-life survey instrument, the Sickness Impact Profile (SIP), is used to complement in-depth interview findings as a way of engaging in data triangulation for the purpose of complementarity (Yauch&Steudel, 2003)

Two frameworks were used for the analysis: the case study and the constant comparative methods. The analytic discussion presented here is informed specifically by the case study analysis. Case study analysis allows for in-depth examples to be brought forth from a rich set of data to explore a specific happening or phenomenon (Mazumdar&Geis, 2001). In this study, the case study analysis was undertaken when identifying qualitative data that explained SIP findings. In this instance, then, cases were not place-based or person-centred but, instead, were the four categories that received the highest mean scores on the SIP (described in greater detail below). Qualitative data from the interviews were then sought out which assisted with explaining these quantitative findings.

The author conducted an interview with participants who also completed a standardised test at the same session.

Qualitative researchers quite often use the first person in their reports.

The author describes the analytic approach as triangulation . . .

. . . and goes on to describe how she achieves it.

FIGURE 8.1 Concurrent use of qualitative and quantitative approaches to data collection. Reprinted from Crooks. Exploring the altered daily geographies and lifeworlds of women living with fibromyalgia syndrome: a mixed method approach. *Social Science & Medicine* 2007, 64 (3): 577–88, © 2007, with permission from Elsevier.

This approach to analysis, in which data from different sources are used to develop a more rounded or complete picture than either could alone, is sometimes called *triangulation* or *data triangulation* (Figure 8.1 and Figure 8.2 for another example). In this second study the researchers used not a concurrent but a *sequential* approach to data collection – using results from a quantitative study to inform sampling for their qualitative study.

This sequential approach can work in either direction. A familiar example is the use of initial qualitative research to identify topics that are later turned into standardised items in a structured questionnaire.

Mixed methods can also be applied to secondary research, and it is becoming increasingly common to see literature reviews that incorporate findings from both qualitative and quantitative research (see Figure 8.3, from a study of how patients understand depression).

Disclosure and sickle cell disorder: A mixed methods study of the young person with sickle cell at school

Simon Martin Dyson, Karl Atkin, Lorraine A. Culley, Sue E. Dyson, Hala Evans, Dave T. Rowley

For this paper the emergent research questions were (in analyzing the survey data) to examine the pattern of disclosure in relation to reported school experiences and (for the interviews) to interpret possible reasons for and against disclosure. As they suggest, we make inferences from each set of data, and report on validation through a triangulation of survey and interview data, though, as Bryman (2007:21) suggests, reflexive analysis on contextual field notes helps us to forge a "negotiated account of the findings" that makes sense of both the quantitative and qualitative data.

The authors asked different questions of their quantative and qualitative data, aiming to integrate the results in their analysis.

They took multiple approaches to sampling, one approach being to interview according to survey (quantative) responses.

Our strategy for research contains key features of mixed methods (Tashakkori&Teddlie, 2003). First, as outlined, we use both quantitative and qualitative data. Second, although the time-scales of the survey questionnaires and the interviews overlapped, the methods were sequenced in that the questionnaire results were used to inform sampling for the interviews by seeking diversity of experience in participants invited to be interviewed (see Glaser & Strauss, 1967). Third, we can specify the relationship between the modes of data collection. Having interviewed the first fifteen interviewees opportunistically, we then selected the next ten based on selecting five who had left school aged 16 and five who had continued to post-compulsory education. We further took responses to a specific questionnaire item on the degree to which young people felt they had been enabled to "catch up" school absences associated with their SCD.

FIGURE 8.2 A sequential approach to data collection is combined with a concurrent approach to analysis to achieve triangulation. Reprinted from Dyson SM, Atkin K, Culley LA, Dyson SE, Evans H, Rowley DT. Disclosure and sickle cell disorder: a mixed methods study of the young person with sickle cell at school. *Social Science & Medicine* 2010, 70: 2036–44, © 2010, with permission from Elsevier.

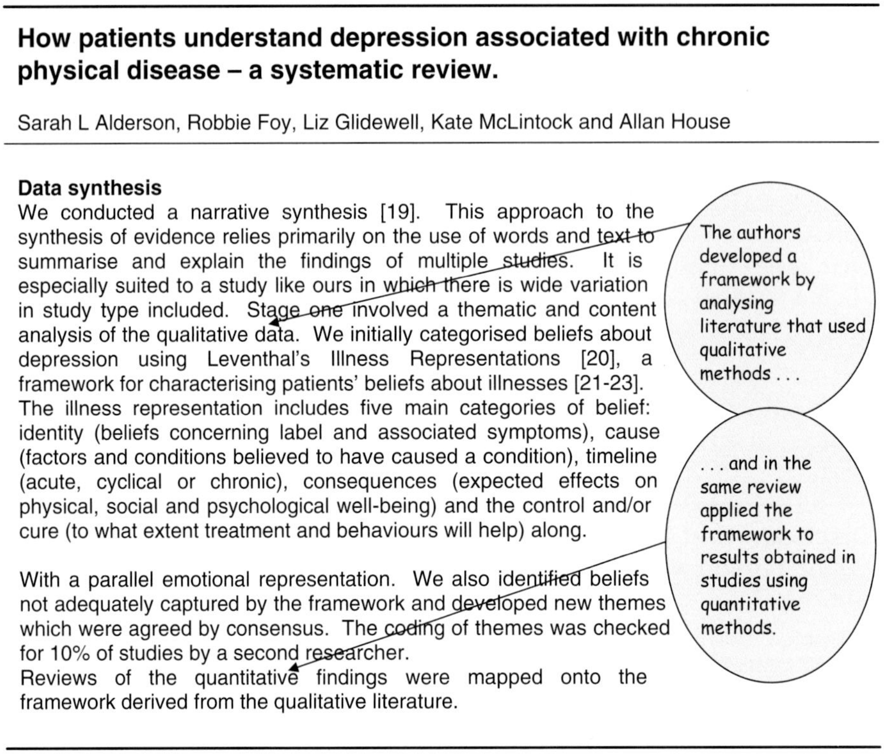

How patients understand depression associated with chronic physical disease – a systematic review.

Sarah L Alderson, Robbie Foy, Liz Glidewell, Kate McLintock and Allan House

Data synthesis

We conducted a narrative synthesis [19]. This approach to the synthesis of evidence relies primarily on the use of words and text to summarise and explain the findings of multiple studies. It is especially suited to a study like ours in which there is wide variation in study type included. Stage one involved a thematic and content analysis of the qualitative data. We initially categorised beliefs about depression using Leventhal's Illness Representations [20], a framework for characterising patients' beliefs about illnesses [21-23]. The illness representation includes five main categories of belief: identity (beliefs concerning label and associated symptoms), cause (factors and conditions believed to have caused a condition), timeline (acute, cyclical or chronic), consequences (expected effects on physical, social and psychological well-being) and the control and/or cure (to what extent treatment and behaviours will help) along.

With a parallel emotional representation. We also identified beliefs not adequately captured by the framework and developed new themes which were agreed by consensus. The coding of themes was checked for 10% of studies by a second researcher.

Reviews of the quantitative findings were mapped onto the framework derived from the qualitative literature.

The authors developed a framework by analysing literature that used qualitative methods . . .

. . . and in the same review applied the framework to results obtained in studies using quantitative methods.

FIGURE 8.3 Results from qualitative and quantitative research studies can be combined in a single literature review and synthesis. Reproduced from Alderson SL, Foy R, Glidewell L, McLintock K, House A. How patients understand depression associated with chronic physical disease – a systematic review. *BMC Family Practice* 2012, 13: 41, © 2012 Alderson *et al.*; licensee BioMed Central Ltd.

III

The Cast: Finding Out About the Subjects of the Research

9

The Research Setting

It can be useful to know where a study is set. *National studies* report results for whole populations. They are often based upon routinely collected data such as the United Kingdom's decennial census or governmental statistics – for example on road traffic fatalities or infectious disease notifications. Well-known examples come from the US Center for Disease Control and Prevention. A number of nationally based studies rely on data that are collected for a specific purpose, such as the United Kingdom's national confidential inquiries, which collect information on all cases of certain types that occur in England and Wales. They include inquiries into peri-operative deaths, maternal deaths, and suicides in psychiatric patients (Figure 9.1). The advantages of studies that are based on national data or on large populations are that the results will apply widely and that they can examine rare problems, as in the example in Figure 9.2. The disadvantages of national studies are that they are expensive and it is difficult to collect more than small amounts of information accurately on each case.

A *community-* or *population-based* study typically might examine differences between different communities, and look for factors in the environment that might explain such differences. In the example illustrated in Figure 9.3 the authors explored the risk of hospital attendance for self-harm in people from different backgrounds, defined according to measures of deprivation and social fragmentation. One weakness of community-based studies is the risk of committing the so-called *ecological fallacy*. So noting that there are higher rates of hospital attendance from areas of high deprivation does not tell you that necessarily it is individuals who are the most deprived who account for those high population rates. In this study, the authors avoided the trap, going on to discuss how their findings point to the need for a population-level intervention targeting high-deprivation areas, not necessarily an intervention targeting deprived individuals.

At a more local level it is common to find studies that are *service-based*, for example, in one hospital or clinic or general practice. The main reasons for doing studies in smaller-scale settings such as hospital clinics are their lower cost and the ability to collect more information accurately. The main disadvantage is that results may not be generalisable – as, for example, with the description of the breast cancer patients outlined in Figure 9.4. Research done in specialist clinics runs the risk of recruiting more severe or complicated cases, or (less obviously) more chronic cases.

Of course every study has to recruit from somewhere and there isn't a perfect answer. What you should look for when you read a paper is a clear description of the setting, including a description of those characteristics that might influence the interpretation of any findings. For example, is a clinic based in a specialist university or teaching hospital, or is a local community-based study recruiting from an especially affluent district? The paper's discussion should revisit this question, reviewing the likelihood of bias resulting from its setting.

Understanding Clinical Papers, Third Edition. David Bowers, Allan House, David Owens and Bridgette Bewick.
© 2014 John Wiley & Sons, Ltd. Published 2014 by John Wiley & Sons, Ltd.

Suicide within 12 months of contact with mental health services; national clinical survey

Louis Appleby, Jenny Shaw, Tim Amos, Ros McDonnell, Catherine Harris, Kerry McCann, Katy Kiernan, Sue Davies, Harriet Bickley, Rebecca Parsons

Introduction

The national confidential inquiry into suicide and homicide by people with mental illness was established in 1992 and has been based at the University of Manchester since 1996. Its aims are to collect detailed clinical data on people who commit suicide or homicide and who have been in contact with mental health services and to recommend changes to clinical practice and policy that will reduce the risk of suicide and homicide by psychiatric patients.

> This national survey is the most recently established of a number of confidential inquiries.

Comprehensive national sample

Information on deaths with a verdict of suicide or an open verdict in a coroner's court was forwarded regularly to the inquiry by the directors of public health in the 105 health authority districts in England and Wales. Open verdicts are often reached in cases of likely suicide and some or all open verdict conventionally included in research on suicide. In this study open verdicts were included unless it was clear that suicide was not considered at inquest – for example, in the cases of children and deaths from unexplained medical causes. These suicides and probable suicides are referred to as suicides in this paper. The sample presented here consists of suicides recorded by directors of public health in the 24 months from 1 April 1996, supplemented with cases recorded as suicide or deaths from undetermined external cause (equivalent to open verdicts) obtained from the Office for National Statistics for the same period.

> Data are collected through official channels which are already established.

FIGURE 9.1 A national survey of deaths by suicide. Reproduced from Appleby L, Shaw J, Amos T, McDonnell R, Harris C, McCann K, *et al*. Suicide within 12 months of contact with mental health services; national clinical survey. *BMJ* 1999, 318: 1235–9, © 1999, with permission from BMJ Publishing Group Ltd.

Sporadic Creutzfeldt-Jakob disease in the United Kingdom: analysis of epidemiological surveillance data for 1970–96

S N Cousens, senior lecturer[a] M Zeidler, research registrar,[b] T F Esmonde, research registrar,[b] R De Silva, research registrar,[b] J W Wilesmith, head of epidemiology department[c] P G Smith, professor of tropical epidemiology and department head,[a] R G Will, consultant neurologist[b]

a Department of Infectious and Tropical Diseases, London School of Hygiene and Tropical Medicine, London WC1E 7HT, b National Creutzfeldt–Jakob Disease Surveillance Unit, Western General Hospital, Edinburgh EH4 2XU, c Central Veterinary Laboratory, Addlestone, Surrey KT15 3NB

Correspondence to: Mr Cousens s.cousens@lshtm.ac.uk

Abstract

Objective: To identify changes in the occurrence of Creutzfeldt-Jakob disease that might be related to the epidemic of bovine spongiform encephalopathy.

Design: Epidemiological surveillance of the United Kingdom population for Creutzfeldt-Jakob disease based on (a) referral of suspected cases by neurologists, neuropathologists, and neurophysiologists and (b) death certificates.

Setting: England and Wales during 1970–84, and whole of the United Kingdom during 1985–96.

Subjects: All 662 patients identified as sporadic cases of Creutzfeldt-Jakob disease.

Only 662 cases were identified from a population of about 50 million surveyed over more than 25 years.

Main outcome measures: Age distribution of patients, age specific time trends of disease, occupational exposure to cattle, potential exposure to causative agent of bovine spongiform encephalopathy.

Results: During 1970–96 there was an increase in the number of sporadic cases of Creutzfeldt-Jakob disease recorded yearly in England and Wales. The greatest increase was among people aged over 70.

FIGURE **9.2** Data from a unit undertaking surveillance of a rare but important disorder. Reproduced from Cousens SN, Zeidler M, Esmonde TF, De Silva R, Wilesmith JW, Smith PG, *et al.* Sporadic Creutzfeldt–Jakob disease in the United Kingdom: analysis of epidemiological surveillance data for 1970–96. *BMJ* 1997, 315: 389–95, © 1997, with permission from BMJ Publishing Group Ltd.

The area-level association between hospital-treated deliberate self-harm, deprivation and social fragmentation in Ireland

Paul Corcoran, Ella Arensman, Ivan J Perry

Annual incidence of hospital-treated deliberate self-harm and level of deprivation and social fragmentation in Ireland by area type, 2002–2004					
	Deliberate self-harm			Deprivation*	Social fragmentation*
	All	Men	Women		
	Rate (95% CI)	Rate (95% CI)	Rate (95% CI)	Mean (SD)	Mean (SD)
Dublin	224 (214 to 233)	189 (176 to 201)	258 (244 to 271)	0.30 (3.12)	3.86 (5.79)
Other cities	301 (288 to 313)	298 (280 to 316)	304 (287 to 322)	1.87 (3.02)	6.01 (6.61)
Urban districts	330 (319 to 341)	279 (265 to 294)	380 (364 to 396)	1.50 (1.03)	3.87 (1.70)
Rural districts	139 (136 to 142)	109 (105 to 113)	172 (167 to 177)	-0.25 (1.14)	-0.69 (1.68)
All	204 (201 to 206)	171 (168 to 175)	237 (233 to 241)	-0.08 (1.57)	0.00 (3.18)
All rates are age-standardised per 100,000.					
*Mean and SD of the electoral division (ED) level of deprivation and social fragmentation. One way analysis of variance, df=3, 3237, p<0.001.					

FIGURE 9.3   Results from a population-based study of self-harm. Reproduced from Corcoran P, Arensman E, Perry IJ. The area-level association between hospital treated deliberate self-harm, deprivation and social fragmentation in Ireland. *Journal of Epidemiology & Community Health* 2007, 61: 1050–5, © 2007, with permission from BMJ Publishing Group Ltd.

Fatigue and psychological distress – exploring the relationship in women treated for breast cancer

B. Bennett, D. Goldstein, A Lloyd, T. Davenport, I. Hickie

Patients and methods

Women following surgical treatment for breast cancer who were either currently receiving adjuvant treatment or who had completed such treatment, were invited to complete two self-report questionnaires (Table 1). The women were recruited from consecutive attendances at the Medical Oncology Centre at the Prince of Wales Hospital, Sydney, Australia. Since the main aim of this cross-sectional study was to investigate the utility of two conceptually different questionnaires, no attempt was made to stratify women according to treatment stage or type. All women were diagnosed with stages I or II (TNM stages: TO – 3NIMO to T2 – 3N0MO) breast cancer [25]. The sample excluded women who were unable to read English, or those with concurrent major medical (e.g., severe cardiac, renal or endocrine disorders) illnesses identified by the clinician. There was no attempt to identify and exclude those with psychological disorders. No patient refused participation. The institutional ethics committee approved the study.

The participants were identified through their attendance at a clinic.

FIGURE 9.4   A service-based study, undertaken in a specialist clinic, of common symptoms. Reprinted from Bennett B, Goldstein D, Lloyd A, Davenport T, Hickie I. Fatigue and psychological distress – exploring the relationship in women treated for breast cancer. *European Journal of Cancer* 2004, 40: 1689–95, © 2004, with permission from Elsevier.

10

Populations and Samples in Quantitative Research

Clinical research often involves a study of a group of people, who are taken to represent a wider group to whom the research might apply. The widest group to whom the research might apply is called the *target population*. It might be, for example, 'All insulin-dependent diabetics aged 15–18 years in the United Kingdom'. It would not be feasible to study all the members of such a target population and it is common therefore to undertake research on a *study population*, such as 'All insulin-dependent diabetics aged 15–18 years who are recorded on a general practice case-register in six participating practices in West Yorkshire'.

Study populations are often drawn from hospital services. They may not be representative if many sufferers from a disorder do not attend hospital (e.g. patients with depression or hypertension). If the majority of sufferers from a disorder do attend a clinic (e.g. babies with epilepsy) the study population may still be atypical if the clinic is a specialist or selective one.

SAMPLING

It is very rarely feasible to include all of the study population, so researchers will often take a *sample* from it, such as 'One in three insulin-dependent diabetics recorded on six general practice case-registers in West Yorkshire'. Sometimes (as in the example in Figure 10.1) a study will use more than one sample.

There are several ways of obtaining a sample from a study population; they are usually called (for obvious reasons) sampling techniques. *Convenience samples* include those whom you encounter and invite to participate, in a haphazard way, for example, by asking colleagues to think of anybody who might be suitable. It is the least satisfactory sampling method, because it may lead to a highly atypical sample, but in ways that are not readily identifiable.

Systematic samples include individuals selected on the basis of some regularly occurring and easily identifiable characteristic, such as first letter of surname, every third patient booked in to see a general practitioner, or consecutive attendees on certain weekdays (Figure 10.2). The problem with this approach is that there may be hidden biases – the people who come to clinic on Mondays may be special in some way that is not easy to spot.

Random samples avoid these potential biases – at least theoretically; some methods are more random than others! For example, the person undertaking the random selection should be unable to influence the process. Suppose you were taking a 'random' sample of patients on your clinic list; you should not be able to influence the procedure to drop any awkward or aggressive patients who happened to come up in the sample. You must be able to tell what sampling method was used before you can decide whether the sample is representative.

Understanding Clinical Papers, Third Edition. David Bowers, Allan House, David Owens and Bridgette Bewick.
© 2014 John Wiley & Sons, Ltd. Published 2014 by John Wiley & Sons, Ltd.

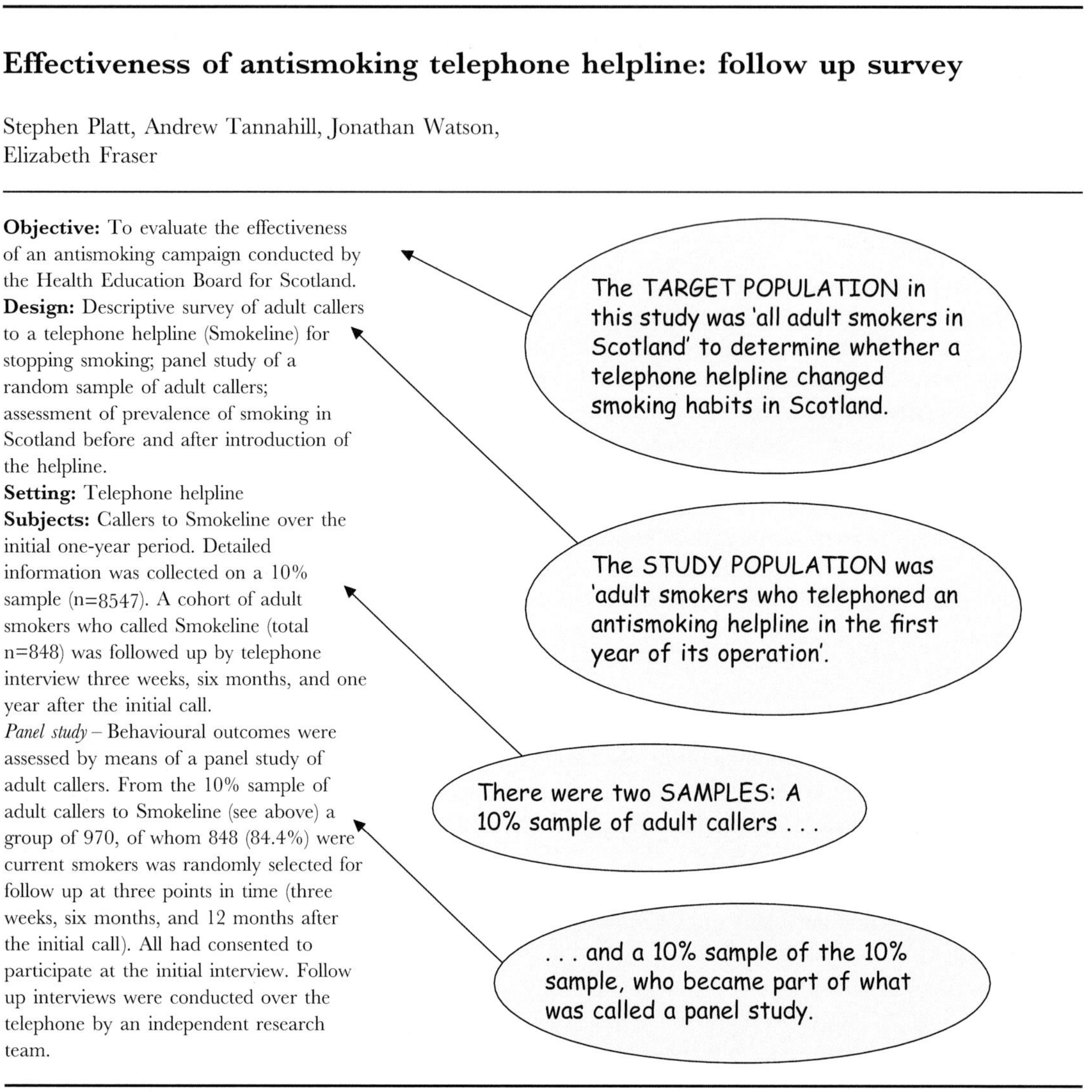

Effectiveness of antismoking telephone helpline: follow up survey

Stephen Platt, Andrew Tannahill, Jonathan Watson,
Elizabeth Fraser

Objective: To evaluate the effectiveness of an antismoking campaign conducted by the Health Education Board for Scotland.
Design: Descriptive survey of adult callers to a telephone helpline (Smokeline) for stopping smoking; panel study of a random sample of adult callers; assessment of prevalence of smoking in Scotland before and after introduction of the helpline.
Setting: Telephone helpline
Subjects: Callers to Smokeline over the initial one-year period. Detailed information was collected on a 10% sample (n=8547). A cohort of adult smokers who called Smokeline (total n=848) was followed up by telephone interview three weeks, six months, and one year after the initial call.
Panel study – Behavioural outcomes were assessed by means of a panel study of adult callers. From the 10% sample of adult callers to Smokeline (see above) a group of 970, of whom 848 (84.4%) were current smokers was randomly selected for follow up at three points in time (three weeks, six months, and 12 months after the initial call). All had consented to participate at the initial interview. Follow up interviews were conducted over the telephone by an independent research team.

The TARGET POPULATION in this study was 'all adult smokers in Scotland' to determine whether a telephone helpline changed smoking habits in Scotland.

The STUDY POPULATION was 'adult smokers who telephoned an antismoking helpline in the first year of its operation'.

There were two SAMPLES: A 10% sample of adult callers . . .

. . . and a 10% sample of the 10% sample, who became part of what was called a panel study.

FIGURE 10.1 A study which describes two random samples. Reproduced from Platt S, Tannahill A, Watson J, Fraser E. Effectiveness of antismoking telephone helpline: follow up survey. *BMJ* 1997, 314: 1371–5, © 1997, with permission from BMJ Publishing Group Ltd.

If you want to know whether any conclusions from a research study can be applied in a different setting (that is, how *generalisable* the results are), you must know the relation between each of these – the target population, the study population, and the sample.

SAMPLE SIZE AND POWER

One other important characteristic of the sample is its size. However well designed and conducted a piece of research is, it may – if the sample is too small – fail to identify important effects which

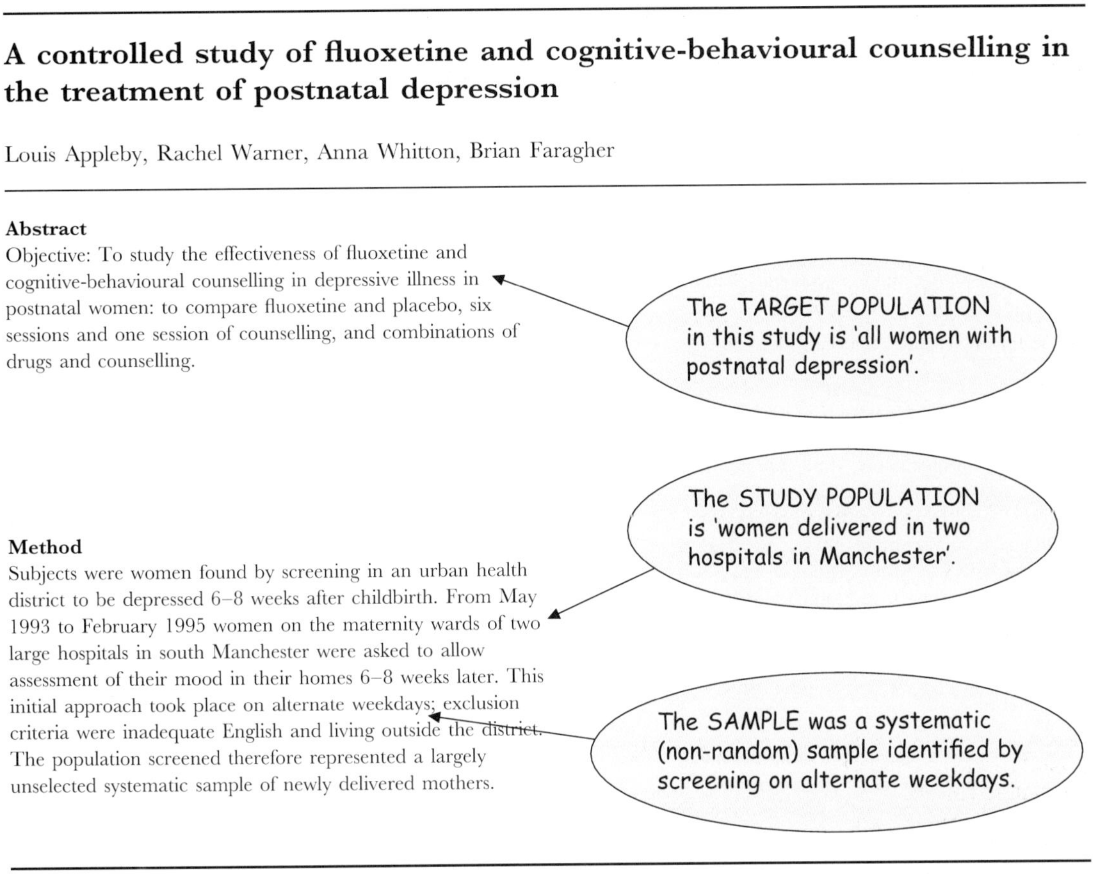

A controlled study of fluoxetine and cognitive-behavioural counselling in the treatment of postnatal depression

Louis Appleby, Rachel Warner, Anna Whitton, Brian Faragher

Abstract

Objective: To study the effectiveness of fluoxetine and cognitive-behavioural counselling in depressive illness in postnatal women: to compare fluoxetine and placebo, six sessions and one session of counselling, and combinations of drugs and counselling.

Method

Subjects were women found by screening in an urban health district to be depressed 6–8 weeks after childbirth. From May 1993 to February 1995 women on the maternity wards of two large hospitals in south Manchester were asked to allow assessment of their mood in their homes 6–8 weeks later. This initial approach took place on alternate weekdays; exclusion criteria were inadequate English and living outside the district. The population screened therefore represented a largely unselected systematic sample of newly delivered mothers.

> The TARGET POPULATION in this study is 'all women with postnatal depression'.

> The STUDY POPULATION is 'women delivered in two hospitals in Manchester'.

> The SAMPLE was a systematic (non-random) sample identified by screening on alternate weekdays.

FIGURE 10.2   A systematic sample of patients attending clinics on particular days. Reproduced from Appleby L, Warner R, Whitton A, Faragher B. A controlled study of fluoxetine and cognitive-behavioural counselling in the treatment of postnatal depression. *BMJ* 1997, 314: 932–5, © 1997, with permission from BMJ Publishing Group Ltd.

are truly present in a population (false-negative results) or obtain a false-positive result by chance (Figure 10.3).

Researchers should therefore give you one of two pieces of information about their sample. If they were able to choose its size, they should explain how they decided what size to adopt to minimise the possibility of errors, presenting a power calculation which indicates the likelihood that their sample was large enough to have avoided giving a false-negative result. On the other hand, they may not have been able to choose sample size for themselves; perhaps there just were not funds available or the time or resources to do more than use a sample that presented itself. In this case, researchers should acknowledge their failing and, by the use of confidence intervals, indicate the uncertainty of their findings.

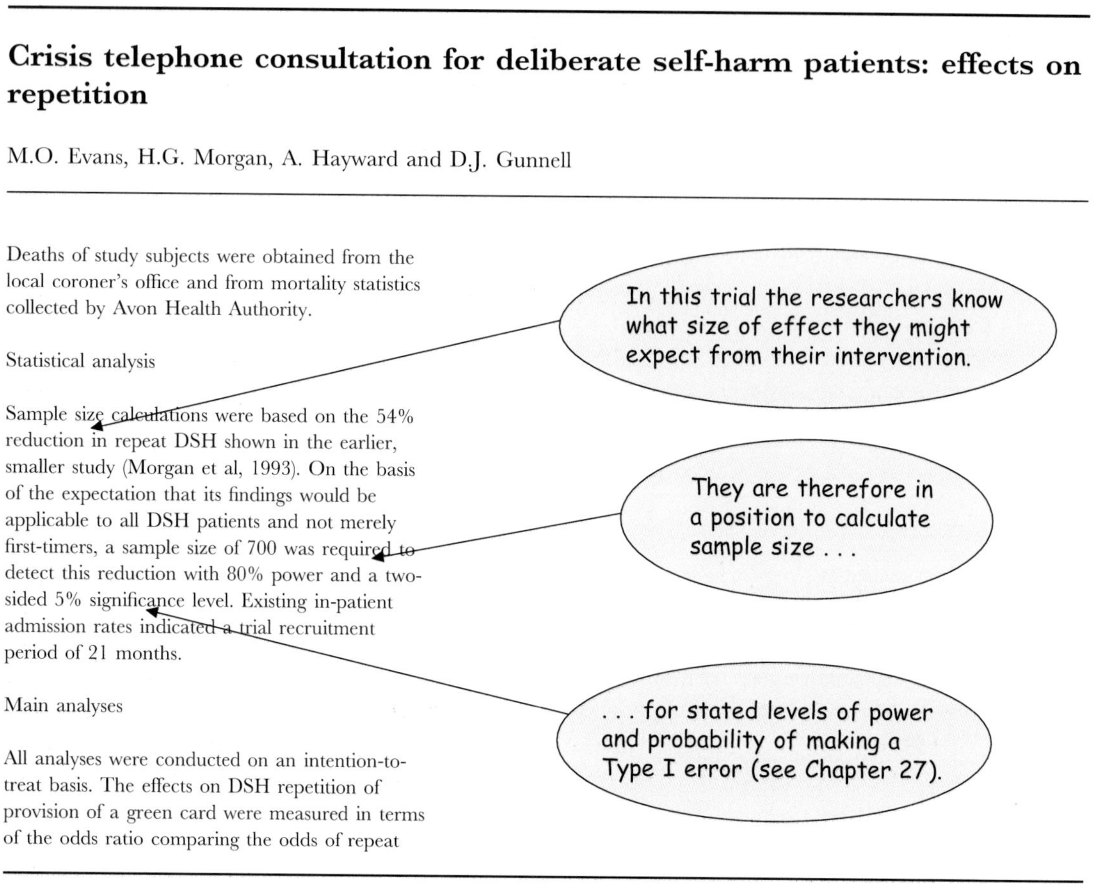

Crisis telephone consultation for deliberate self-harm patients: effects on repetition

M.O. Evans, H.G. Morgan, A. Hayward and D.J. Gunnell

Deaths of study subjects were obtained from the local coroner's office and from mortality statistics collected by Avon Health Authority.

Statistical analysis

Sample size calculations were based on the 54% reduction in repeat DSH shown in the earlier, smaller study (Morgan et al, 1993). On the basis of the expectation that its findings would be applicable to all DSH patients and not merely first-timers, a sample size of 700 was required to detect this reduction with 80% power and a two-sided 5% significance level. Existing in-patient admission rates indicated a trial recruitment period of 21 months.

Main analyses

All analyses were conducted on an intention-to-treat basis. The effects on DSH repetition of provision of a green card were measured in terms of the odds ratio comparing the odds of repeat

In this trial the researchers know what size of effect they might expect from their intervention.

They are therefore in a position to calculate sample size . . .

. . . for stated levels of power and probability of making a Type I error (see Chapter 27).

FIGURE 10.3 Sample size calculation in a clinical trial. Reproduced from Evans MO, Morgan HG, Hayward A, Gunnell DJ. Crisis telephone consultation for deliberate self-harm patients: effects on repetition. *British Journal of Psychiatry* 1999, 175: 23–7, © 1999, with permission from the Royal College of Psychiatrists.

11

The Sample in Qualitative Research

If you have read anything about qualitative research then you will know there are two obvious differences between the samples used in qualitative and those used in quantitate research. First, they are not designed to be *representative* in the statistical sense, although they may be *typical* of a certain group. Second, and most strikingly for many, is how small the sample size usually is. What is the explanation for these two observations?

THE NATURE OF SAMPLES IN QUALITATIVE RESEARCH

The commonest approach is usually called *purposive sampling*. Let us take an example. Suppose you wanted to ask a question like: 'What do people think about whether hospitals should provide chaplaincy services, and if they support the idea then what do they think those services should do?'. You might want to concentrate on interviewing people from different faith backgrounds, or with different personal experiences of illness, because you suspect that these characteristics will influence the opinions people hold. So you might go out and seek deliberately (purposively) some Christians, or Jews, or Muslims, or some people who had been seriously ill in hospital or had a family member who had died in hospital. Depending on your exact question, you might aim:

- To interview a group of people all with the same characteristics, say only Jews – an *homogeneous sample*.
- To interview a range of people chosen to capture as wide a range as possible of the characteristics you think are relevant, so-called *maximum diversity* sampling.
- To interview people who represent *extreme cases* – campaigners, for example.

In the paper outlined in Figure 11.1, taken from a study of the constructions by midwives of breast milk and breast-feeding, the authors describe two studies. In their observational study, they sampled for *diversity* in training and clinical experience; in their interview study, they sampled for *homogeneity*, seeking only senior staff with managerial or other experience.

A particular type of purposive sampling is referred to as *theoretical*. It means simply that the aim of choosing a sample is to test a particular theory. In our experience it is uncommon in health research. Frequently, qualitative researchers are not terribly specific about how they obtained a sample and one is left concluding that what they have – by design or by default – is *an opportunistic or convenience sample*. This may matter a great deal, but it may matter less than it does for some quantitative studies – if all that is needed is a reasonably broad or typical set of responders.

Understanding Clinical Papers, Third Edition. David Bowers, Allan House, David Owens and Bridgette Bewick.
© 2014 John Wiley & Sons, Ltd. Published 2014 by John Wiley & Sons, Ltd.

Liquid gold from the milk bar: Constructions of breastmilk and breastfeeding women in the language and practices of midwives

E. Burns, V. Schmied, J. Fenwick, A. Sheehan

Participants
Midwives
A total of 76 midwives participated in this study. Thirty six midwives participated in the postnatal observational component, nine midwives in the antenatal parenting education component, and 11 midwives participated in interviews. Demographic details were collected from midwives who participated in the antenatal and postnatal observations. At site 1 four of the 18 midwives who participated in observations had additional lactation consultant qualifications whilst at site 2 ten of the 18 midwives held these qualifications. The average years of midwifery experience was 12 at site 1 and 15 at site 2. The range of midwifery experience spanned from one-year Batchelor of Midwifery student through to a lactation consultant with 43 years of midwifery experience (see Burns, 2011)

The authors conducted an initial observational study of midwives with a diverse range of experiences.

Interviews with senior staff
At each PI 1 collected individual interviews with senior members of the postnatal team. These data were gathered to gain an insight into the dominant organisational discourses and disposition towards breastfeeding support. In total, 11 interviews were conducted with senior staff, including managers, midwifery educators, senior lactation consultants and senior clinicians. The interviews ranged from 23 min to 70 min. These interview data provided greater depth of understanding about the managerial and organisational factors impacting upon the provision of postnatal breastfeeding support. All interviews were transcribed verbatim.

In an interview study, the researchers concentrated on a small number of professionals who were senior in their careers.

FIGURE 11.1   Sampling purposively – for diversity in an observational study and for shared characteristics in an interviewing study. Reprinted from Burns E, Schmied V, Fenwick J, Sheehan A. Liquid gold from the milk bar: constructions of breastmilk and breastfeeding women in the language and practices of midwives. *Social Science & Medicine* 2012, 75: 1737–45, © 2012, with permission from Elsevier.

SAMPLE SIZE IN QUALITATIVE RESEARCH

The sample for qualitative research is not based on statistical ideas of representativeness, but on the need to collect certain types of information from certain types of people. Thus, the question to ask about sample size is: 'Have the researchers included enough participants to ensure that all the data they want can reasonably be collected?'.

   The answer to this question is not easy to specify and typically it involves a judgement by the reader, who has to ask himself or herself: 'Is it likely that the researchers have missed anything important by including too few participants, or too few of a certain type?'. The researchers themselves may not have known how many participants they needed at the start of their project and have dealt with their uncertainty by going on until they stopped obtaining new information. This is sometimes called achieving *data saturation* (see Figure 11.2, taken from a study of the uptake of screening for bowel cancer). Our experience is that authors rather rarely define exactly how they arrived at the decision that they had achieved data saturation.

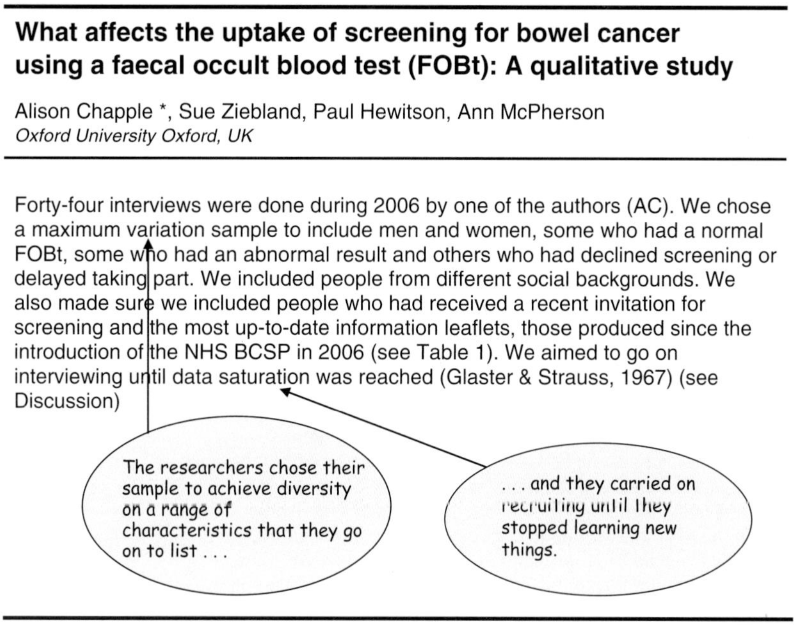

What affects the uptake of screening for bowel cancer using a faecal occult blood test (FOBt): A qualitative study

Alison Chapple *, Sue Ziebland, Paul Hewitson, Ann McPherson
Oxford University Oxford, UK

Forty-four interviews were done during 2006 by one of the authors (AC). We chose a maximum variation sample to include men and women, some who had a normal FOBt, some who had an abnormal result and others who had declined screening or delayed taking part. We included people from different social backgrounds. We also made sure we included people who had received a recent invitation for screening and the most up-to-date information leaflets, those produced since the introduction of the NHS BCSP in 2006 (see Table 1). We aimed to go on interviewing until data saturation was reached (Glaster & Strauss, 1967) (see Discussion)

The researchers chose their sample to achieve diversity on a range of characteristics that they go on to list . . .

. . . and they carried on recruiting until they stopped learning new things.

FIGURE 11.2   Sample characteristics chosen for maximum variation and sample size chosen to ensure data saturation. Reprinted from Chapple A, Ziebland S, Hewitson P, McPherson A. What affects the uptake of screening for bowel cancer using a faecal occult blood test (FOBt): a qualitative study. *Social Science & Medicine* 2008, 66: 2425–35, © 2008, with permission from Elsevier.

Another way to view sample size in qualitative research is to ask yourself about the *unit of analysis*. A very common approach is to explore attitudes, beliefs, or knowledge. When it is, then the unit of analysis is likely to be each expressed attitude and not the person from whom that attitude is elicited. So the real sample size may be larger than the apparent size. Figure 11.3 gives an illustration. Here, the researchers interviewed only 15 people with chronic lung disease, but from them they elicited 65 examples of the challenges posed by living with the disease – what they called 'dilemma stories' – and it was these that formed the focus of their study.

SAMPLING FOR QUALITATIVE RESEARCH

You will often find two other pieces of information and they relate to how the researchers identified their sample. First, you may find reference to a *sampling frame*, which sounds very technical, but is in fact just another name for the study population from which the sample was drawn. Second, researchers often construct a *sampling matrix*, which again sounds complex, but is not; you can think of it like a table listing the desired characteristics of participants and assigning quotas to each cell in the table. For example, in our example in Figure 11.2, the corresponding sampling matrix might have looked like the 2×4 table shown in Figure 11.4.

The researchers would assign numbers (a quota) to each cell. We do not know if they did and sometimes researchers fill up a table like this as they go along – as a check on how they are doing in achieving variation in their sample – but for now we are simply illustrating the term.

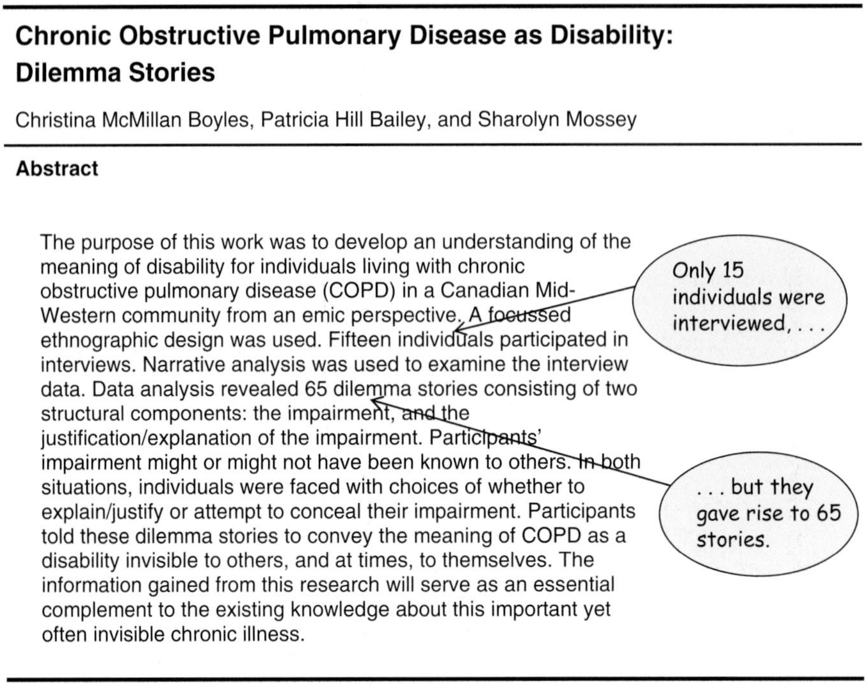

Chronic Obstructive Pulmonary Disease as Disability: Dilemma Stories

Christina McMillan Boyles, Patricia Hill Bailey, and Sharolyn Mossey

Abstract

The purpose of this work was to develop an understanding of the meaning of disability for individuals living with chronic obstructive pulmonary disease (COPD) in a Canadian Mid-Western community from an emic perspective. A focussed ethnographic design was used. Fifteen individuals participated in interviews. Narrative analysis was used to examine the interview data. Data analysis revealed 65 dilemma stories consisting of two structural components: the impairment, and the justification/explanation of the impairment. Participants' impairment might or might not have been known to others. In both situations, individuals were faced with choices of whether to explain/justify or attempt to conceal their impairment. Participants told these dilemma stories to convey the meaning of COPD as a disability invisible to others, and at times, to themselves. The information gained from this research will serve as an essential complement to the existing knowledge about this important yet often invisible chronic illness.

Only 15 individuals were interviewed, . . .

. . . but they gave rise to 65 stories.

FIGURE **11.3** Clarifying the unit of analysis: not 15 participants, but 65 'dilemma stories'. Reproduced from Boyles CM, Bailey PH, Mossey S. Chronic obstructive pulmonary disease as disability: dilemma stories. *Qualitative Health Research* 2011, 21 (2): 187–98, © 2011 SAGE Publications. Reprinted by permission of SAGE Publications.

	Men	Women
FOBt +		
FOBt −		
Declined Screen		
Delayed Screen		

FIGURE **11.4** Example of a sampling matrix; in this case one which might have been used in conjunction with Figure 11.2.

12

Identifying and Defining Cases

Once a means of obtaining a sample has been decided, researchers often want to limit the characteristics of individuals included in the sample. They will usually do so by applying inclusion and exclusion criteria.

Inclusion criteria often include an age range or, for example, the meeting of diagnostic criteria for a particular clinical condition. *Case definition* is aided by the use of standardised criteria. An example is the International Classification of Diseases (http://www.who.int/classifications/icd). A paper should, where appropriate, always make it clear what criteria were used for case definition.

Exclusion criteria are the other side of the coin. They are the criteria which will lead a participant to be dropped from the study, even though they are in the sample and meet the inclusion criteria. In Figure 9.4, for example, one exclusion criterion was not speaking English. Exclusion criteria may lead to a homogenous, clearly defined group of participants, but one which bears little relation to the real clinical world, so that generalisation is difficult. For example, a clinical trial of a new drug for the treatment of dementia excluded patients who had any psychiatric history, any neurological disorder, or any other significant physical illness (Figure 12.1). Since many dementia sufferers have one or other comorbidity, it may not be easy to decide how applicable the trial's results would be in clinical practice.

Once the inclusion and exclusion criteria have been established, they need to be applied to the sample population, to identify and exclude participants for the study. For example, it may be that the sample will be screened for a condition, with a more detailed second evaluation for participants who screened positive. This process may lead to problems if it is inaccurate or biased. For example, if screening involves filling out a questionnaire, then illiterate participants will not be able to participate unless special arrangements are made.

The final characteristic which determines the nature of participants in a study is their willingness to participate (that is, to join the study) and their willingness to remain in the study once recruited. We can break these down into:

- *Refusals* are those who decline to participate when they are approached for consent.
- *Dropouts* are those who consent and start the study, but do not complete it.
- *Losses to follow-up* are those on whom outcome data are not obtained; they are often, but not always, dropouts.

If any of these groups is large in relation to the sample it can seriously bias a study, since those who agree to participate in, and complete, a study are not necessarily the same as those who refuse or drop out.

It can be helpful in working out what happened to all the participants in a study if the authors' account includes a flow chart, as in Figure 12.2.

Understanding Clinical Papers, Third Edition. David Bowers, Allan House, David Owens and Bridgette Bewick.
© 2014 John Wiley & Sons, Ltd. Published 2014 by John Wiley & Sons, Ltd.

A 24-week, double-blind, placebo-controlled trial of donepezil in patients with Alzheimer's disease

S.L. Rogers, PhD; M.R. Farlow, MD; R.S. Doody, MD, PhD; R. Mohs, PhD; L.T. Friedhoff, MD, PhD; for the Donepezil Study Group

Methods

Patient population. Patients eligible for this study had a diagnosis of uncomplication AD. These men and women of any race aged 50 years or older showed no evidence of insulin-dependent diabetes mellitus or other endocrine disorders; asthma or obstructive pulmonary disease; or clinically significant uncontrolled gastrointestinal, hepatic, or cardiovascular diseases. The diagnosis of probable AD was made according to criteria outlined by the National Institute of Neurological and Communicative Disorders and Alzheimer's Disease and Related Disorders Association (NINCDS-ADRDA), with patients also fitting DSM-III-R illness categories of 290.000 or 290.10, with no clinical or laboratory evidence of a cause other than AD for their dementia. Patients had scores on the Mini-Mental State Examination (MMSE) of 10 to 26, and a Clinical Dementia Rating (CDR) score of 1 (mild dementia) or 2 (moderate dementia) at both screening and baseline. Patients who were known to be hypersensitive to ChE inhibitors or had been taking tacrine and/or other investigational medications within 1 month of baseline were excluded. Concomitant medications such as anticholinergics, anticonvulsants, antidepressants, and antipsychotics were not allowed during the course of this study. Drugs with CNS activity were either prohibited or partially restricted. All other medications were permitted. Patients were required to have a reliable caregiver. Written informed consent was obtained from both the patient and from their caregiver.

> Exclusion criteria were relative youth or the presence of other physical illnesses.

> Inclusion criteria were based on case definition and scores on measures of intellectual impairment.

> Further exclusions were applied to restrict the use of other drugs during the trial . . .

> . . . and a further inclusion criterion was the presence of a caregiver.

FIGURE 12.1 Inclusion and exclusion criteria applied to recruits into a trial of a new drug for the treatment of dementia. Reproduced from Rogers SL, Farlow MR, Doody RS, Mohs R, Friedhoff LT, for the Donepezil Study Group. A 24-week, double-blind, placebo-controlled trial of donepezil in patients with Alzheimer's disease. *Neurology* 1998, 50: 136–45, with permission from Wolters Kluwer Health.

Effect of consumption of food cooked in iron pots on iron status and growth of young children: a randomised trial

Abdulaziz A Adish, Steven A Esrey, Theresa W Gyorkos, Johanne Jean-Baptiste, Arezoo Rojhani

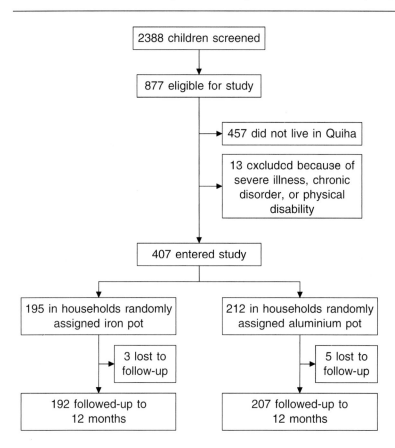

FIGURE 12.2   Flow chart describing the cases included in a randomised controlled trial. Reprinted from *The Lancet* 353: Adish AA, Esrey SA, Gyorkos TW, Jean-Baptiste J, Rojhani A. Effect of consumption of food cooked in iron pots on iron status and growth of young children: a randomised trial. 1999; 712–16, © 1999, with permission from Elsevier.

13

Controls and Comparisons

Often, results from a particular sample make sense only when they can be compared with those from another. For example, knowing the incidence rate of new-variant CJD (Creutzfeldt–Jakob disease) in the United Kingdom is interesting in its own right, but it might also be interesting to know the rate in other European countries. People may develop lung cancer even when they do not smoke, but live with somebody who does. But do they develop lung cancer more often than non-smokers who don't live with a smoker?

There are several ways by which authors might obtain comparison data for use in their own study. A common example is the use of 'normal ranges' for tests. This is especially useful when comparison data would be difficult to collect. For example, in the study illustrated in Figure 13.1, the researchers were interested in comparing health-related quality of life in long-term head and neck cancer survivors with general population norms.

Sometimes it is common sense to use normal ranges. We cannot check the population range of haemoglobin afresh for every study that reports it! On the other hand, published norms may be misleading if they were obtained a long time ago or from a very different population. This became such a problem with the most widely used IQ testing battery (the Weschler Adult Intelligence Scales (WAIS)) that the whole measure was redesigned and applied to a new population so that an up-to-date range of reference values could be produced. The Tanner charts widely used to judge children's growth have been revised in the same way. There are, however, many published results which are not so up-to-date.

A second approach is to use an historical comparison group, so that results produced now are compared with those produced some time previously. The problem with this approach is that it really isn't possible to explain any differences between the 'then and now' groups, because so many things may have changed in the time between the two studies.

The third and commonest approach is therefore to obtain a comparison group from the same population as the sample and study both at the same time. The comparison group may be identified in a systematic way. For example, suppose the main study is concerned with outcome of hospital admission for myocardial infarction among Asian men, then we might construct a comparison group by taking the next two non-Asian men with myocardial infarction admitted after each Asian participant included in our study.

In some studies the comparison subjects might be taken entirely at random from the same population as the sample.

One particular type of comparison subject is a *control*, who is somebody who comes from the same population as the subjects, but does *not* have the condition which defines the subjects. That condition might be:

- A *disease*, such as cancer – as in a case-control study (Chapter 6), where cases and controls come from the same population, but only cases have the disorder of interest.

Understanding Clinical Papers, Third Edition. David Bowers, Allan House, David Owens and Bridgette Bewick.
© 2014 John Wiley & Sons, Ltd. Published 2014 by John Wiley & Sons, Ltd.

Health-related quality of life in long-term head and neck cancer survivors: a comparison with general population norms

E Hammerlid and C Taft

Table 5 A comparison between the female and male head and neck cancer patients and Norwegian population values

	Female		Male	
	Cancer patients	Population sample	Cancer patients	Population sample
n	42	142	93	134
Age	mean 60	60–69	mean 63	60–69
Functional scales*				
Physical functioning	89 (82–96)	78	85 (80–89)	89
Role functioning	87 (78–96)	89	83 (77–89)	90
Social functioning	91 (85–97)	83	86 (81–90)	81
Emotional functioning	85 (79–91)	83	86 (82–90)	85
Cognitive functioning	91 (86–96)	86	86 (83–96)	83
Global quality of life	74 (66–81)	69	73 (69–78)	74
Symptom scale/single items**				
Fatigue	18 (10–25)	33	24 (20–29)	24
Pain	12 (5–18)	32	16 (12–21)	21
Nausea and vomiting	2 (0–4)	4	3 (1–4)	2
Dyspnoe	10 (4–16)	20	20 (15–25)	16
Insomnia	18 (9–26)	33	18 (13–23)	19
Loss of appetite	15 (6–23)	6	10 (5–15)	4
Constipation	15 (5–23)	16	9 (5–15)	9
Diarrhoea	2 (0–4)	9	5 (2–18)	8
Financial difficulties	9 (3–15)	12	12 (6–17)	13

Note: *Higher score means better functioning. ** Higher score means more problems.
n = number of patients.

FIGURE 13.1 Comparison results from a clinical population with published population norms for the same measure. Reprinted by permission from Macmillan Publishers Ltd: Hammerlid E, Taft C. Health-related quality of life in long-term head and neck cancer survivors: a comparison with general population norms. *British Journal of Cancer* 2001, 84 (2): 149–156, © 2001.

- Exposure to a *risk*, such as smoking or hypertension – as in a cohort analytic study (Chapter 6), where controls are defined as those who have not been exposed to the risk of interest.
- Exposure to a *treatment* – as in a randomised controlled trial, where the controls receive either no treatment or placebo (Chapter 7).

There is no reason why researchers should restrict themselves to one control group and in more complex studies they may choose two or more, as in the example shown in Figure 13.2.

Sometimes simply taking a control sample at random isn't enough. For example, suppose a group of researchers wanted to study the health needs of recent immigrants, to find out if they were greater than the local population. Recent immigrants tend to be predominantly young people, while a random sample from the native population would contain all ages. There would be difficulties comparing the health of two groups whose average age was different.

This is a particular example of a common problem known as *confounding*. What happens is that a variable (called a *confounder*) is associated with both exposure and outcome in a study. In this example, age is a confounder – it is associated with being an immigrant and with health-care needs. Confounders cause problems because they can make it look as if there is a direct association between variables when

Health of UK servicemen who served in Persian Gulf War

Catherine Unwin, Nick Blatchley, William Coker, Susan Fery, Matthew Hotopf, Lis Hull, Khalida Ismail, Ian Palmer, Anthony David, Simon Wessley

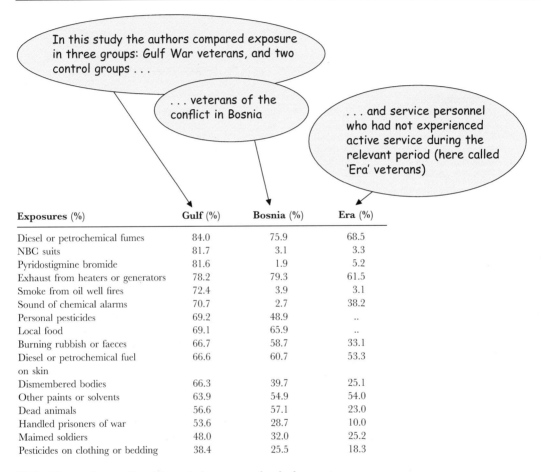

In this study the authors compared exposure in three groups: Gulf War veterans, and two control groups . . .

. . . veterans of the conflict in Bosnia

. . . and service personnel who had not experienced active service during the relevant period (here called 'Era' veterans)

Exposures (%)	Gulf (%)	Bosnia (%)	Era (%)
Diesel or petrochemical fumes	84.0	75.9	68.5
NBC suits	81.7	3.1	3.3
Pyridostigmine bromide	81.6	1.9	5.2
Exhaust from heaters or generators	78.2	79.3	61.5
Smoke from oil well fires	72.4	3.9	3.1
Sound of chemical alarms	70.7	2.7	38.2
Personal pesticides	69.2	48.9	..
Local food	69.1	65.9	..
Burning rubbish or faeces	66.7	58.7	33.1
Diesel or petrochemical fuel on skin	66.6	60.7	53.3
Dismembered bodies	66.3	39.7	25.1
Other paints or solvents	63.9	54.9	54.0
Dead animals	56.6	57.1	23.0
Handled prisoners of war	53.6	28.7	10.0
Maimed soldiers	48.0	32.0	25.2
Pesticides on clothing or bedding	38.4	25.5	18.3

Table: **15 most frequently self-reported exposures by deployment**

FIGURE 13.2   A study using two control groups. Reprinted from *The Lancet* 353: Unwin C, Blatchley N, Coker W, Fery S, Hotopf M, Hull L, *et al*. Health of UK servicemen who served in the Persian Gulf War. 1999; 169–78, © 1999, with permission from Elsevier.

there is not really. Alternatively, confounding may mask an association which is really present. For example, if we compared immigrants with the total native population, we might miss a link between ill-health and immigrant status: the immigrants may seem as healthy as the natives but would not be *if we took their age into account* (see also Chapter 30). This sort of *negative confounding* is much less common than confounding which leads to an apparent association between two variables which are not directly associated.

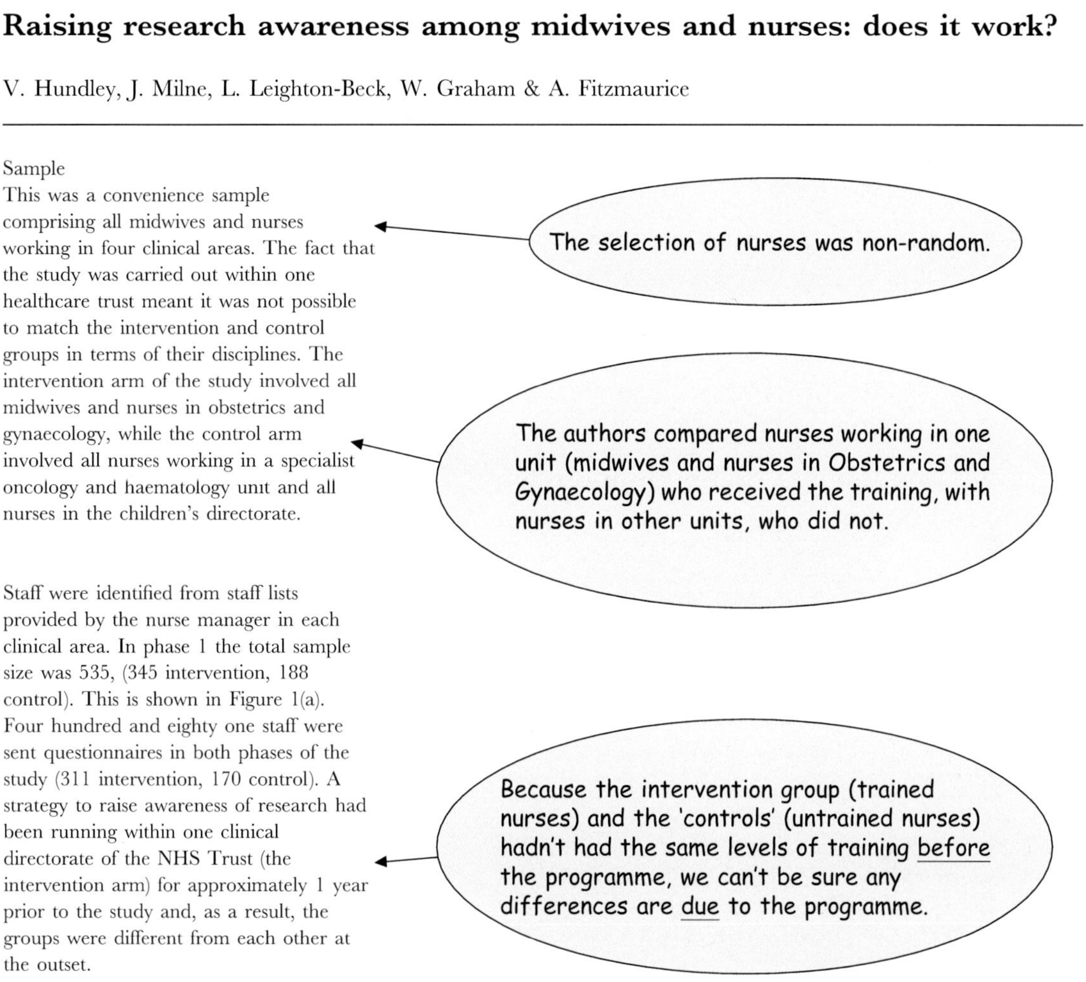

Raising research awareness among midwives and nurses: does it work?

V. Hundley, J. Milne, L. Leighton-Beck, W. Graham & A. Fitzmaurice

Sample
This was a convenience sample comprising all midwives and nurses working in four clinical areas. The fact that the study was carried out within one healthcare trust meant it was not possible to match the intervention and control groups in terms of their disciplines. The intervention arm of the study involved all midwives and nurses in obstetrics and gynaecology, while the control arm involved all nurses working in a specialist oncology and haematology unit and all nurses in the children's directorate.

The selection of nurses was non-random.

The authors compared nurses working in one unit (midwives and nurses in Obstetrics and Gynaecology) who received the training, with nurses in other units, who did not.

Staff were identified from staff lists provided by the nurse manager in each clinical area. In phase 1 the total sample size was 535, (345 intervention, 188 control). This is shown in Figure 1(a). Four hundred and eighty one staff were sent questionnaires in both phases of the study (311 intervention, 170 control). A strategy to raise awareness of research had been running within one clinical directorate of the NHS Trust (the intervention arm) for approximately 1 year prior to the study and, as a result, the groups were different from each other at the outset.

Because the intervention group (trained nurses) and the 'controls' (untrained nurses) hadn't had the same levels of training <u>before</u> the programme, we can't be sure any differences are <u>due</u> to the programme.

FIGURE 13.3 Non-random selection of intervention and control groups in a trial. Reproduced from Hundley (2000) with permission from John Wiley & Sons.

One way round confounding is to take a random sample and then adjust for the effects of a confounder such as age in the analysis (see Chapters 30 and 31). Another approach is to take a *matched sample* of controls, in which only controls are included who are (say) of the same sex and same age as the subjects.

Controls are not always randomly selected, as in the example in Figure 13.3.

Finally, check whether the authors have used enough controls and if they have justified the size of the control group – which is just as important as sample size in the main study group. There's nothing magic about having the same number of controls as cases; in fact, it is often a good idea to have more controls than cases (particularly if the number of cases is small) because it increases the *power* of the study (Chapter 10).

IV

Establishing the Facts:
Starting with Basic Observations

14

Identifying the Characteristics of Quantitative Data

Clinical papers contain the results from the analysis of data. Somewhere near the beginning of most quantitative papers you will find a *baseline table*, which summarises the principal features of the participants in the study, based on both demographic and clinical data. We will deal with theses summary measures in detail in Chapter 15, but the choices that the authors make as to which measures are the most appropriate will depend on two main factors:

- The *types* of variables (and thus the types of data) involved.
- How the data are distributed – in other words, their *shape*. By 'shape' we mean: are most of the values bunched up together in the middle of their possible range? Do they tend to be clustered together at the top or at the bottom of the range? Are they spread out fairly evenly over the whole range?

When you read a clinical paper you will want to know, have the authors used methods of analysis appropriate to the type of data concerned? Let us deal with that question first.

TYPES OF VARIABLE – TYPES OF DATA

There are four types of variables:

- *Nominal categorical variables* (e.g. gender, blood type, etc.). These variables produce nominal data. Each data value is allocated to a category (e.g. the category 'Male' or the category 'Female'). Importantly, these categories *cannot* be arranged into any meaningful order.
- *Ordinal categorical variables* (e.g. levels of pain, degree of satisfaction), which produce ordinal data. Each value is similarly allocated to a category (e.g. the categories: '0 (no pain)', '1 (some pain)', '2 (a lot of pain)', '3 (excruciating pain)'). Notice, however, that in contrast to nominal data, ordinal categories *can* be put into some meaningful order. It is important to note that ordinal 'numeric' values, such as the above pain scores, are *not* true numbers. We cannot properly measure pain, or any ordinal variable for that matter, we can only *assess* values by judgment, observation, questioning, physical examination, and so on. It's this non-numeric quality of ordinal data which makes some statistical procedures inappropriate (like calculating a mean). However, as we will see in Chapter 15, there are appropriate methods for dealing with these sorts of data.
- *Metric continuous variables* (e.g. such as weight (g), serum cholesterol (mmol/1), time in ICU (days)) produce metric continuous data. These data result from the proper *measurement* of things. In contrast to categorical data, metric data *are* true numbers. This means that, unlike with ordinal data, we can legitimately perform arithmetic operations on this type of data.

Understanding Clinical Papers, Third Edition. David Bowers, Allan House, David Owens and Bridgette Bewick.
© 2014 John Wiley & Sons, Ltd. Published 2014 by John Wiley & Sons, Ltd.

- *Metric discrete variables* (e.g. parity (numbers of previous births), mortality (number of deaths), etc.) produce metric discrete data. These data arise from *counting* things. They are also true numbers (and invariably whole numbers – *integers*, to be technical)

IDENTIFYING DATA TYPE

Figure 14.1 might help you to identify data type. One distinguishing feature of metric data is that they will have units of measurement attached to them (including numbers of things). For example, 10.5 *kg*, 12 *hours*, 1.6 *metres*, 140 *outpatients*, six *deaths*, and so on. Categorical data do not. A baby is said to have an Apgar score of just 8, not eight 'Apgars'.

Let us see some examples from practice. In the first of the studies below (Figure 14.2), the authors have used a number of different data types to summarize the basic characteristics of the two groups of children who participated in a trial of the effectiveness of two head-lice lotions. Note that the use of the ' + ' signs in the evaluation of infestation is not meant to correspond to any *exact* number. These are ordinal measures: ' + + +' is greater than ' + +', ' + +' is greater than ' + ', and so on. The *number* of live nits could have been recorded as discrete metric data, but the difficulty of counting them exactly makes this impracticable.

In the next example, the authors were comparing the use of a Foley catheter versus vaginal prostaglandin E_2 gel for induction of labour at term. Their baseline table is shown in Figure 14.3. This table displays all four types of variable. Notice in particular that although parity data are metric discrete, the authors have 'ordinalised' the third category into ' ≥ 2'. All we can say about women in this category is that their parity is greater than that of women in categories '0' and '1', but not by exactly how much.

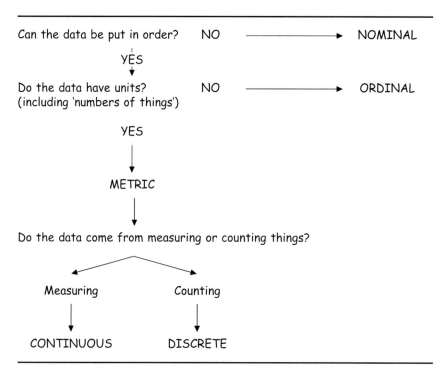

FIGURE **14.1** Types of data.

Controlled study of malathion and *d*-phenothrin lotions for *Pediculus humanus* var *capitis*-infested schoolchildren

Olivier Chosidow, Claude Chastang, Caroline Brue, Elisabeth Bouvet, Mohand Izri, Nicole Monteny, Sylvie Bastuji-Garin, Jean-Jacques Rousset, Jean Revuz

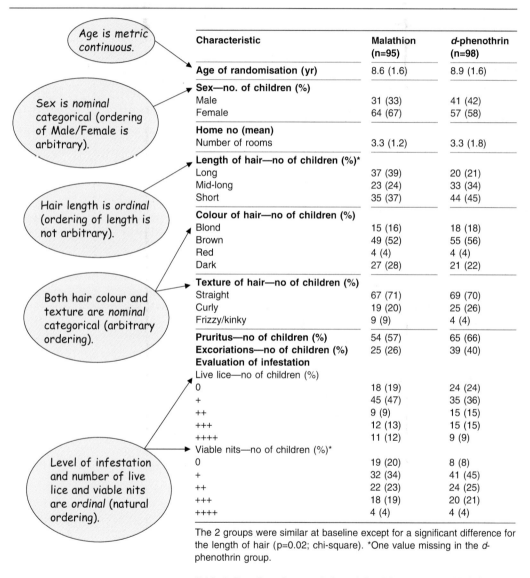

Characteristic	Malathion (n=95)	*d*-phenothrin (n=98)
Age of randomisation (yr)	8.6 (1.6)	8.9 (1.6)
Sex—no. of children (%)		
Male	31 (33)	41 (42)
Female	64 (67)	57 (58)
Home no (mean)		
Number of rooms	3.3 (1.2)	3.3 (1.8)
Length of hair—no of children (%)*		
Long	37 (39)	20 (21)
Mid-long	23 (24)	33 (34)
Short	35 (37)	44 (45)
Colour of hair—no of children (%)		
Blond	15 (16)	18 (18)
Brown	49 (52)	55 (56)
Red	4 (4)	4 (4)
Dark	27 (28)	21 (22)
Texture of hair—no of children (%)		
Straight	67 (71)	69 (70)
Curly	19 (20)	25 (26)
Frizzy/kinky	9 (9)	4 (4)
Pruritus—no of children (%)	54 (57)	65 (66)
Excoriations—no of children (%)	25 (26)	39 (40)
Evaluation of infestation		
Live lice—no of children (%)		
0	18 (19)	24 (24)
+	45 (47)	35 (36)
++	9 (9)	15 (15)
+++	12 (13)	15 (15)
++++	11 (12)	9 (9)
Viable nits—no of children (%)*		
0	19 (20)	8 (8)
+	32 (34)	41 (45)
++	22 (23)	24 (25)
+++	18 (19)	20 (21)
++++	4 (4)	4 (4)

The 2 groups were similar at baseline except for a significant difference for the length of hair (p=0.02; chi-square). *One value missing in the *d*-phenothrin group.

Table 2: **Baseline characteristics of the *P humanus capitis*-infested schoolchildren assigned to receive malathion or *d*-phenothrin lotion**

FIGURE 14.2   Types of data used to describe the baseline characteristics of subjects in a nitlotion study. Reprinted from *The Lancet* 344: Chosidow O, Chastang C, Brue C, Bouvet E, Izri M, Monteny N, *et al*. Controlled study of malathion and *d*-phenothrin lotions for *Pediculus humanus* var *capitis*-infected schoolchildren. 1994; 1724–9, © 1994, with permission from Elsevier.

Foley catheter versus vaginal prostaglandin E2 gel for induction of labour at term (PROBAAT trial): an open-label, randomised controlled trial

Marta Jozwiak, Katrien Oude Rengerink, Marjan Benthem, Erik van Beek, Marja GK Dijksterhuis, Irene M de Graaf, Marloes E van Huizen, Martijn A Oudijk, Dimitri NM Papatsonis, Denise AM Perquin, Martina Porath, Joris AM van der Post, Robbert JP Rijnders, Hubertina CJ Scheepers, Marc EA Spaanderman, Maria G van Pampus, Jan Willem de Leeuw, Ben WJ Mol, Kitty WM Bloemenkamp, for the PROBAAT Study Group

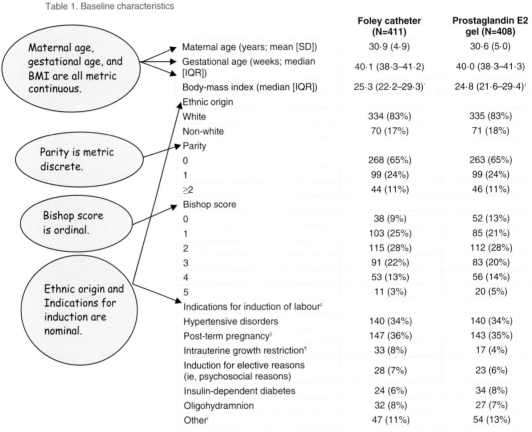

Table 1. Baseline characteristics

	Foley catheter (N=411)	Prostaglandin E2 gel (N=408)
Maternal age (years; mean [SD])	30·9 (4·9)	30·6 (5·0)
Gestational age (weeks; median [IQR])	40·1 (38·3–41·2)	40·0 (38·3–41·3)
Body-mass index (median [IQR])	25·3 (22·2–29·3)*	24·8 (21·6–29·4)†
Ethnic origin		
White	334 (83%)	335 (83%)
Non-white	70 (17%)	71 (18%)
Parity		
0	268 (65%)	263 (65%)
1	99 (24%)	99 (24%)
≥2	44 (11%)	46 (11%)
Bishop score		
0	38 (9%)	52 (13%)
1	103 (25%)	85 (21%)
2	115 (28%)	112 (28%)
3	91 (22%)	83 (20%)
4	53 (13%)	56 (14%)
5	11 (3%)	20 (5%)
Indications for induction of labour‡		
Hypertensive disorders	140 (34%)	140 (34%)
Post-term pregnancy§	147 (36%)	143 (35%)
Intrauterine growth restriction¶	33 (8%)	17 (4%)
Induction for elective reasons (ie, psychosocial reasons)	28 (7%)	23 (6%)
Insulin-dependent diabetes	24 (6%)	34 (8%)
Oligohydramnion	32 (8%)	27 (7%)
Other‖	47 (11%)	54 (13%)

Data are n (%) unless otherwise indicated.

*10% missing values (52 of 411 participants).

†8% missing values (34 of 408 participants).

‡More than one indication possible.

§Defined according to local hospital protocol for induction of labour, which in most cases was a gestational age ≥41 weeks.

¶Defined as estimated fetal weight <10th percentile.

‖In this group, decreased fetal movement, maternal disease, and obstetric cholestasis were seen most often.

Figure 14.3 Types of data used in a study comparing Foley catheter versus prostaglandin E_2 gel for the induction of labour at term. Reprinted from *The Lancet* 378: Jozwiak M, Oude Rengerink K, Benthem M, van Beek E, Dijksterhuis MGK, de Graaf IM, *et al.* Foley catheter versus vaginal prostaglandin E_2 gel for induction of labour at term (PROBAAT trial): an open-label, randomised controlled trial for the PROBAAT Study Group. 2011; 2095–103, © 2011, with permission from Elsevier.

SHAPES OF DISTRIBUTIONS

We will see reasons why the distributional shape of the data is important in a moment, but for now the four distributional shapes most commonly found with clinical data are:

- *Negatively (or left-) skewed* Most of the values will lie in the top half of the range, with progressively fewer and fewer values 'tailing' off towards the lower end.
- *Positively (or right-) skewed* Most of the values lie in the bottom half of the range, with a longer 'tail' towards the upper end.
- *Uniform* The values here are spread fairly evenly across the whole range.
- *Mound or hump-shaped* Most of the values are clustered around the middle of the range, with progressively fewer and fewer values tailing off towards both ends of the range.

We need a particular mention of what is called the *Normal distribution* (dear to the hearts of statisticians everywhere) which is a symmetric bell-shaped distribution, such as that for birthweights in Figure 14.4. Note that it is good practice always to capitalize the word *Normal* to distinguish it from the word *normal*, used in a more general sense of *usual* or not abnormal. It is important to know something about

Are clinical criteria just proxies for socioeconomic status? A study of low birth weight in Jamaica

John W Peabody, Paul J Gertler

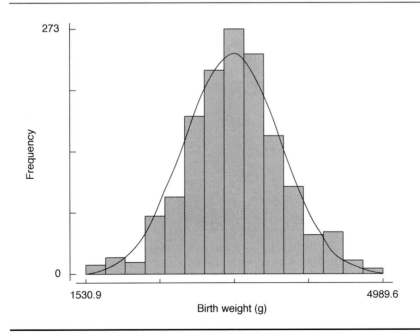

FIGURE **14.4** Normally distributed Jamaican birthweight data. Reproduced from Peabody JW, Gertler PJ. Are clinical criteria just proxies for socioeconomic status? A study of low birth weight in Jamaica. *Journal of Epidemiology and Community Health* 1997, 51: 90–5, © 1997, with permission from BMJ Publishing Group Ltd.

distributional shape because many statistical procedures depend on the assumptions made about this feature of the data. For example, some procedures should be used only on data which are Normally distributed.

The obvious question arises, how do authors (and we as readers) find out what shape any particular set of data has? In particular, are the data Normally distributed (or approximately so)? One way is to draw a *histogram* of the data (see Chapter 36 for material on charts, but Figure 14.4 is an example of a histogram) and assess the shape visually ('eyeballing'). There are also analytic methods for assessing Normality, but they are not frequently reported. If authors have not provided any evidence on distributional shape you should expect them to play safe, assume a non-Normal distribution, and choose a suitable procedure.

In the next example, the authors were investigating the adequacy of hormone replacement therapy for the prevention of osteoporosis and they measured serum E_2 levels in a cross-section of 45 patients who were using transdermal E_2 preparations. Figure 14.5 is the authors' histogram of serum E_2 levels. We can

---

Adequacy of hormone replacement therapy for osteoporosis prevention assessed by serum oestradiol measurement, and the degree of association with menopausal symptoms

M RODGERS
J E MILLER

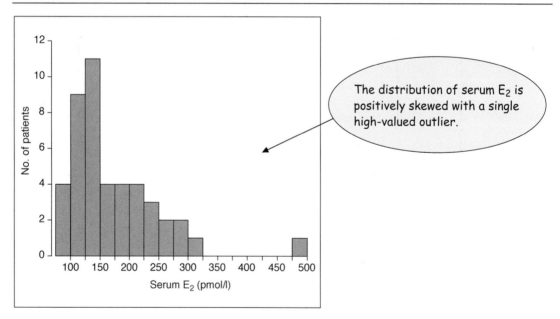

Figure 1. Frequency distribution of serum E_2 levels (pmol/l) in 45 patients on transdermal E_2 preparations.

FIGURE 14.5 Positively skewed distribution of serum E_2 levels, with a single outlier. Reprinted from Rodgers M, Miller JE. Adequacy of hormone replacement therapy for osteoporosis prevention assessed by serum oestradiol measurement, and the degree of association with menopausal symptoms. *British Journal of General Practice* 1997, 47: 161–6, with permission from the Royal College of General Practitioners.

see that the values tend to cluster in the lower end of the range. The right tail is longer than the left so the distribution is positively skewed (and certainly not Normal). Notice the single high-valued outlier (*outliers are values that lie a considerable distance from the broad mass of values*).

To sum up, if data are to be analysed, authors need first to identify the type of data involved and then determine the shape of their distribution. You will not always see references to data type and less so for evidence on distributional shape. As a reader, however, you need to be able to identify what data types are involved, if only to satisfy yourself that the most appropriate techniques have been used. If reference is made to either of these aspects of the data, you will probably find them in the Methods/Statistical Analysis section. Here are four brief examples from published papers in which the authors indicate that they have taken distribution and variable type into account in deciding on their methods of analysis (note that we have yet to encounter – but will do so later in the book – the methods mentioned):

> Statistical analysis. The distribution of baseline ulcer area and baseline ulcer duration were highly skewed, so we used the logarithm of baseline ulcer area and ulcer duration in the subsequent analysis.
>
> (*Watson* et al., *2011*)

> Statistical analysis. To compare the distributions of data between the two study groups, we used the *t* test for continuous variables if the data were normally distributed, and the Mann–Whitney *U*-test for data that were not normally distributed. We used the Kolmogorov–Smirnov algorithm to identify whether variables had a normal distribution.
>
> (*Kobayashi* et al., *2012*)

> Statistical analysis. Because of skewed distributions, we report medians and interquartile ranges along with Mann–Whitney test.
>
> (*Lowe* et al., *2010*)

> We examined strength and IQ for normality by testing for skewness and kurtosis. Variables that deviated significantly from a normal distribution were subject to a transformation before further analysis.
>
> (*Subramanian* et al., *2011*)

In this chapter you have seen how important it is for authors to identify both data types and distributional shapes if they are to use the most appropriate methods of analysis. So much for the theory. In Chapter 15 you will see some good and bad examples of appropriateness in the analysis of data.

15

Summarising the Characteristics of Quantitative Data

As we noted in Chapter 14, near the beginning of most quantitative research papers you will find information, in the form of a *baseline table*, about the participants in the study. These tables will generally include some *summary measures*, both of the *location* and of the *spread* (or dispersion) of the sample data.

A summary measure of location (sometimes referred to as a measure of central tendency) is the single value around which the data appear to mass or *locate*. A summary measure of spread is a value which indicates how much the data are spread out. In this chapter we will see how the choices which authors make between the various summary measures of location and spread are affected by the type of data in question and their distributional shape – both of which we examined in Chapter 14. When you read a clinical paper you will want to know that the authors have used the most appropriate summary measures for the data in question. We will start with measures of location.

SUMMARY MEASURES OF LOCATION

There are three principal measures of location that you will see authors using:

- The *mean* (properly called the *arithmetic mean*, to distinguish it from other types of mean, e.g. the geometric mean, which very rarely crop up in the main journals). This is what we all otherwise know as the *average* – the sum of the values divided by their number. So we can think of the mean as a summary measure of 'average-ness'.
- The *median*. This is the *middle* value, after all the values have been arranged in ascending order. Thus half of the values will be smaller than the median value and half larger. In this sense, the median is a summary measure of 'central-ness'.
- The *mode*, used only with categorical data, and rarely encountered in research papers, identifies the category with the highest frequency.

Let us see how the choice made by authors between the first two measures is influenced by data type and distributional shape:

- *Metric data.* Authors should quote either the mean or the median. The latter may be preferred if the data are skewed or otherwise not-symmetrical, since the mean is affected by distributional shape (particularly by outliers) and may not be thought representative of the broad mass of the data.
- *Ordinal data.* Authors should quote the median but not the mean. This is because (see Chapter 14) ordinal data are not truly numeric.
- *Nominal data.* The mode can be used as a measure of location for nominal data, but is rarely seen.

Understanding Clinical Papers, Third Edition. David Bowers, Allan House, David Owens and Bridgette Bewick.
© 2014 John Wiley & Sons, Ltd. Published 2014 by John Wiley & Sons, Ltd.

In addition to these three measures, authors will usually describe, in the baseline table, the proportions or percentages of values in each category (e.g. the percentages of male and female participants).

SUMMARY MEASURES OF SPREAD

There are three principal measures available:

- The *standard deviation* (often abbreviated as SD or s.d.). This can be thought of as the average distance of all the data values from their collective mean. The bigger the spread the bigger, the average distance from the mean, hence the bigger the value of the standard deviation.
- The *range*. This is the distance from the smallest value to the largest value.
- The *interquartile range* (sometimes abbreviated as IQR). This is a measure of the difference between that value *below* which a quarter of the values lie (known as the *first quartile* or the 25th percentile) and that value above which a quarter of the values lie (known as the third quartile or the 75th percentile). The interquartile range is thus a measure of the spread of the *middle 50% of values*.

The choice of the most appropriate measure is again influenced by data type and distributional shape.

For *metric data*, authors can appropriately use either the standard deviation or the interquartile range. As with the choice between mean and median, the interquartile range may be preferred if the data are skewed or otherwise not symmetrical, since the standard deviation is affected by distributional shape (particularly by outliers, even though the rest of the distribution might be quite narrowly spread) and may not be thought representative of the broad mass of the data.

On occasion, you may see authors quoting the *range* as a measure of the spread of their data. We discuss the range and its shortcomings in the following section.

For *ordinal data*, the choice is between the range and the interquartile range, but not the standard deviation – once again this is because ordinal data are not truly numeric. The interquartile range is a stable measure – not much affected by distributional shape, but the range is very sensitive to the presence of any outliers. This instability makes the range unsuitable as a measure of spread in most circumstances. In addition to the range and interquartile range, you will sometimes see authors quoting other spread measures, such as from the 10th percentile to the 90th percentile.

These ideas are illustrated in Figure 15.1, which shows the quartiles and interquartile range for some hypothetical systolic blood pressure data.

To sum up:

- If the data are *metric*, the *standard deviation* is most appropriate as a summary measure of spread (unless the data are skewed, in which case the interquartile range might be considered).
- If the data are *ordinal*, the *interquartile range* (or the *range*) is most appropriate, not the standard deviation.

Note that the mean should *always* be paired with the standard deviation, the median with the interquartile range or range.

Although summary measures of spread for *nominal* data do exist (for some examples, see Bowers, 2008) they have not found common usage.

As an example from practice, Figure 15.2 is from a study to determine whether a blockade of epidural analgesia (bupivacaine) administered before limb amputation reduced post-amputation pain. One group of patients received the bupivacaine blockade, the other (control) group received saline. The authors' first table describes the baseline characteristics of both groups of patients.

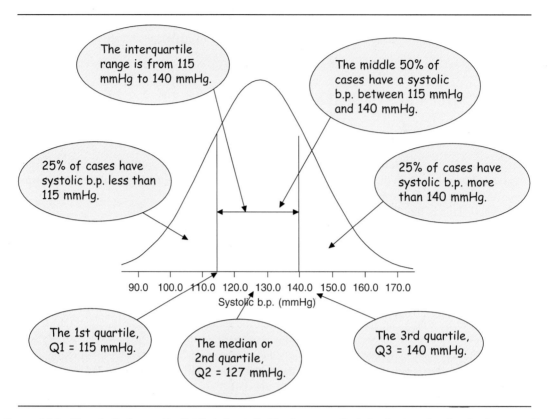

FIGURE 15.1 Hypothetical normally distributed systolic blood pressure (b.p) distribution, showing the three quartile values and the interquartile range.

Notice that the authors use the mean and standard deviation to summarize age (metric data), but the median and the interquartile range to summarize daily opioid consumption at admission, which is also metric. This may be because they suspected that the data were skewed and wanted more representative measures than the mean and standard deviation would provide, or they particularly wanted a summary measure which captured 'central-ness'.

Their opioid consumption results show that the median daily level of opioid used at admission in the blockade group (those having the bupivacaine) was 50 mg. In other words, half of the group had an opioid consumption less than 50 mg and half had more. The interquartile range for this group was from 20 to 68.8 mg. That is, a quarter of this group consumed less than 20 mg, a quarter consumed more than 68.8 mg, and the remaining middle 50% used an amount which varied between these two figures. As can be seen, the control group on average used far less opioids, a median of only 30 mg, although the spread in levels of usage was higher (5–62.5 mg).

The baseline table will usually contain (as is the case above) more than the summary measures discussed here. We see that information on the proportion of males and females in each group is also given, as well as other facts relating to the health of the subjects (whether diabetic, history of previous stroke, previous amputation, etc.). What information authors consider relevant and choose to present will depend, of course, on the nature of the study.

In the final example the authors investigated the prognostic factors for recovery from back pain. Their baseline table is shown in Figure 15.3. They have used the median and range as summary measures for duration of index episode, though the data are metric, possibly because of a skewed distribution or perhaps

Randomised trial of epidural bupivacaine and morphine in prevention of stump and phantom pain in lower-limb amputation

Lone Nikolajsen, Susanne Ilkjaer, Jørgen H Christensen, Karsten Krøner, Troels S Jensen

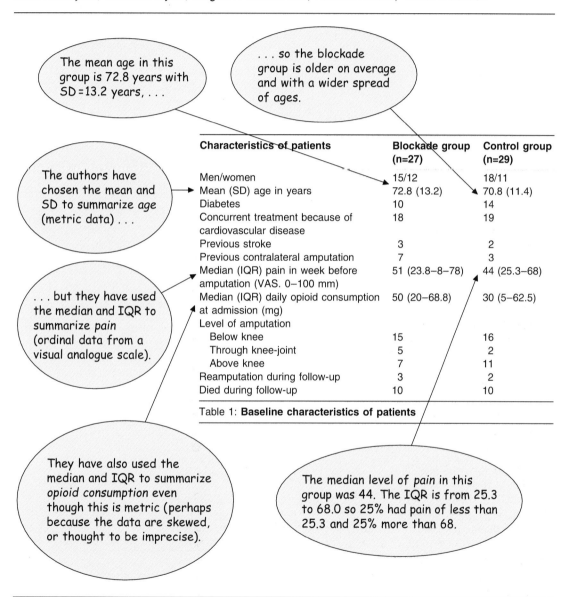

The mean age in this group is 72.8 years with SD = 13.2 years, . . .

. . . so the blockade group is older on average and with a wider spread of ages.

The authors have chosen the mean and SD to summarize *age* (metric data) . . .

. . . but they have used the median and IQR to summarize *pain* (ordinal data from a visual analogue scale).

They have also used the median and IQR to summarize *opioid consumption* even though this is metric (perhaps because the data are skewed, or thought to be imprecise).

The median level of *pain* in this group was 44. The IQR is from 25.3 to 68.0 so 25% had pain of less than 25.3 and 25% more than 68.

Characteristics of patients	Blockade group (n=27)	Control group (n=29)
Men/women	15/12	18/11
Mean (SD) age in years	72.8 (13.2)	70.8 (11.4)
Diabetes	10	14
Concurrent treatment because of cardiovascular disease	18	19
Previous stroke	3	2
Previous contralateral amputation	7	3
Median (IQR) pain in week before amputation (VAS. 0–100 mm)	51 (23.8–8–78)	44 (25.3–68)
Median (IQR) daily opioid consumption at admission (mg)	50 (20–68.8)	30 (5–62.5)
Level of amputation		
Below knee	15	16
Through knee-joint	5	2
Above knee	7	11
Reamputation during follow-up	3	2
Died during follow-up	10	10

Table 1: **Baseline characteristics of patients**

FIGURE 15.2 Baseline characteristics in a post-operative stump pain study. Reprinted from *The Lancet* 350: Nikolajsen L, Ilkjaer S, Christensen JH, Krøner K, Jensen TS. Randomised trial of epidural bupivacaine and morphine in prevention of stump and phantom pain in lower-limb amputation. 1998; 1353–7, © 1998, with permission from Elsevier.

Clinical course and prognostic factors in acute low back pain: an inception cohort study in primary care practice

J Coste, G Delecoeuillerie, A Cohen de Lara, J M Le Parc, J B Paolaggi

The authors use the mean and SD for age (metric), . . .

. . . and the median and range for duration of episode (metric), perhaps because data are unreliable.

The median duration of the index episode was 26 hours. The shortest duration was 1.5 hours, the longest 70 hours . . .

. . . but they *inappropriately* use the mean and SD for both pain and disability questionnaire score (both ordinal). Median and IQR would have been more appropriate.

TABLE I—*Baseline characteristics of subjects (n=103) at entry to study. Except where stated otherwise, values are numbers (percentages) of subjects*

	Value
Sociodemographic variables:	
Mean (SD) age (years)	46.5 (14.3)
Male sex	62 (60)
French nationality	92 (89)
Manual worker	29 (28)
Employed at entry	75 (73)
Back pain history:	
One or more previous acute episodes	63 (61)
Previous chronic (>3 months) episode of low back pain	8 (8)
Prior back surgery	0
Median (minimum, maximum) duration of index episode (hours)	26 (1.5, 70)
Sudden onset (<2 minutes)	36 (35)
Pain and disability variables:	
Mean (SD) initial visual analogue scale score	6.6 (1.8)
Constant pain at night	16 (16)
Pain aggravated by impulsion	44 (43)
Pain aggravated by moving back	99 (96)
Pain worse on standing	67 (95)
Pain worse on lying	27 (26)
Unable to stand even briefly	18 (17)
Mean (SD) initial disability questionnaire score[†]	12.1 (5.6)
Physical findings:	
Limited passive movements	72 (70)
Catch	61 (59)
Straight leg raising <75°	31 (30)
Psychosocial variables:	
DSM-III-R diagnosis	12 (12)
Depression	5 (5)
Generalised anxiety	7 (7)
Compensation status[‡]	9 (9)
Job difficulty (heavy labour)	16 (16)
Poor job satisfaction	34 (33)

[†] If able to stand.
[‡] Invariably awarded in France for pain occurring at work.

FIGURE 15.3 Baseline characteristics in an acute back pain study. Reproduced from Coste J, Delecoeuillerie G, Cohen de Lara A, Le Parc JM, Paolaggi JB. Clinical course and prognostic factors in acute low back pain: an inception cohort study in primary care practice. *BMJ* 1994, 308: 577–80, © 1994, with permission from BMJ Publishing Group Ltd.

because they believed that patient recall of episode duration was likely to be imprecise and preferred to treat it as if it would yield ordinal data.

They have *inappropriately* used the mean and standard deviation as summary measures both for the pain scores and the disability questionnaire scores, both of which are ordinal with short scales (see Chapter 14). More appropriate would have been the median and the interquartile range. (Note: this is also true of the summary results for deprivation scores and social fragmentation scores presented in Figure 9.3).

When you read a clinical paper containing summary measures of location and spread, you should be able to tell if they are appropriate for the types of data involved and their distributional shapes.

The choice of suitable *summary* measures for sample data is not the only decision influenced by the type of data and their distributional shape. As we will see in later chapters, these two factors also have a crucial role in making appropriate choices in many other areas of statistical analysis. Hypothesis testing, which we will consider in Chapter 27, is just one example.

16

Identifying and Summarising the Characteristics of Qualitative Data

When you begin searching for published qualitative health research, the most common types of qualitative data uncovered are likely to be text from interview transcripts. There are, however, many methods of collecting qualitative data (participant and non-participant observation; group interviews; published texts and artefacts) and therefore data might include written text (interview transcripts, public documents, blog postings), images (photos or drawings), or visual recordings (YouTube clips). Compared to quantitative data, qualitative data will normally:

- Be relatively *unstructured* (not constrained by pre-determined categories or numerical values).
- Deal with *meaning* (rather than quantifying an aspect of social life but rather on a qualitative assessment).

The data collected will be determined by the aims of the research and the aspect of health to be investigated. An example of a description of the focus and boundaries of research that investigated health-care professions' encounters with patients' aggression is given in Figure 16.1.

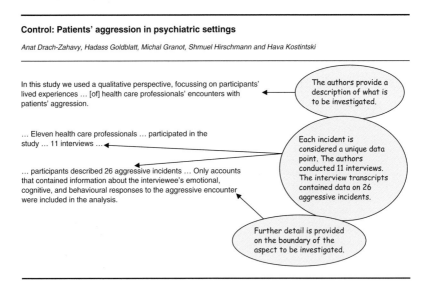

Control: Patients' aggression in psychiatric settings

Anat Drach-Zahavy, Hadass Goldblatt, Michal Granot, Shmuel Hirschmann and Hava Kostintski

In this study we used a qualitative perspective, focussing on participants' lived experiences … [of] health care professionals' encounters with patients' aggression.

The authors provide a description of what is to be investigated.

… Eleven health care professionals … participated in the study … 11 interviews …

… participants described 26 aggressive incidents … Only accounts that contained information about the interviewee's emotional, cognitive, and behavioural responses to the aggressive encounter were included in the analysis.

Each incident is considered a unique data point. The authors conducted 11 interviews. The interview transcripts contained data on 26 aggressive incidents.

Further detail is provided on the boundary of the aspect to be investigated.

Figure 16.1   A study of patients' aggression, where the boundaries of the data to be collected were defined by the health-care being investigated. Reproduced from Drach-Zahavy A, Goldblatt H, Granot M, Hirschmann S, Kostintski H. Control: patients' aggression in psychiatric settings. *Qualitative Health Research* 2012, 22 (1): 43–53, © 2012 SAGE Publications. Reprinted by permission of SAGE Publications.

How units of analysis are defined is, in part, dictated by the philosophical and theoretical perspectives underpinning the research design (we touched upon this in Chapter 11 – see Figure 11.3). It is beyond the scope of this text to explore these dimensions, but for an in-depth discussion see Hesse-Biber and Leavy (2011). Within published papers you often see evidence of authors' underlying perspectives. Of interest to us, in understanding how to identify characteristics of qualitative data, is how authors describe their data and what detail they provide on how units of analysis were decided upon. How authors describe data which was included in an investigation of neighbourhood influences on physical activity is illustrated in Figure 16.2.

Not all material encountered or generated during the research process is necessarily used in the analysis. In some instances material that could be included as data in one study is instead used for an alternate purpose in another. For example, there may be instances when images (generated by participants) are used as a means to elicit interview material and are not included as 'data' to be analysed. See Figure 16.3.

We have considered examples that have participant (e.g. Figure 16.2) or incident of interest (e.g. Figure 16.1) as the unit of analysis. Another relatively common unit of analysis within published papers is significant utterance, phrase, or sentence. An example is shown in Figure 16.4.

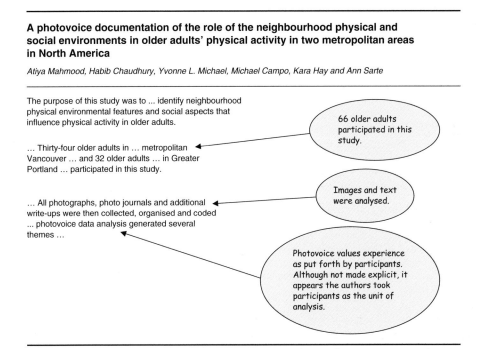

A photovoice documentation of the role of the neighbourhood physical and social environments in older adults' physical activity in two metropolitan areas in North America

Atiya Mahmood, Habib Chaudhury, Yvonne L. Michael, Michael Campo, Kara Hay and Ann Sarte

The purpose of this study was to ... identify neighbourhood physical environmental features and social aspects that influence physical activity in older adults.

66 older adults participated in this study.

... Thirty-four older adults in ... metropolitan Vancouver ... and 32 older adults ... in Greater Portland ... participated in this study.

Images and text were analysed.

... All photographs, photo journals and additional write-ups were then collected, organised and coded ... photovoice data analysis generated several themes ...

Photovoice values experience as put forth by participants. Although not made explicit, it appears the authors took participants as the unit of analysis.

FIGURE 16.2   A study of neighbourhood influences on physical activity in older adults: how authors described their data. (Photovoice is a method that usually involves participants taking photos that represent their experience/point of view. These photos can then be used to facilitate discussion and develop narratives.) Reprinted from Mahmood A, Chaudhury H, Michael YL, Campo M, Hay K, Sarte A. A photovoice documentation of the role of neighbourhood physical and social environments in older adults' physical activity in two metropolitan areas in North America. *Social Science and Medicine* 2012, 74: 1180–92, © 2012, with permission from Elsevier.

Qualitative research using photo-elicitation to explore the role of food in family relationships among obese adolescents

Jonathan Lachal, Mario Speranza, Oliver Taieb, Bruno Falissard, Herve Lefevre, Maire-Rose Moro, Anne Revah-Levy

… this article aims to explore how family and food interact …

… the present study … semi-structured interviews, with photo elicitation tool. The photograph is provided by the subject, and used as the basis for the interview …

Images generated by participants formed part of the interview…

… all interviews were audio-recorded … transcribed verbatim … and analysed using IPA …

… but the images were not included as data to be analysed.

FIGURE 16.3 Reprinted from Lachal J, Speranza M, Taieb O, Falissard B, Lefevre H, Moro M-R, *et al.* Qualitative research using photo-elicitation to explore the role of food in family relationships among obese adolescents. *Appetite* 2012, 58: 1099–1105, © 2012, with permission from Elsevier.

Cognitive representations of AIDS: A phenomenological study

Elizabeth H. Anderson and Margaret Hull Spencer

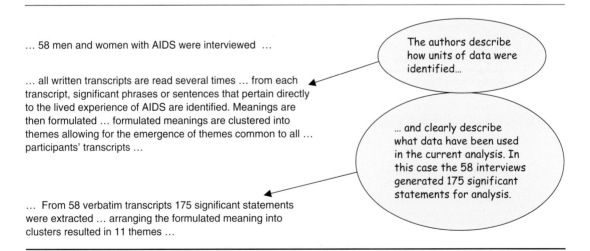

… 58 men and women with AIDS were interviewed …

… all written transcripts are read several times … from each transcript, significant phrases or sentences that pertain directly to the lived experience of AIDS are identified. Meanings are then formulated … formulated meanings are clustered into themes allowing for the emergence of themes common to all … participants' transcripts …

The authors describe how units of data were identified…

… and clearly describe what data have been used in the current analysis. In this case the 58 interviews generated 175 significant statements for analysis.

… From 58 verbatim transcripts 175 significant statements were extracted … arranging the formulated meaning into clusters resulted in 11 themes …

FIGURE 16.4 The unit of analysis may be a significant utterance, phrase, or sentence. Reproduced from Anderson EH, Spencer MH. Cognitive representations of AIDS: a phenomenological study. *Qualitative Health Research* 2002, 12: 1338–52, © 2002 SAGE Publications. Reprinted by permission of SAGE Publications.

17

Measuring the Characteristics of Participants: Quantitative

Chapter 12 dealt with the issue of inclusion and exclusion criteria for study participants – who is in and who is out. Once the sample has been assembled according to these criteria, you need to know about their characteristics, so that you can judge how close the study participants are to the patients or clients in your practice. If the study sets out to draw comparisons between two or more groups you will want to know whether the groups are sufficiently comparable.

The extracts in Figure 17.1 from a clinical trial examining one form of social care (called 'case management') in long-term and severe mental illness provide a fairly typical illustration of this two-stage research process:

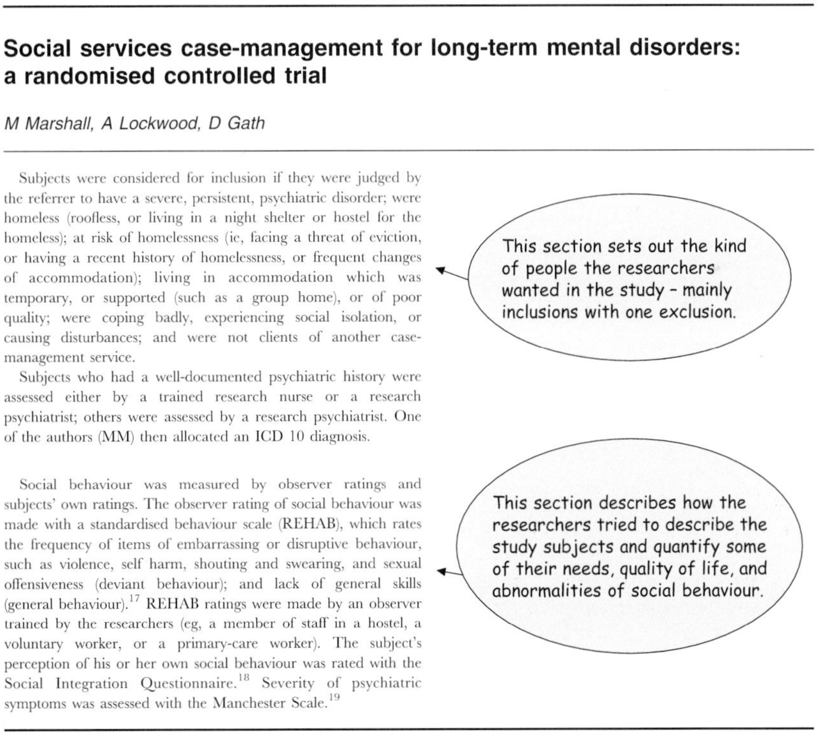

Social services case-management for long-term mental disorders: a randomised controlled trial

M Marshall, A Lockwood, D Gath

Subjects were considered for inclusion if they were judged by the referrer to have a severe, persistent, psychiatric disorder; were homeless (roofless, or living in a night shelter or hostel for the homeless); at risk of homelessness (ie, facing a threat of eviction, or having a recent history of homelessness, or frequent changes of accommodation); living in accommodation which was temporary, or supported (such as a group home), or of poor quality; were coping badly, experiencing social isolation, or causing disturbances; and were not clients of another case-management service.

Subjects who had a well-documented psychiatric history were assessed either by a trained research nurse or a research psychiatrist; others were assessed by a research psychiatrist. One of the authors (MM) then allocated an ICD 10 diagnosis.

> This section sets out the kind of people the researchers wanted in the study – mainly inclusions with one exclusion.

Social behaviour was measured by observer ratings and subjects' own ratings. The observer rating of social behaviour was made with a standardised behaviour scale (REHAB), which rates the frequency of items of embarrassing or disruptive behaviour, such as violence, self harm, shouting and swearing, and sexual offensiveness (deviant behaviour); and lack of general skills (general behaviour).[17] REHAB ratings were made by an observer trained by the researchers (eg, a member of staff in a hostel, a voluntary worker, or a primary-care worker). The subject's perception of his or her own social behaviour was rated with the Social Integration Questionnaire.[18] Severity of psychiatric symptoms was assessed with the Manchester Scale.[19]

> This section describes how the researchers tried to describe the study subjects and quantify some of their needs, quality of life, and abnormalities of social behaviour.

FIGURE 17.1 Extracts from a clinical trial, describing inclusions, exclusions, and some of the baseline measure. Reprinted from *The Lancet* 345: Marshall M, Lockwood A, Gath D. Social services case-management for long-term mental disorders: a randomised controlled trial. 1995; 409–12, © 1995, with permission from Elsevier.

Understanding Clinical Papers, Third Edition. David Bowers, Allan House, David Owens and Bridgette Bewick.
© 2014 John Wiley & Sons, Ltd. Published 2014 by John Wiley & Sons, Ltd.

These measures are sometimes called *baseline* measures, because they are taken at the start of the study, or *casemix* measures, because they describe the mix of cases in the study. You need them not only to check the relevance of the study to your patients or clients, but also, if it is a follow-up study, as a baseline that can be used later to see how much, if at all, they have improved or deteriorated.

In many papers these initial findings are set out in the first table of the results section – showing us the consequences of the inclusion and exclusion process and of sampling. The table shown in Figure 17.2 comes from the 'case management' trial illustrated above.

Social services case-management for long-term mental disorders: a randomised controlled trial

M Marshall, A Lockwood, D Gath

	Control group (n=40)		Case-management (n=40)	
	No	%	No	%
Age grouping				
20–29	4	10.0	4	10.0
30–39	6	15.4	11	28.2
40–49	16	40.0	6	15.4
50–59	5	12.5	9	22.5
60+	9	22.5	9	22.5
Sex				
Male	34	85.0	34	85.0
Female	6	15.0	6	15.0
History				
Illness >1 year	40	100	40	100
Previous psychiatric admission	34	85.0	34	85.0
In contact with psychiatric services	25	62.5	21	52.5
ICD 10 diagnosis				
Schizophrenia and related disorders	32	80.0	27	67.5
Mood disorders	3	7.5	6	15.0
Personality disorder	2	5.0	3	7.5
Neurotic disorders	1	2.5	3	7.5
Organic disorders	2	5.0	1	2.5
Housing status				
Hostels for the homeless	18	45.0	20	50.0
Staffed group homes	7	17.5	4	10.0
Unstaffed group home	5	12.5	5	12.5
Night shelter or sleeping rough	4	10.0	3	7.5
Supported flat	3	7.5	3	7.5
Own flat	2	5.0	3	7.5
Poor quality bedsit	0	0.0	2	5.0
With family	1	2.5	0	0.0

In the case of this trial comparing two treatments, the table needs to show how similar or different the two groups were before the study interventions began.

As it turns out, there are differences. For example, a greater proportion of the case-management group have mood disorders or neurosis and fewer of them are in contact with psychiatric services.

Table 1: **Characteristics of subjects**

FIGURE 17.2 Baseline or casemix measures from a clinical trial. Reprinted from *The Lancet* 345: Marshall M, Lockwood A, Gath D. Social services case-management for long-term mental disorders: a randomised controlled trial. 1995; 409–12, © 1995, with permission from Elsevier.

INFORMATION AND MEASUREMENT BIAS

Many assessments – like those in the case management study – allow for some subjective judgement by the researcher who is trying to rate participants. Consequently, the researcher's own attitudes (rather than just the characteristics of the participants) could sway his or her judgement.

This sort of bias is especially likely when researchers are undertaking follow-up assessments in cohort studies or clinical trials. After all, many researchers undertake their investigations because they reckon that a new intervention is a winner or that a particular exposure is a cause of disease. Picture yourself rating outcome; how could you prevent your prior opinions about the treatment, or exposure to some risk, from influencing your measurements?

Study participants too are influenced by knowing whether they received active or placebo treatment, or old versus new interventions, or whether a study is designed to show a link between a certain exposure and an outcome. First, knowledge about the treatment or exposure will often affect participants' *judgements* about their symptoms or their experience of disability. Second, the same knowledge can have impact upon their *expression* or *description* of symptoms or disability when they are being rated.

For this reason researchers often take steps to conceal from the person doing the rating which group the participant has been allocated to or drawn from. This process is referred to as '*blinding*' or '*masking*' the rater. In clinical trials, the participant can easily reveal which treatment they received to a rater who is supposed to be blinded to treatment status. For these reasons, attempts are routinely made to blind participants as well as raters whenever feasible. This process of blinding researcher and participant is referred to as a *double-blind* procedure; *single-blind* referring to situations where one party is aware (usually the participant). but the other is not.

It can be relatively easy to double-blind some drug treatment studies, especially where the manufacturer assists the research by producing and supplying placebo or alternative drugs with identical appearance. Even so, different side-effect profiles mean that clinically aware raters can (or think that they can) readily determine which participants had which treatments. Many psychological therapies and surgical procedures are not amenable to double-blind techniques. Nevertheless, researchers such as those in the example in Figure 17.3 go to great lengths to achieve as much blinding as possible in rigorous efforts to reduce measurement biases.

In cohort or case-control studies, where the two groups of participants are not allocated to interventions, the blinding technique is applicable – but not always possible. Sometimes researchers make remarkably strenuous efforts to achieve blinding of raters, occasionally going to such lengths as to transcribe interviews, so as to remove any visual or verbal clues as to which group the participant belonged, and arranging for the rating of these transcripts.

Those asked to extract information from case notes or other routine records may also, on occasions, be blinded to whether the record belongs to a member of the case group or the control group (in a case-control study) or in the group exposed or unexposed to the risk factor (in a cohort analytic study); one such situation is shown in Figure 17.4. The reason for this masking is that evidence about research bias has shown that the distortions that may result from unblinded studies can be large enough to bring about false findings, either exaggerating or wrongly minimising the true study results.

BIAS ARISING FROM MISSING VALUES

However careful researchers are, it is all-but-inevitable that there will be missing values in their data. It may be that participants fail to complete a particular questionnaire, for example, or decline to answer certain questions. In studies that involve some follow-up, there is the additional problem that not all of the original sample may be available for subsequent assessments. This can lead to biased results, if the missing values are not randomly distributed. That is, if certain participants (say women, or the elderly, or people

Electroconvulsive therapy: results in depressive illness from the Leicestershire trial

S BRANDON, P COWLEY, C McDONALD, P NEVILLE, R PALMER, S WELLSTOOD-EASON

After the initial assessment each patient was allocated a code number and regardless of diagnosis allocated according to previously determined random numbers to receive treatment or placebo (simulated treatment). Elaborate arrangements ensured that research and nursing staff had no opportunity to discover which group the patients were in. Treatment was carried out in "sealed off" electroconvulsive therapy units and administered by a member of the research team who had no access to any other information on the patient. Nurses and anaesthetists had no contact with the patients outside the electroconvulsive therapy suite and were "sworn to secrecy." Other nursing staff had no access to patients during or after treatment until the patient was able to enter the recovery room. We could find no evidence of any breach of security.

In the treatment room all patients received a standard anaesthetic of methohexitone and suxamethonium at a dosage related to body weight (1 mg methohexitone/kg, 0.5 mg suxamethonium/kg). No atropine was used, and oxygenation was maintained throughout. An Ectron Mark IV electroconvulsive therapy machine was used with bilateral temporal

> Even patients who did not receive ECT were anaesthetized, and the treatment suite was closed to all but research staff sworn to secrecy.

FIGURE 17.3   Blinding patients and staff so that measures made later can be masked as to the allocation of subjects to treatment groups. ECT = electroconvulsive therapy. Reproduced from Brandon S, Cowley P, McDonald C, Neville P, Palmer R, Wellstood-Eason S. Electroconvulsive therapy: results in depressive illness from the Leicestershire trial. *BMJ* 1984, 288: 23–6, © 1984, with permission from BMJ Publishing Group Ltd.

with alcohol dependence, or people assigned to treatment A rather than treatment B) are less likely to complete the measures than others, then the results of the study may be systematically distorted by the absence of data from those participants. What can the researchers do?

First, they could simply give you data for those measures (or those participants) for which the data are available. This can be a little confusing if the numbers keep changing, but at least it can help you 'track' the data collection process in the study. Second, researchers can *impute* results for the missing values or participants. They might do this, for example, by assuming that a missing value was the same as the average for that value in the sample. Statisticians have developed increasingly clever methods for accurate imputation of missing values and this procedure may be alluded to or described in detail in the research report.

Particularly in relation to follow-up studies, researchers have a third option. Suppose they are conducting a study in which assessments are made at baseline and at 3-monthly intervals for a year, so there should be results available for each participant at 0, 3, 6, 9, and 12 months. For obvious reasons, it is the values at later follow-ups that are more likely to be missing. The researchers can decide to assume that each missing value is the same as the last one actually obtained for that participant – the so-called *last-observation-carried-forward* (Figure 17.5). So if a participant misses (say) her 9- and 12-month follow-up

Prenatal ultrasound examinations and risk of childhood leukaemia: case-control study

Estelle Naumburg, Rino Bellocco, Sven Cnattingius, Per Hall, Anders Ekbom.

Concerns over a possible association between exposure to ultrasound in utero and an increased risk of childhood malignancies have not been substantiated, but previous studies have been hampered by low statistical power or based on interviews with the parents done retrospectively, or both. To assess the impact of ultrasound and the risks of childhood lymphatic and myeloid leukaemia, we performed a nationwide population based case-control study using prospectively assembled data on prenatal exposure to ultrasound.

Subjects, methods, and results

The cases in this study comprised all children born and diagnosed as having leukaemia between 1973 and 1989 and reported to the nationwide Swedish registers of birth, cancer, and causes of death – in all, 752 cases. One control was randomly selected for each child with leukaemia from the Swedish Birth Registry and matched by sex and year and month of birth. The study was restricted to cases and controls without Down's syndrome (n=731), and medical records of 652 (89%) matched case-control pairs could be retrieved (578 cases with lymphatic leukaemia and 74 with myeloid leukaemia).

Altogether, 361 (48%) of the children with leukaemia had developed it before the age of 4, and 21 children were born in twin pregnancies. Information on exposure was extracted from antenatal, obstetric, and other standardised medical records by one of us (EN), who was blind to whether the child was a case or control. Conditional logistic regression was performed to study the association between prenatal exposure to ultrasound and childhood leukaemia (lymphatic and myeloid leukaemia). Maximum likelihood methods were used to estimate the odds ratio and 95% confidence intervals.

Blinding is about masking group membership from people carrying out any kind of measurement; casenote information is a common target of blinding procedures – for all the same reasons as in direct rating of live participants.

FIGURE 17.4   Blinding people who are extracting casenote information to the participants' group membership (cases or controls). Reproduced from Naumburg E, Bellocco R, Cnattingius S, Hall P, Ekbom A. Prenatal ultrasound examinations and risk of childhood leukaemia: case-control study. *BMJ* 2000, 320: 282–3, © 2000, with permission from BMJ Publishing Group Ltd.

assessments, then the missing values are assumed to be the same as those which *were* obtained at the 6-month assessment.

Missing values in a randomised controlled trial present particular problems. Researchers may simply present results for those participants on whom they have all assessments, but we know these *trial completers* are not the same as all participants (they tend to do better than trial dropouts). An alternative is to provide results for all *trial entrants*, with missing values for the dropouts imputed. This is known as *intention-to-treat analysis* (see Chapter 7).

A 24-week, double-blind, placebo-controlled trial of donepezil in patients with Alzheimer's disease

S.L. Rogers, PhD; M.R. Farlow, MD; R.S. Doody, MD, PhD; R. Mohs, PhD; L.T. Friedhoff, MD, PhD; for the Donepezil Study Group

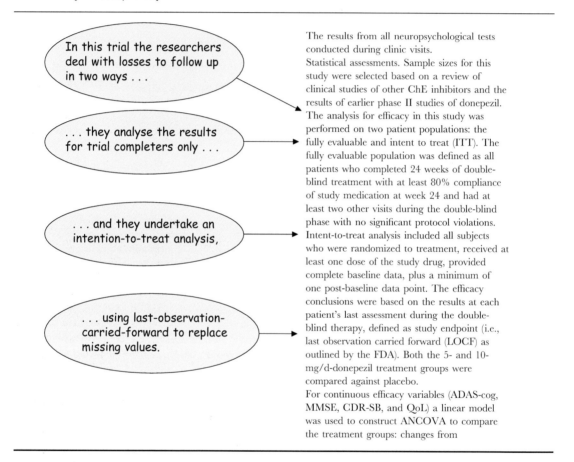

In this trial the researchers deal with losses to follow up in two ways . . .

. . . they analyse the results for trial completers only . . .

. . . and they undertake an intention-to-treat analysis,

. . . using last-observation-carried-forward to replace missing values.

The results from all neuropsychological tests conducted during clinic visits.
Statistical assessments. Sample sizes for this study were selected based on a review of clinical studies of other ChE inhibitors and the results of earlier phase II studies of donepezil. The analysis for efficacy in this study was performed on two patient populations: the fully evaluable and intent to treat (ITT). The fully evaluable population was defined as all patients who completed 24 weeks of double-blind treatment with at least 80% compliance of study medication at week 24 and had at least two other visits during the double-blind phase with no significant protocol violations. Intent-to-treat analysis included all subjects who were randomized to treatment, received at least one dose of the study drug, provided complete baseline data, plus a minimum of one post-baseline data point. The efficacy conclusions were based on the results at each patient's last assessment during the double-blind therapy, defined as study endpoint (i.e., last observation carried forward (LOCF) as outlined by the FDA). Both the 5- and 10-mg/d-donepezil treatment groups were compared against placebo.
For continuous efficacy variables (ADAS-cog, MMSE, CDR-SB, and QoL) a linear model was used to construct ANCOVA to compare the treatment groups: changes from

FIGURE 17.5   Dealing with missing values in a clinical trial. Reproduced from Rogers SL, Farlow MR, Doody RS, Mohs R, Friedhoff LT, for the Donepezil Study Group. A 24-week, double-blind, placebo-controlled trial of donepezil in patients with Alzheimer's disease. *Neurology* 1998, 50: 136–45, with permission from Wolters Kluwer Health.

In Figure 17.5, which comes from a clinical trial evaluating a new anti-dementia drug, the authors explain how they have dealt with missing values at follow-up.

Whichever approach researchers take, you should be able to find an estimate of the possible impact on their results. In other words, they should tell you what effect missing values might have had, and how their results might have been different, if either there were no missing values or they had made different assumptions when imputing the missing values. This sort of calculation is often called a *sensitivity analysis*.

18

Measuring the Characteristics of Participants: Qualitative

Qualitative health research normally seeks to understand the meanings individuals use to explain and make sense of their experiences. The characteristics of the participants and of the researchers are central to understanding the boundaries of the experiences represented in any piece of research.

Qualitative researchers want to include within their sample diverse and varied ways of understanding a given phenomenon, such that the diversity captured is similar to that found within the target population.

As implied in Chapter 11, qualitative research usually uses *non-probability samples* for selecting participants. To allow the reader to evaluate critically whether or not the sample obtained is fit for purpose, qualitative papers should include a description of the characteristics of participants (e.g. see Figure 18.1).

In addition, qualitative researchers normally recognise the role of the researcher within the research process and hence characteristics of the researchers should also be described (again, see Figure 18.1).

In published papers you should see a description of the characteristics of participants and researchers. The information should include sufficient detail to enable you to appraise whether the diversity captured in the sample represents the diversity of experiences in the population of interest. Characteristics of participants do not need to be representative of the target population in order to capture diversity of experience. For example, the proportion of males within a sample does not need to be representative of the proportion of males within the population of interest – what is important is to ensure that the sample captures the diversity of views likely to be found within the male population.

Qualitative researchers differ on the extent to which they believe that findings from their research should have relevance to samples and contexts wider than the original piece of research. It is beyond the scope of this chapter to discuss the issue of generalisation in detail; the position taken by a researcher relates to their *epistemological* (how knowledge is acquired) and *ontological* (what can be known) viewpoint. Generally, however, it is accepted that qualitative health research should have an application wider than the individual study: the extent to which findings might have relevance to other groups of individuals, settings, and conditions may be considered by the author. Generalisablity is often linked to characteristics of the participants. Consideration might include an appraisal of the extent to which the characteristics of the sample enable findings to be generalised to the population and/or setting of interest. Generalisation might also include an appraisal of whether findings can be transferred to other populations/settings not considered within the study. See Figure 18.2, from a study of the experiences of parents of children with traumatic brain injury, where the authors point out the limitations of their study in terms of generalisability.

Understanding Clinical Papers, Third Edition. David Bowers, Allan House, David Owens and Bridgette Bewick.
© 2014 John Wiley & Sons, Ltd. Published 2014 by John Wiley & Sons, Ltd.

Toward caring for oneself in a life of intense ups and downs: A reflexive-collaborative exploration of recovery in bipolar disorder

Veseth, M., Binder, PE., Borg, M. And Davidson, L.

The aim ... was to investigate and explore the lived experiences of improvement in bipolar disorder ...

The characteristics of researchers are clearly described.

All authors have clinical experience with psychotherapy and other mental health care treatment ... [and] hold interest in and have experience with qualitative research ... a group of 12 service users with first-hand experience of mood disorders joined this study as co-researchers ...

The characteristics of participants are clearly described. The authors go on to describe the sample in terms of employment, relationships, and children.

Thirteen participants, 7 women and 6 men, were included in the study. Their ages ranged from 27-64 years, with a mean age of 47 years. All participants were living in the western part of Norway. They reported both bipolar I and bipolar II diagnosis.

...our [i.e. researchers] preconceptions offer a position that enables us to understand our participants' experiences ... we believe there is added value in bringing together professional and service user perspectives ... even though the researchers and co-researchers in the present study formed a research team with a multitude of diverging experiences ... we are all in close proximity to the study field ... it is plausible to imagine that researchers with more distance from the field ... would identify other important aspects of the processes of recovery ...

The authors provide an appraisal of the strengths and limitations afforded by their own position.

... another methodological limitation is the small and relatively homogeneous group of participants; ... all adult, ethnic Norwegians ... all had struggled with mental health problems at approximately the same period of time, and received help ... from the same mental health system ...

The boundaries of experiences represented by participant stories are explained. Explanations refer directly to the characteristics of the sample. Here authors are commenting on the limited applicability of their findings.

FIGURE 18.1 Description of the characteristics of participants in a study of recovery from bipolar disorder. Reproduced from Veseth M, Binder PE, Borg M, Davidson L. Toward caring for oneself in a life of intense ups and downs: a reflexive-collaborative exploration of recovery in bipolar disorder. *Qualitative Health Research* 2012, 22 (1): 119–33, © 2012 SAGE Publications. Reprinted by permission of SAGE Publications.

Parents' experiences following children's moderate to severe traumatic brain injury: A clash of cultures

Roscigno, C.I. and Swanson, K.M.

The purpose ... to describe the common experiences of a sample of English-speaking parents from across the United States following their ... child's ... traumatic brain injury.

> Here authors describe how this research positioned the researcher within the research process.

Bracketing or consciously striving to set aside a priori knowledge is an important tenant of descriptive phenomenology ... bracketing encourages the investigator to become aware of his or her a priori knowledge and biases ... [and] reflect on how these factors could potentially bias interpretations and take measures to suspend premature conclusions.

> This section sets out the kind of families the researchers wanted in the study.

... families were recruited from across the United States from 2005 to 2007 ... recruitment was primarily aimed at recruited a diverse group of children. We believed that a sample reflecting diversity of the children would also result in a diverse group of parents with varied experiences. To be included, children needed to be (a) 6 to 18 years of age at time of injury; (b) categorized with moderate to sever traumatic brain injury...; (c) able to participate in an interview process; (d) between 4 months and 3 years postinjury ast the time the parents were enrolled; (f) fluent in English; (g) able to assent or consent ...; (h) living with at least one parent or legal guardian who was willing to be interviewed separately ...

> The authors go on to describe their sample in terms of who was interviewed.

... final sample consisted of 42 parents from 37 familes ... from 13 of the 50 United States ...

...these findings were derived from a sample ... limited in racial, ethnic, and language diversity; hence caution should be used when applying findings ...

> The boundaries of experiences represented by participant stories are explained. Explanations refer directly to the characteristics of the sample. Here the author is saying something about the extent to which they believe findings from this sample could be transferred to the population.

FIGURE 18.2 Diversity as a characteristic of the participants in a study of the experience of the parents of children who had suffered a traumatic brain injury. Reproduced from Roscigno CI, Swanson KM. Parents' experiences following children's moderate to severe traumatic brain injury: a clash of cultures. *Qualitative Health Research* 2011, 21 (10): 1413–26, © 2011 SAGE Publications. Reprinted by permission of SAGE Publications.

Measuring the Characteristics of Measures

Making an accurate diagnosis is crucial in health-care. The measures used to attempt a correct diagnosis vary, ranging from simple observation to quite complex procedures or tests. In this chapter we are going to discuss some of the important characteristics of these diagnostic measures as an aid to understanding what you may see in clinical papers.

THE MEASURES

Researchers generally use four separate but related measures when they present the accuracy of a diagnostic test:

- *Sensitivity*: the percentage of those patients *with* the condition whom the test correctly identifies as having it. In other words, the percentage of true positives.
- *Specificity*: the percentage of those patients *without* the condition whom the test correctly identifies as not having it. In other words, the percentage of true negatives.
- *Positive predictive value (PPV)*: the percentage (or proportion) of patients whom the test identifies as having the condition who do have it.
- *Negative predictive value (NPV)*: the percentage (or proportion) of patients whom the test does not identify as having the condition who do not have it.

Clearly, the PPV and NPV diagnostics are clinically more useful. Typically, as a clinician, you want to know the chances of a patient having the condition if they return a positive test result (positive predictive value), rather than whether they will give a positive test result if they are known to have the condition (sensitivity). Notice that since the sensitivity of a test depends on the condition being present, and the specificity depends on the condition being absent, then both of these measures are largely unaffected by the prevalence of the condition. This is not true for PPV and NPV which are markedly affected by prevalence.

In an ideal world we would like a test which had 100% sensitivity and 100% specificity, but sadly this is not possible in practice. There is an optimal (but never perfect) value for the trade-off between sensitivity and specificity, which gives the best results for both measures, although this will also be influenced by the nature of the condition. For example, a diagnostic test for acute myocardial infarction using serum creatine kinase (CK)-BB concentration needs as high a sensitivity as possible so that immediate action (aspirin, streptokinase, etc.) can be taken. A high specificity is not so crucial since counter-measures are not likely to harm patients (although it might cause them some alarm). On the other hand, if surgery is the required option for those identified as having some condition, then we would obviously want a very high (preferably 100%) specificity. In our example, choosing an appropriate trade-off value of CK-BB is thus fairly crucial. The idea is illustrated in Figure 19.1, taken from a study investigating the possible use of serum tyrosine hydroxylase (STH) activity (mU/l), as an indicator of melanoma. The STH activity

Understanding Clinical Papers, Third Edition. David Bowers, Allan House, David Owens and Bridgette Bewick.
© 2014 John Wiley & Sons, Ltd. Published 2014 by John Wiley & Sons, Ltd.

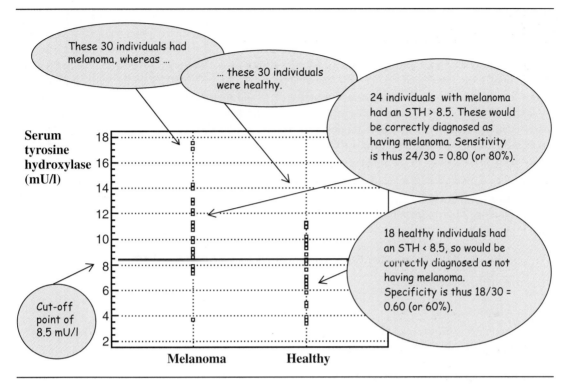

FIGURE 19.1 Diagnostic plot for the serum tyrosine hydroxylase (STH) activity data, indicating the cut-off point of 8.5 mU/l. Reprinted from Ros-Bullón MR, Sánchez-Pedreño P, Martínez-Liarte JH. Serum tyrosine hydroxylase activity is increased in melanoma patients. An ROC curve analysis. *Cancer Letters* 1998, 129 (2): 151–5, © 1998, with permission from Elsevier.

levels in 30 healthy and 30 melanoma patients are shown, with an optimal cut-off value of 8.5 mU/l (derived using a *receiver operating characteristic* (ROC) curve, described below). As you can see, for the 30 individuals with melanoma, this cut-off value correctly identifies 24 of them as having melanoma (STH > 8.5). Sensitivity is thus $24/30 = 0.80$ (or 80%). Among the 30 healthy individuals, 18 had STH < 8.5, so would be correctly diagnosed as not having melanoma. Specificity is thus $18/30 = 0.60$ (or 60%). Notice though that six individuals with melanoma would be mis-diagnosed as being healthy and 12 healthy individuals would be diagnosed as having melanoma. Increasing or decreasing the cut-off value will always cause the sensitivity to decrease and the specificity to increase, respectively. What one hand giveth, the other hand taketh away. We will return to this trade-off question in a moment.

What does all this mean? When you read papers containing diagnostic test studies, you would like to see information on all four diagnostic measures, along with their confidence intervals. If the measure being used for the tests is ordinal or metric, there should be some evidence that various trade-off points have been explored. You also need some information on the prevalence of the condition in the population concerned, particularly if the test is to be used in wider (potentially different) populations.

THE SENSITIVITY VERSUS SPECIFICITY TRADE-OFF – THE RECEIVER OPERATING CHARACTERISTIC (ROC) CURVE

To return to the sensitivity versus specificity trade-off question. As previously noted, what we would really like is a test that gives only true positives (i.e. no false negatives, implying a sensitivity of 1 (or 100%)) and only true negatives (i.e. no false positives, such that $(1 - \text{specificity}) = 0$). One popular method for finding the optimum trade-off point is to draw a ROC curve. This is a plot, for each trade-off point, of sensitivity (i.e. the true positive rate) on the vertical axis against $(1 - \text{specificity})$ (i.e. the false-positive rate) on the horizontal axis. The only plot of trade-off points which will give us both a sensitivity of 1 (no false negatives) and a specificity of 1 (no false positives, i.e. $1 - \text{specificity} = 0$) is a line which goes up the vertical axis to the top left-hand corner (corresponding to a sensitivity of 1) and then across the top of the graph to where $(1 - \text{specificity}) = 1$. The total area of this rectangular shape is then $1 \times 1 = 1$. We call this the *area under the curve* (AUC). Note that a test which produces as many false positives as true positives (i.e. a test with no discriminatory power) would give a ROC curve which lay on the 45° diagonal from the origin (see Figure 19.2, from a study of the diagnostic criteria for pre-diabetes and its progression to diabetes).

HbA$_{1c}$ 5.7-6.4% and impaired fasting plasma glucose for diagnosis of prediabetes and risk of progression to diabetes in Japan (TOPICS 3): a longitudinal cohort study

• Yoriko Heianza, Shigeko Hara, Yasuji Arase, Kazumi Saito, Kazuya Fujiwara, Hiroshi Tsuji, Satoru Kodama, Shiun Dong Hsieh, Yasumichi Mori, Prof Hitoshi Shimano, Nobuhiro Yamada, Kinori Kosaka, Hirohito Sone

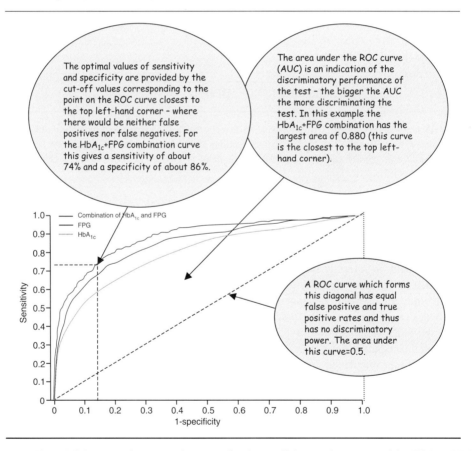

FIGURE 19.2 Three ROC curves from a study to predict future diabetes when assessed by HbA$_{1c}$ 5.7%–6.4% criterion, by FPG, and by a combination of HbA1c and FPG. Reprinted from *The Lancet* 378: Heianza Y, Hara S, Arase Y, Saito K, Fujiwara K, Tsuji H, *et al*. HbA$_{1c}$ 5.7-6.4% and impaired fasting plasma glucose for diagnosis of prediabetes and risk of progression to diabetes in Japan (TOPICS 3): a longitudinal cohort study. 2011 (9786); 147–55, © 2011, with permission from Elsevier.

The optimal trade-off (i.e. the trade-off point which minimizes the sum of false positives plus false negatives) thus corresponds to that point on the curve which lies closest to the top left-hand corner, because this is the trade-off value that combines the highest sensitivity (the smallest false-negative rate) with the highest specificity (the smallest false-positive rate). The closer the ROC curve is to the top left-hand corner, the larger the AUC. If authors are describing the choice between more than one available test (e.g. they may be comparing the performance of a new test with a 'gold standard' test which is assumed to give the correct result) they will be looking for the test with the largest AUC. When you are reading a paper which contains one or more ROC curves you will want to see a value for each AUC, together with its confidence interval.

To see how this works in practice, consider Figure 19.2 again, which shows the ROC curves for three possible tests for the diagnosis of pre-diabetes. The tests assess the levels of the new glycated haemoglobin (HbA_{1c}) 5.7–6.4% criterion, the FPG (fasting plasma glucose) criterion of 5.6–6.9 mmol/l, and a combination of both. As you can see, the combination test (HbA_{1c} with FPG) is closer to the top left-hand corner than either HbA_{1c} or FPG separately. The AUC and 95% confidence intervals for the three ROC curves are: for HbA_{1c}, AUC = 0.795 (0.767–0.822); for FPG, AUC = 0.846 (0.821–0.870); and for the combination of HbA_{1c} and FPG, AUC = 0.880 (0.859–0.901).

As a final point, note that if a test uses a nominal (yes/no) measure (e.g. blood in stool (Y/N), pain when urinating (Y/N), etc.), then there can be no trade-off between sensitivity and specificity.

20

Measurement Scales

Clinical papers will frequently report the analysis of data produced by a *measurement scale*. Less frequently you will come across papers which describe the development of a new scale. In this chapter, we are going to say something about measurement scales and point out what you as a reader should look out for.

WHY DO WE NEED THEM?

In Chapter 14, we outlined the difference between categorical data and metric data. Metric variables (such as weight, waiting time, number of deaths) can be *properly measured*. However, this is not true for categorical variables such as levels of pain or anxiety, degree of well-being, ethnic origin, gender, and so on; these have to be *assessed* in some way. For some variables, such as ethnicity or gender, this can be done with simple questioning. For other variables, like level of satisfaction, degree of general health, whether experiencing post-natal depression or not, and so on, a more complex approach is usually needed. This will often mean the use of an appropriate measurement scale.

WHAT ARE MEASUREMENT SCALES?

A measurement scale (also referred to as an *instrument*) will usually be based on a questionnaire, or a physical or visual examination, or a mix of these methods; in any case the end result is a score. For example, the Glasgow Coma Scale has just three questions or *items* – degrees of eye opening, of verbal response, and of motor response. Possible scores range from 3 (deep coma or death) to 15 (fully awake). Note that in measurement scales the word 'item' is used rather than the word 'question', since the scale may not consist entirely of questions; some observational or measurement elements may be included.

Some measurement scales are short and reasonably straightforward, some are longer and more complex, and may consist of a number of *dimensions*, each one of which may have one or more items. You can think of each dimension of a scale as a distinct aspect of the condition being measured. For example, a scale to measure general well-being might have three dimensions: physical well-being, mental well-being, and social well-being, the level of each one of which may elicited by means of several questions or items.

We can illustrate these ideas with the study of back pain (Figure 15.3). Values for the demographic variables (age, gender, and nationality) will have been elicited from the patient. However, the pain, and psychosocial scores, will have been derived using appropriate measurement scales.

Understanding Clinical Papers, Third Edition. David Bowers, Allan House, David Owens and Bridgette Bewick.
© 2014 John Wiley & Sons, Ltd. Published 2014 by John Wiley & Sons, Ltd.

WHEN AUTHORS USE DATA FROM MEASUREMENT SCALES

When authors make use of data derived from a measurement scale they should at least provide the name of the scale in the Methods section and give full source details in the references at the end of the paper. The authors of a study of cognitive decline satisfy this requirement. In their Methods section they provide a detailed and comprehensive account of the tests used to measure five cognitive function items. For example, for the verbal fluency item they say:

> We used two measures of verbal fluency: phonemic and semantic. Participants were asked to recall in writing as many words beginning with 'S' (phonemic fluency) and as many animal names (semantic fluency) as they could. One minute was allowed for each test; the observed range for these tests was 0–35.
>
> *(Singh-Manoux* et al., *2012)*

Full source references to all scales used were provided in the References section.

DEVELOPMENT OF A NEW MEASUREMENT SCALE

You may encounter papers devoted to the development of a new scale. Scale development can be a complex and lengthy process, so what follows is a brief summary.

Researchers will develop a new scale if there is no existing scale that meets their needs. For example, Figure 20.1 is an extract from a paper in which the authors justified the development of a new scale to measure the stigma relating to sexually transmitted infections among women, because they considered that there was no suitable existing scale.

Comparing doctor- and nurse-led care in sexual health clinics: patient satisfaction questionnaire

Miles K, Penny N, Power R and Mercy D

… the National Strategy for Sexual Health and HIV proposes that nurses have an expanding role as specialists and consultants for the management of sexually transmitted infections (STIs) .... . However, there is no evidence demonstrating the acceptance of nurses as first-line providers in the speciality of sexual health, or genitourinary medicine (GUM). This paper therefore focuses on an empirical study that aims to develop a *valid and reliable* measure of patient satisfaction that would be used to compare care provided for female patients at nurse-led or doctor-led clinics at a GUM clinic. (our italics)

These authors developed a new scale because there was no existing scale covering this area.

FIGURE 20.1 Development of new scale because there was no suitable existing scale. Reproduced from Miles K, Penny N, Power R, Mercy D (2002) with permission from John Wiley & Sons.

Development and validation of a core outcome measure for palliative care: the palliative care outcome scale

Hearn J, and Higginson IJ

Quality of life and outcome measures for patients with advanced illness need to be able to assess the key goals of palliative care. Various outcome measures and systems for evaluating palliative care have been developed in recent years. [author then lists a number of such scales].... none of these systematically covers all those domains considered important to palliative care. .... The aim of this study was to develop a core outcome measure for patients with advanced cancer and their families which would cover more than either physical symptoms or quality of life, but remain brief and simple to administer.

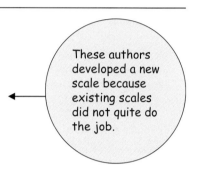

These authors developed a new scale because existing scales did not quite do the job.

FIGURE 20.2   Development of new scale because the existing scale did not quite do the job. Reproduced from Hearn J, Higginson IJ, on behalf of the Palliative Care Core Audit Project Advisory Group. Development and validation of a core outcome measure for palliative care: the palliative care outcome scale. *Quality in Health Care* 1999, 8: 219–27, © 1999, with permission from BMJ Publishing Group Ltd.

Sometimes a new scale is developed because an existing scale is in some way unsuitable – perhaps too long, too expensive, too invasive, or maybe does not quite measure what researchers need to measure. Figure 20.2 is taken from a paper reporting the development of a new palliative care outcome scale because existing scales did not quite do the job.

SCALE CONSTRUCTION

The construction of a new measurement scale will consist of a number of stages:

- Careful consideration of the condition in question. What is it? How does it arise? How is it manifest? Talking to patients and those familiar and experienced with the condition will be part of this process.
- Research of the literature and examination of any existing scales covering the same or similar conditions.
- The first two stages lead to a tentative initial selection of items which cover the domain of the condition (some of these items may be borrowed from existing scales).
- Once a set of items has been identified, these will need to be put into question form. The authors might refer to questions being put in some specific format. For example, the authors of a paper describing the development of a new scale to measure the attitudes and beliefs of patients towards hyperlipidaemia and its treatments, report that: 'Response categories used a 5-point *Likert scale* to assess the degree to which physicians agreed or disagreed with each attitudinal statement'. (*Foley, Vasey & Markson, 2003*)
- The questions are then organised into an appropriate order and structure – and hence into a scale.
- A draft of the scale can then be passed back to the experienced colleagues who can check that all important aspects of the condition are covered by the suggested items and make suggestions to plug any existing gaps. The object is parsimony (i.e. just enough items to cover the domain adequately, but no more).

- The new scale will then have to be road-tested to ensure that it possesses a number of properties desirable in any scale (see below).

The Likert scale quoted above is one of a number of possible ways of framing questions. Readers who want to know more can use a search engine which will reveal many sources offering details of questionnaire design and types of questions.

When they are choosing scale items, you may see authors reporting their use of factor (or principal component) analysis. These methods are a little too complex to discuss in any detail here, but briefly, *factor* (or *principal component*) analysis is a procedure for identifying a smaller number of underlying variables, known as *constructs*, from a larger set of variables.

DESIRABLE PROPERTIES OF SCALES

When you read a clinical paper describing the development of a new scale, the authors need to demonstrate that their scale has a number of properties, without which the scale will be of little value. For example, Figure 20.3 is extracted from a paper which describes the development of a scale to measure children's emotional responses during medical procedures, and refers to the necessity for a scale to have the properties of validity and reliability. Clearly these properties are (along with other qualities) extremely important, and we want here to provide at least an outline of these and some other desirable scale properties. We will do this assuming the scale is questionnaire-based, which many scales are (other than the most simple). Note that there is some inconsistency in the literature in the use of some of the terms. When authors claim reliability and repeatability for a measure they have used, you might wish to check their quoted sources to determine which of the following properties have in fact been established.

Scale Validity

Put simply, *validity* is the ability of a scale to measure what it is supposed to measure, no more and no less. You will see references to a number of different 'types' of validity, the most important of which we will now briefly describe.

Children's Emotional Manifestation Scale: Development and Testing

Ho Cheung W and Lopez V

Therefore there is a need for preoperative interventions that can minimise children's anxiety and enhance their ability to cope with surgery. First, however, to evaluate the effectiveness of preoperative interventions, the availability of a *valid and reliable* instrument that accurately documents the manifestation of children's emotions towards stressful medical procedures is crucial. Regrettably, the existing literature lacks an assessment tool with effective properties. (our italics)

It is important that any measurement scale is both valid and reliable.

FIGURE 20.3   The scale properties of validity and reliability in a scale to measure children's emotions. Reproduced from Ho Cheung W, Lopez V. (2003) with permission from John Wiley & Sons.

Face Validity

If a scale appears on the surface to be measuring what it is supposed to be measuring, and does so with simple, relevant, and unambiguous questions, then it is said to have the property of *face validity*. This property is thought to increase the level of compliance of those completing the questionnaire.

Clinical papers may report a number of ways in which face validity might be checked. Many researchers use *reading* simplicity. For example, to quote again from the hyperlipidaemia medication adherence paper (see above), the scale questions were evaluated and:

> This activity resulted in the re-wording, and sometimes the elimination, of poorly or awkwardly worded items, or items that were judged to be poor representatives of their constructs. The items as a whole were also reviewed in terms of readability. The Flesch–Kinkaid reading grade level rated the final survey at a 8th grade level. (Foley, Vasey & Markson, 2003)

And from the paper on the development of a satisfaction questionnaire for patients attending a sexual health clinic (Figure 20.1):

> The second draft of the questionnaire was tested for face validity with nine patients of various ethnic origins and ages. Difficult questions were reworded and ambiguous questions excluded.
>
> (*Miles* et al., 2002)

Content Validity

Roughly speaking, a scale has *content validity* if there are enough items in the scale to address adequately the domain of the construct (the aspect of the condition) in question. In other words, all the items in the scale are relevant to the construct and all aspects of the construct are covered by the items in the scale. A scale with content validity measures what it is supposed to measure (and it does not measure what it is not supposed to).

Ensuring that a scale has content validity needs careful item selection and is part of the scale development process. Some authors might demonstrate that their scale has this property. How? One accepted method is to ask a number of experienced specialists to review the scale and rate the relevancy of each item. For example, in their paper describing the development of their Children's Emotional Manifestation Scale (Figure 20.3), content validity is demonstrated as follows:

> Content validity was established by six nurse experts rating of each item on a four-point scale (from $1 =$ not relevant to $4 =$ very relevant). The Content Validity Index (CVI), the % of the total number of items rated by the experts as either 3 or 4, was 96%. A CVI score of 80% or higher is generally considered to have good content validity.
>
> (*Ho Cheung and Lopez, 2003*)

Criterion and Concurrent Validity

Suppose there exists a well-established, highly thought of 'gold standard' scale, used to measure post-natal depression. We can call this 'gold standard' scale the *criterion scale* – it's the *benchmark* against which we can assess the performance of any other scale which claims to measure post-natal depression. But let's assume that this 'gold standard' criterion scale is long (i.e. has many questions and/or procedures), and is thus time-consuming and expensive to administer. We would be happy if a new, simpler, and shorter scale could be developed which could be shown to measure post-natal depression just as well (or perhaps almost as well) as the 'gold standard' scale. The crucial question is, how can we judge the efficacy of this new scale? One possibility would be to employ the 'gold standard' scale to get post-natal depression scores from a group of new mothers, and at about the same time (which is the *concurrent* bit) use the new scale against a matching group of recent mothers to get their post-natal depression scores. If there is a strong association between the two sets of scores (i.e. women who score high on one scale also score high on the other scale, and those who score low on one scale also score low on the other, etc.), then we have demonstrated the concurrent validity of the new scale. We would be justified in claiming that the new scale is an acceptable substitute for the 'gold standard' scale (provided it is otherwise satisfactory), and is cheaper and quicker to administer.

In this context, the association between the two scales is usually measured using a correlation coefficient. We will deal with correlation in considerable detail in Chapter 28, but a few words here might be helpful. Two variables are said to be *positively* associated if high values of one variable tend to correspond with high values of the other variable, and low values with low values. Conversely, if *high* values of one variable tend to correspond with *low* values of the other variable then the two variables are said to be *negatively* associated. We can measure the strength of any possible association by calculating a correlation coefficient which can vary from -1 (negative correlation), through 0, to $+1$ (positive correlation). Values closer to 1 (or -1) indicate stronger association than values closer to 0.

Thus authors might demonstrate that their new scale has concurrent validity by showing that their new scale is strongly associated with the 'gold standard' scale – if an alternative 'gold standard' scale is available. Figure 20.4 describes a test for concurrent validity by the authors of the Behavioural

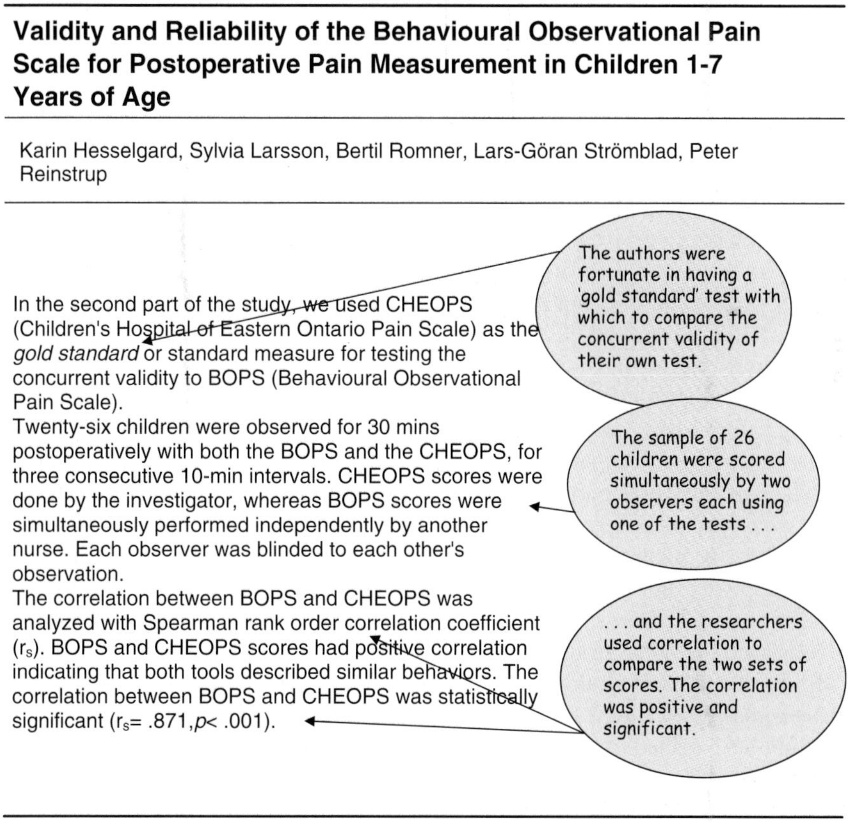

Validity and Reliability of the Behavioural Observational Pain Scale for Postoperative Pain Measurement in Children 1-7 Years of Age

Karin Hesselgard, Sylvia Larsson, Bertil Romner, Lars-Göran Strömblad, Peter Reinstrup

In the second part of the study, we used CHEOPS (Children's Hospital of Eastern Ontario Pain Scale) as the *gold standard* or standard measure for testing the concurrent validity to BOPS (Behavioural Observational Pain Scale).

Twenty-six children were observed for 30 mins postoperatively with both the BOPS and the CHEOPS, for three consecutive 10-min intervals. CHEOPS scores were done by the investigator, whereas BOPS scores were simultaneously performed independently by another nurse. Each observer was blinded to each other's observation.

The correlation between BOPS and CHEOPS was analyzed with Spearman rank order correlation coefficient (r_s). BOPS and CHEOPS scores had positive correlation indicating that both tools described similar behaviors. The correlation between BOPS and CHEOPS was statistically significant ($r_s = .871, p < .001$).

The authors were fortunate in having a 'gold standard' test with which to compare the concurrent validity of their own test.

The sample of 26 children were scored simultaneously by two observers each using one of the tests . . .

. . . and the researchers used correlation to compare the two sets of scores. The correlation was positive and significant.

FIGURE 20.4 Testing for concurrent validity in a children's post-operative pain scale by comparing with a 'gold standard' test. The researchers used correlation to compare the scores. Reproduced from Hesselgard K, Larsson S, Romner B, Strömblad L-G, Reinstrup P. Validity and reliability of the Behavioural Observational Pain Scale for postoperative pain measurement in children 1–7 years of age. *Pediatric Critical Care Medicine* 2007, 8 (2): 102–8, with permission from Wolters Kluwer Health.

Observational Pain Scale (BOPS), used for post-operative pain measurement in children, in which they compare their scale with the 'gold standard' Children's Hospital of Eastern Ontario Pain Scale (CHEOPS).

Unfortunately a 'gold standard' test is not always available. For example, on the development of a patient satisfaction questionnaire for patients at a sexual health clinic (Figure 20.1), the authors comment:

> Concurrent validity could involve the questionnaire being administered alongside an existing measure to determine whether there was a strong correlation between the two. Since no measure of satisfaction relevant to sexual health was identified, a comparative measure against another scale was not possible.
>
> (*Miles* et al., *2002*)

Authors may sometimes mention a variant of criterion validity known as *predictive validity*. This scale property relates to situations where the criterion, against which we want to judge our new scale, may not be available until some time has passed. We are using the scale in a predictive sense. For example, we may have a scale which indicates something that can only be confirmed (or not) with a biopsy. If the usual situation prevails – no suitable criterion scale exists – then predictive validity obviously cannot be established. In these circumstances, researchers may turn to construct validity.

Construct Validity

We know that we cannot directly measure things such as anxiety, well-being, the likelihood of pressure sores, and the like, in the same way we can measure weight or systolic blood pressure. We can of course *assess* the various *surface* manifestations of, say, anxiety (e.g. sweaty palms, restlessness, nausea, etc.) without too much difficulty. Conditions such as anxiety, well-being, or pain are known as *constructs* and many scales have been developed to measure them (we are now using the word 'measure' in the sense of 'assess the degree or level of'). Construct validity refers to the degree to which a scale measures the construct it is supposed to and does not measure any aspects of a different construct. In other words, the scale must provide a true assessment of the existence and level of the construct in question. If authors of a clinical paper are describing the development of a new scale, they should demonstrate that their scale has construct validity. There are a number of ways in which they can do this.

One possibility is for them to form hypotheses about the responses of subjects to their new scale and demonstrate that these hypotheses are satisfied. These hypotheses might include a comparison of their scale with an existing scale which purports to measure the same construct (e.g. by examining correlations between scores, which should be reasonably high). Conversely, they may compare their scale with another scale which should *not* be related. These would be expected to produce non-significant or even negative correlations (e.g. applying an anxiety scale to calm and relaxed individuals).

Another possibility is for authors to apply the new scale to two groups: one group believed to have the condition or construct, the other group not (this approach is known as the *method of extreme groups*). The group with the condition should produce high scores on the new scale, the group without, low scores. A further possibility might be to give a therapeutic intervention to the same two dissimilar groups, who might be expected to react differently if the scale has successfully discriminated between them.

As an example of the scale comparison method of establishing construct validity, Figure 20.5 is from a study into the use of the SF-36 scale to measure the general health of post-stroke patients (the authors claiming that this application of SF-36 was unexplored). The authors compared their proposed scale with a number of other scales, first making hypotheses about the expected correlations. Figure 20.6 shows the authors' comment taken from their results section. They do not comment further as to whether or not they feel these results establish construct validity.

Psychometric properties of the SF-36 in the early post-stroke phase

Hagen S, Bugge C and Alexander H

Construct validity was assessed by examining the relationship between the eight SF-36 subscores and the scores on other standard outcome measures: the Barthel Activities of Daily Living (ADL) Index, the Canadian Neurological Scale (CNS), and the Mini-Mental State Examination (MMSE). …. On the basis of the content of the questions it was hypothesised that there would be positive bivariate correlations between all SF-36 subscores and the Barthel Index, MMSE and CNS. … The latter three instruments, used here for validation purposes, all measure some aspect of physical or cognitive ability which should be associated, directly or indirectly, with elements of health status measured within the SF-36. More specifically, we would expect only low to moderate correlations between SF-36 scores and the MMSE as the SF-36 items do not directly address cognitive problems. In general, higher correlation coefficients would be expected in relation to the Barthel Index and the CNS which address physical aspects of health and related disability. The highest correlations might be expected between Physical Functioning, Role Limitation – Physical, General Health, and Social Functioning scores and both the Barthel and CNS. Moderate correlations might be expected between Bodily Pain, Vitality, and Role Limitation – Emotional scores and the Barthel Index and CNS. It was expected that Mental Health scores would be weakly correlated with the Barthel Index, CNS and MMSE scores. Spearman's rank correlations were used to test for associations.

The authors of this paper tested for the construct validity of SF-36 in post-stroke patients by comparing SF-36 scores with the Barthel ADL Index, the MMSE, and the Canadian Neurological Scale. They hypothesised various levels of correlation between SF-36 and these three other scales.

FIGURE 20.5   Demonstrating construct validity, from a paper on the use of SF-36 with post-stroke patients. (Note: Physical Functioning, Role Limitation – Physical, General Health, Social Functioning, Bodily Pain, Vitality, Role Limitation – Emotional, and Mental Health, are all dimensions of SF-36.) Reproduced from Hagen S, Bugge C, Alexander H. (2003) with permission from John Wiley & Sons.

   As a final comment, it is important to note that a scale developed for some particular population, even with large and representative samples, and whose validity has been satisfactorily demonstrated (we might describe it as being *internally* valid), may not be *externally* valid (i.e. it may not be valid when applied to some different population).

RELIABILITY

Even before the validity of a new scale is established, its *reliability* must first be demonstrated. Simply put, reliability means that the scale has the property of *repeatability or reproducibility*. You can administer it any number of times and it will always give consistent results. In other words, when a reliable scale is applied to a group of individuals by a single observer at two different times, or by two observers at the

Psychometric properties of the SF-36 in the early post-stroke phase

Hagen S, Bugge C and Alexander H

The strongest correlations were found between SF-36 scores and the Barthel Index and CNS, as hypothesised. The highest of these were with Physical Functioning and Social Functioning as expected; however, correlations with Role Limitations – Physical was markedly lower ... . Correlations with Mental Health scores were stronger than expected for both the Barthel Index and CNS. Correlations between SF-36 and MMSE scores were moderate for Physical Functioning and Mental Health and weaker for the remaining subscales, as expected.

The results of the author's comparisons of their scale and three other scales as a measure of construct validity.

FIGURE 20.6   Authors' comment on the correlations between scale scores from the paper shown in Figure 20.5 on the use of the SF-36 scale with post-stroke patients. Reproduced from Hagen S, Bugge C, Alexander H. (2003) with permission from John Wiley & Sons.

same time, it will produce *similar* scores. The crucial word here is 'similar'. How close do the scores have to be before they can be judged to be similar and the scale thus said to be reliable?

The authors of any scale development paper should demonstrate that their scale is reliable. You are unlikely to see anything like a 'reliability coefficient' quoted. Instead, authors may report a number of reliability-associated measures, the more important ones which we describe briefly below. As you will see, the similarity between scores can be judged in a number of ways.

Internal Consistency – Cronbach's Alpha (α)

Internal consistency is one measure thought to reflect the reliability of a scale. You might expect that a scale addressing some underlying construct will have a number of similar items. For example, the Geriatric Depression Scale (GDS) has questions like, 'Have you dropped many of your activities and interests?', 'Do you feel that your life is empty?', 'Do you often feel helpless?', and so on. These questions are tapping into the same construct. It seems reasonable to expect that if the test is reliable, then the scores by a group of patients on one of these items will be correlated with their scores on other, similar, items.

Such correlations are said to measure *internal consistency* and one common method of measuring this correlation is with *Cronbach's* α. To be acceptable, α should have a value above 0.7. One problem with α is that it is dependent on the number of items in the scale. Increase the number of items and α will increase (although the actual inter-item correlations may not have changed!). A second problem is that α takes no account of variation from observer to observer, or from one time period to another, and is thus likely to exaggerate reliability.

As an example from the literature, the authors of a paper describing the development of a scale to measure the attitudes of nurses working with acute mental health patients, the Attitudes Towards Acute Mental Health Scale (ATAMHS), reported the reliability of their scale as follows:

> The sample obtained for this study was greater than the 100 participants regarded as the minimum to ensure reliability of the statistical procedures . . . . The ATAMHS had a coefficient alpha of 0.72, which indicated reasonable reliability.
>
> (*Baker* et al., *2005*)

Similarly, the authors of the post-stroke SF-36 study, referred to earlier, reported the reliability of the SF-36 scale thus:

> The reliability of the SF-36 was assessed in terms of its internal consistency. . . . all values of Cronbach's α exceeded the generally accepted criterion of 0.7. This would tend to indicate a high level of correlation among items within the same subscale, and correspondingly good reliability.
>
> *(Hagen* et al.*, 2003)*

Internal consistency can also be thought of as a measure of the *homogeneity* of a scale. By this, we mean that all the items in a scale should be addressing different aspects of the same underlying construct and not different constructs. For example, if we are measuring some particular phobia, then all the scale items should relate in some way to different aspects of this phobia, not to other phobias or other general anxieties or fears. The implication of homogeneity is that all the items should correlate to some extent with each other and should also correlate with the total scale score. As you have just seen, this is the basis of measures of internal consistency. This notion leads to the idea of *split-half reliability*. This involves splitting the scale items randomly into two equal halves and then correlating the two halves. If the scale is internally consistent, then the two halves should be strongly correlated and hence reliable.

Stability

The *stability* of a measurement scale is a further measure of its reliability. This is the capacity of a scale to give similar scores in the following situations:

- When administered to a particular group of individuals at different time periods – *test–retest reliability*.
- When administered by two different observers – *inter-observer reliability*.
- When administered by the same observer at two different time periods – *intra-observer reliability*.

As far as test–retest reliability is concerned, the clinical paper should tell you how long the interval is between the first administration of the test and the second – 2 to 14 days is usual, although longer periods might be acceptable depending on the condition being measured.

All three of these forms of stability-reliability are probably best measured by the *intra-class correlation coefficient* (ICC). In practice, perhaps because the ICC is not always readily computable, authors may present a value either for a correlation coefficient, or for Cohen's chance-adjusted coefficient of agreement, kappa (κ), which we will discuss in more detail in Chapter 23. Briefly, κ measures the agreement between two sets of scores discounting any element of agreement expected to have arisen by chance.

An example of test–retest stability (and hence scale reliability) which uses κ is shown in Figure 20.7. This is from a study into the reproducibility of a scale to assess environmental sensitivity in individuals exposed to a range of substances in the environment.

Figure 20.8 is an example of test–retest stability which uses correlation. This is from the previously quoted study on a scale to measure patient satisfaction with nurse-led sexual health clinics (Figure 20.1).

A value of 0.95 for Pearson's correlation coefficient indicates a very strong association between the original scores and the retest scores. Note, however, that the sample size is very small which makes for unreliable results and, in addition, as you will see in Chapter 28, for ordinal data such as these, Spearman's correlation coefficient is more appropriate.

Reproducibility of the University of Toronto Self-administered Questionnaire Used to Assess Environmental Sensitivity

McKeown-Eyssen GE, Sokoloff ER, Jazmaji V, Marshall LM and Baines CJ

Reproducibility of the questionnaire was assessed by comparing responses from people who completed it on two different occasions. .... Within 5-7 months of returning the first questionnaire 200 respondents were randomly selected to receive the questionnaire a second time .... Kappa statistics were statistically significant for all systems (13 body systems were monitored), and were above 0.4 for 11 of 13 systems, indicating good levels of agreement. (and thus of test–retest reliability)

These authors used κ to measure the test–retest stability (and thus the reliability) of their environment sensitivity scale.

The first three lines of the authors' results are shown below:

Body system	% observed agreement	kappa	95% CI
Eye	88.8	0.57	0.37, 0.76
Ear	79.1	0.53	0.38, 0.68
Nose	89.6	0.36	0.13, 0.62

FIGURE 20.7 Using κ to examine the test–retest (reliability) property of scale. Reproduced from McKeown-Eyssen GE, Sokoloff ER, Jazmaji V, Marshall LM, Baines CJ. Reproducibility of the University of Toronto self-administered questionnaire used to assess environmental sensitivity. *American Journal of Epidemiology* 2000, 151: 1216–22, by permission of Oxford University Press.

Comparing doctors and nurse-led care in sexual health clinics: patient satisfaction questionaire

Miles K, Perry N, Power R and Mercy D

Phase 6 – test-retest stability

The final questionnaire consisted of 34 statements. It was re-administered (n=28) in the clinic, and 13 women agreed to receive a second postal questionnaire. .... with a mean of 13.75 days between first and second questionnaires . The second questionnaire was used to confirm stability, using a test-retest analysis. .... A Pearson correlation between the original and re-test scores was 0.95 (p<0.001), demonstrating questionnaire stability.

These authors used Pearson correlation to measure the test–retest stability (and thus the reliability) of their patient satisfaction scale.

FIGURE 20.8 Using correlation to examine the test–retest (reliability) property of a patient satisfaction scale for use in sexual health clinics. Reproduced from Miles K, Penny N, Power R, Mercy D (2002) with permission from John Wiley & Sons.

SENSITIVITY TO CHANGE – SCALE RESPONSIVENESS

If we are interested in the effect of some therapeutic intervention on a group of individuals experiencing some condition, then we want the scale that measures that condition to be sensitive to any change due to the intervention. In other words we want the scale to be able to capture the *treatment effect*. We call this the *sensitivity-to-change* or *responsiveness* property of the scale. In any paper describing the development of such a scale the authors should demonstrate that it has this property.

One way that they might do this is to measure changes over some time period using both their new scale and some other comparable scales. Ideally, these comparisons will be not only with scales which might be expected to reflect similar change, but also with scales which should not. What actual method is used for the comparison will depend on the particular circumstances (e.g. on the nature of the data), but correlation is one possibility.

Notice that there is a tension between the sensitivity-to-change property of a scale and the idea of test–retest reliability. Clearly, the latter is not appropriate for conditions where there is likely to be change over the short term, particularly where any therapeutic intervention is envisaged, and certainly not during the test–retest interval.

As an example of scale sensitivity to change we can return again to the study using SF-36 with post-stroke patients (Figure 20.4). One of the stated aims of this study was, 'To examine the reliability, validity and *sensitivity to change* of the SF-36 in patients in the early post-stroke period' (our italics). SF-36 scores were measured at 1, 3, and 6 months post-stroke. Figure 20.9 is an extract from that paper in which the authors used Wilcoxon's matched-pairs test to compare median change scores between a number of SF-36 subscales, and the Barthel ADL Index (see Chapter 25), the Canadian Neurological Scale (CNS), and the Mini-Mental State Examination (MMSE). The authors concluded that, 'Sensitivity to change was poorer in the later stages of the study'.

THE USE OF RECEIVER OPERATING CHARACTERISTIC CURVES WITH SCALE SCORES

Finally, authors may mention the use of the *receiver operating characteristic* (ROC) curve in conjunction with their newly developed scale as a way of determining optimum trade-off points for the scores obtained from it. The use of ROC curves and the sensitivity/specificity of trade-off scores were described in Chapter 19.

Psychometric properties of the SF-36 in the early post-stroke phase

Hagen S, Bugge C and Alexander H

Significant improvements were seen between 1 and 3 months in all SF-36 subscores except Bodily Pain, General Health, and Mental Health. Similarly there were significant improvements in Barthel Index, CNS and MMSE scores. There were no significant changes in SF-36 scores between 3 and 6 months while, of the three comparison measures, the CNS and MMSE both showed significant improvement. …. Between 3 and 6 months, none of the SF-36 subscales appeared to be responsive to change.

The authors measured sensitivity to change of SF-36 in post-stroke patients by comparing change over time in SF-36 with change in three other scales.

FIGURE 20.9 Sensitivity to change of SF-36 in post-stroke patients. Reproduced from Hagen S, Bugge C, Alexander H. (2003) with permission from John Wiley & Sons.

21

Exploring and Explaining: Topic Guides

Perhaps the most common qualitative research method for the collection of data is the interview. There are different forms of interviews. For example, one study may use face-to-face in-depth interviews, while another may use focus group discussions (see Chapter 4). Some studies seek to evaluate or investigate an event, while others aim to explore participant views of a given phenomenon. Interviews that seek to understand participants' views of their own experience generally use a relatively unstructured format. On those occasions when the study aims to *compare* participants' accounts, the interview format will be more structured. Who sets the interview agenda also varies between studies. For some studies the topics to be covered within the interview will largely be predetermined by the researcher, while in others the content to be covered will be primarily driven by the participant. Figure 21.1 (from a study aimed at determining the

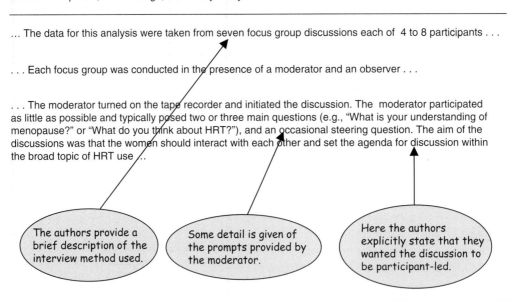

What is this thing called Hormone Replacement Therapy? Discursive construction of medication in situated practice

Christine Stephens, Claire Budge, and Jenny Carryer

... The data for this analysis were taken from seven focus group discussions each of 4 to 8 participants . . .

. . . Each focus group was conducted in the presence of a moderator and an observer . . .

. . . The moderator turned on the tape recorder and initiated the discussion. The moderator participated as little as possible and typically posed two or three main questions (e.g., "What is your understanding of menopause?" or "What do you think about HRT?"), and an occasional steering question. The aim of the discussions was that the women should interact with each other and set the agenda for discussion within the broad topic of HRT use . .

The authors provide a brief description of the interview method used.

Some detail is given of the prompts provided by the moderator.

Here the authors explicitly state that they wanted the discussion to be participant-led.

FIGURE 21.1   Use of focus groups in a participant-led study on the views of women towards HRT. Reproduced from Stephens C, Budge, C, Carryer J. What is this thing called hormone replacement therapy? Discursive construction of medication in situation practice. *Qualitative Health Research* 2002, 12: 347–359, © 2002 SAGE Publications. Reprinted by permission of SAGE Publications.

Qualitative research using photo-elicitation to explore the role of food in family relationships among obese adolescents

Jonathan Lachal, Mario Speranza, Olivier Taieb, Bruno Falissard, Herve Lefevre, QUALIGRAMH, Marie-Rose Moro, Anne Revah-Levy

… investigation of the place of food within family relationships among obese adolescents …

> Here authors describe the aim of the study …

…study was conducted by way of semi-structured interviews, with photo elicitation tool.

> … and go on to describe what methods were used to elicit data. In this study a photo was used as a prompt.

The photograph is provided by the subject, and used as the basis for the interview, enabling the verbal material to be steered and also enriched.

Preliminary interviews were conducted with the adolescents to faciliate contact during the recorded interview … the young people were provided with a disposible digital camera and asked to take photograph with the following instructions:

> Here it might seem like the participant has the potential to steer the interview by providing a photo of their choice …

"We want you to take a photograph of the table after a family meal. It should be taken before the table is cleared. There should not be anyone visible in the photograph … you will choose just one [photograph] to comment on … in the interview"

> … but here we learn that the photograph is to be taken following instructions that guide the participant towards a particular image.

The interviews were semi-structured, with an open-ended approach … the investigators had a set of questions on an interview schedule …

> The authors explain that an interview schedule was used …

. . .there was an endeavor to enter the … social world of the respondents … respondents consequently shared more closely in the direction taken by the interview and could introduce an issue that investigators had not thought of. Respondents were viewed as experiential experts … and were allowed opportunity to tell their own story… investigators were free to probe interesting areas … and could follow respondents interests …

> … but that the researcher could deviate from the five questions provided in the interview schedule. So this study uses prompts provided by the participant (i.e. the photo) and by theresearcher. (i.e. scheduled questions).

… interviews started with description and commentary on the meal photographs …

> It appears that the interview was intended to follow a given structure.

FIGURE 21.2 Use of a predetermined set of questions (a topic guide) in a study of food, family relationships, and adolescent obesity. Reprinted from Lachal J, Speranza M, Taieb O, Falissard B, Lefevre H, Moro M-R, *et al.* Qualitative research using photo-elicitation to explore the role of food in family relationships among obese adolescents. *Appetite* 2012, 58: 1099–105, © 2012, with permission from Elsevier.

views of a group of women to hormone replacement therapy (HRT)) provides an example of where the participants set the agenda of the focus group's discussion of HRT (See Figure 21); the intention was for the researcher (known as the moderator) to have minimum input.

Interviews will differ in the degree of structure imposed, flexibility of researcher and/or participant to deviate from the content, and focus on description of 'factual information' versus exploring participants' experience. All interviews, however, share the characteristic of being shaped by the research objectives. The researcher will usually construct a *topic guide* for the interview. This is the document that provides information on the content to be covered within the interview. The topic guide provides documentation of the key issues and areas of discussion. Often the topic guide will provide a structure (e.g. order of topics to be covered) and prompts that can be used to guide the interview conversation. In Figure 21.2 a photograph provided by the participants acted as a prompt, but the researchers had a set of questions (their topic guide) about adolescent obesity, to which they wanted participants to respond, although participants could also raise material of their own.

V

Establishing More of the Facts:
Some Common Ways of Describing Results

22

Fractions, Proportions, and Rates

Researchers often present their findings as raw numbers, but it may be that more sense is conveyed when the raw number becomes some kind of fraction. Probably the most widely used fractions in health research are *proportions*. Proportions are fractions in which the numerator (the bit on the top) is a subset of the denominator (remember that in the fraction $\frac{3}{4}$, 3 is called the numerator and 4 is called the denominator). For example, $\frac{3}{4}$ could mean 3 out of 4; if so, then it is a proportion. Proportions can be useful because they allow various judgements and comparisons that are not possible with raw numbers.

If, for example, the annual number of adults who attend an Emergency Department after harming themselves (usually by self-poisoning with medicines of some kind) rises from 850 to 1350 over a 5-year period, the rise is by more than 50%. However, the number of adults in the catchment population may have also risen over the same period. Consequently, when the yearly proportions of adults attending are calculated, the apparent increase in self-harm might be much smaller – perhaps rising from 280 per 100 000 to 350 per 100 000. In health research a common explanation for an increase in denominator is an alteration in the catchment population served by the hospital (perhaps, in this example, when a nearby Emergency Department closed down).

A more complex fraction commonly used in research is a *rate*. A rate has a numerator, a denominator, and a stated time period (e.g. 18.2 suicides per 100 000 males aged 15 or over per year was the approximate suicide rate in the United Kingdom in 2011). One widely used rate in clinical epidemiology is the *inception rate* (also known as *incidence*) of a disease – referring to the rate of new cases arising. If the inception rate for schizophrenia were around 1 per 10 000 people per year then a city of half a million people might expect 50 new cases each year. Motor neurone disease has a much lower estimated incidence: around 2 per 100 000 per year.

The *prevalence* of a disease usually refers to the number of existing cases at the time of counting; it therefore includes those who have long since developed the disease as well as more recent cases. For long-lasting conditions prevalence is much higher than incidence. For example, motor neurone disease has a prevalence of around 7 per 100 000. Chronic but not life-threatening diseases such as rheumatoid arthritis have even larger differences between incidence and prevalence. Because it is not defined by duration, prevalence is not really a rate but a proportion – although it is not unusual to see it mistakenly referred to as 'prevalence rate'.

Sometimes you will see a prevalence described as a *period prevalence* or a *point prevalence*. If we collected all of the cases present in a particular population at one point in time (sometimes called a *census date*), that would give us a point prevalence. If we collected all the cases that were evident during a particular period of time, say a month or a year, that would give us a period prevalence. Period prevalence will include all new cases arising in that period as well as well as all cases that existed at the start of the period and extend into it. For relatively chronic and stable conditions (for example multiple sclerosis like, say), point prevalence is a good measure, while for more transient disorders (for example back pain bad enough to lead to time off work), a period prevalence may give a better measure of burden to the community.

Self-harm in England: a tale of three cities

Mulicentre study of self-harm

Keith Hawton, Helen Bergen, Deborah Casey, Sue Simkin, Ben Palmer, Jayne Cooper, Nav Kapur, Judith Horrocks, Allan House, Rachel Lilley, Rachel Noble, David Owens

■ **Abstract** *Background* Self-harm is a major healthcare problem in the United Kingdom, but monitoring of hospital presentations has largely been done separately in single centres. Multicentre monitoring of self-harm has been established as a result of the National Suicide Prevention Strategy for England. *Method* Data on self-harm presentations to general hospitals in Oxford (one hospital), Manchester (three hospitals) and Leeds (two hospitals), collected through monitoring systems in each centre, were analysed for the 18-month period March 2000 to August 2001. *Results* The findings were based on 7344 persons who presented following 10,498 episodes of self-harm. Gender and age patterns were similar in the three centres, 57.0% of patients being female and two-thirds (62.9%) under 35 years of age. The largest numbers by age groups were 15–19 year-old females and 20–24 year-old males. The female to male ratio decreased with age. Rates of self-harm were higher in Manchester than Oxford or Leeds, in keeping with local suicide rates. The proportion of patients receiving a specialist psychosocial assessment varied between centres and was strongly associated with admission to the general hospital. Approximately 80% of self-harm involved self-poisoning. Overdoses of paracetamol, the most frequent method, were more common in younger age groups, antidepressants in middle age groups, and benzodiazepines and sedatives in older age groups. Alcohol was involved in more than half (54.9%) of assessed episodes. The

These two age-and-sex-specific rates reveal a key finding: in both females and males, people who attend hospital due to self-harm are young, with females younger than males.

Rates are compared across the three cities in the monitoring study. Raw numbers for each city would be misleading because the three cities are unequal in size.

We need these simple *proportions* rather than raw numbers to judge whether there are important points to be made about method of self-harm and about alcohol consumption.

FIGURE 22.1 Summary of a descriptive study setting out rates and proportions. Reproduced from Hawton K, Bergen H, Casey D, Simkin S, Palmer B, Cooper J, *et al.* (2007) with kind permission of Springer Science + Business Media.

Figure 22.1 is part of the Abstract of a study about trends in self-harm. The study is full of raw numbers that have been turned into various proportions and rates. In practice we often want to examine rates according to a variety of denominators. In the text (but not shown here in the Abstract) these authors describe for each of the three cities the rates in males and in females ('sex-specific rates') and, referred to in Figure 22.1, rates for '15–19 year-old females' and for '20–24 year-old males' ('age- and sex-specific rates').

In the next two chapters we are going to look at some fractions that are particularly prevalent in clinical papers.

23

Risks and Odds

If you toss a coin you know the chance of it coming down heads. People use various ways to express this chance (Figure 23.1) . Notice that, strangely, the ways of describing the chance split into those that yield a numerical result of 0.5 and those with a numerical result of 1. This is because in practice we use two quite different fractions to express chance: *risk* and *odds*. For most of us, risk accords with the way we think in our everyday lives and is much the easier to understand. Researchers, however, calculate and tell readers about chance in terms of risks *and* odds, so this chapter sets out the principles of both of these concepts.

Suppose you tossed a coin twice and it came down once as a head and once as a tail. This is represented in Figure 23.2, and looking at this illustration, you might reasonably say that the *risk* (or probability) of tossing a head is: heads (1) divided by the total of heads and tails (2), which comes out at $1/2 = 0.5$. The risk can be described as a fraction in which the numerator corresponds to the number of times an event occurs while the denominator corresponds to the total number of possible events. The *odds* of tossing a head, however, is rather different: you divide heads (1) by tails (1) – which comes out at $1/1 = 1$. The odds, therefore, can be described as a fraction in which the numerator corresponds to the number of times an event occurs while the denominator corresponds to the number of times an event does not occur. If you look back at Figure 23.1 you should now be able to make sense of the two sets of terms: the terms in the left-hand column refer to risk, those on the right to odds.

One in two	Evens
Fifty per cent (50%)	One-to-one
0.5	Fifty-fifty
A half	Equal chance
Expressed numerically as 0.5	Expressed numerically as 1

FIGURE 23.1 Terminology in common use when describing the chance of tossing a head.

	Number of throws
Heads	1
Tails	1
TOTAL	2

FIGURE 23.2 A plausible result from two tosses of a coin.

Understanding Clinical Papers, Third Edition. David Bowers, Allan House, David Owens and Bridgette Bewick.
© 2014 John Wiley & Sons, Ltd. Published 2014 by John Wiley & Sons, Ltd.

RISK

In clinical research, risk has the same meaning as *probability*; the terminology has been heavily influenced by public health academics who have concentrated on the concept of *risk factors* causing disease. One consequence of risk and probability being synonyms is that it is accepted practice to refer to the risk of bad or good events occurring. For example, researchers may calculate and tell you the risk of getting better from a disease; in epidemiological terms risk does not necessarily carry the connotation of danger.

ODDS

Odds is (or *odds are*; it is accepted practice to speak of odds as plural or singular) another *bona fide* method of expressing chance. Although most people find risk the easier to think about, odds has several properties

---

Change in social status and risk of low birth weight in Denmark: population based cohort study

Olga Basso, Jørn Olsen, Anne Mette T Johansen, Kaare Christensen

---

Abstract

Objective: To estimate the risk of having a low birth-weight infant associated with changes in social, environmental, and genetic factors.

Design: Population based, historical cohort study using the Danish medical birth registry and Statistic Denmark's fertility database.

Subjects: All women who had a low birthweight infant (<2500 g) (index birth) and a subsequent liveborn infant (outcome birth) in Denmark between 1980 and 1992 (exposed cohort, n = 11 069) and a random sample of the population who gave birth to an infant weighing ≥2500 g and to a subsequent liveborn infant (unexposed cohort, n = 10 211).

Main outcome measures: Risk of having a low birthweight infant in the outcome birth as a function of changes in male partner, area of residence, type of job, and social status between the two births.

Results: Women in the exposed cohort showed a high risk (18.5%) of having a subsequent low birthweight infant while women in the unexposed cohort had a risk of 2.8%. After adjustment for initial social status, a decline in social status increased the absolute risk of having a low birthweight infant by about 5% in both cohorts, though this was significantly only in the unexposed cohort. Change of male partner did not modify the risk of low birth weight in either cohort.

Conclusion: Having had a low birthweight infant and a decline in social status are strong risk factors for having a low birthweight infant subsequently.

Here the researchers are interested in the risk of a subsequent low birthweight infant if a previous childbirth was of low weight.

They determine this risk and compare it with the equivalent risk in a general population sample.

FIGURE 23.3   Determining risk in a cohort study. Reproduced from Basso O, Olsen J, Johansen AMT, Christensen K. Change in social status and risk of low birth weight in Denmark: population based cohort study. *BMJ* 1997, 315: 1498–502, © 1997, with permission from BMJ Publishing Group Ltd.

Helicobacter pylori infection and mortality from ischaemic heart disease: negative result from a large, prospective study

N J Wald, M R Law, J K Morris, A M Bagnall

Abstract

Objective—To determine whether there is an independent association between *Helicobacter pylori* infection of the stomach and ischaemic heart disease.
Design—Prospective study with measurement of IgG antibody titres specific to *H pylori* on stored serum samples from 648 men who died from ischaemic heart disease and 1296 age matched controls who did not (nested case-control design).
Subjects—21 520 professional men aged 35–64 who attended the British United Provident Association (BUPA) medical centre in London between 1975 and 1982 for routine medical examination.
Main outcome measure—Death from ischaemic heart disease.
Results—The odds of death from ischaemic heart disease in men with *H pylori* infection relative to that in men without infection was 1.06 (95% confidence interval 0.86 to 1.31). In a separate group of 206 people attending the centre, plasma fibrinogen was virtually the same in those who were positive for *H pylori* (2.62 g/l) and those who were negative (2.64 g/l).

Men with or without *Helicobacter pylori* infection are compared as to their odds of developing a myocardial infarction. The authors chose to compare the two odds, but could as easily have calculated the two risks (one for each group) and compared those.

The authors divide the two odds to find the value 1.06: the odds of death for men with the disease relative to the odds of death for men without the disease. This is the odds ratio (discussed in Chapter 24).

FIGURE 23.4   Determining odds (expressed as one odds relative to another) in a cohort study. Reproduced from Wald NJ, Law MR, Morris JK, Bagnall AM. *Helicobacter pylori* infection and mortality from ischaemic heart disease: negative result from a large, prospective study. *BMJ* 1997, 315: 1199–201, © 1997, with permission from BMJ Publishing Group Ltd.

that are invaluable to epidemiologists and statisticians. It is not important here to go into why odds is such a useful measure, but one of the main reasons is explained in Chapter 24, where we describe the calculation and uses of *risk ratios* and *odds ratios*.

Extracts from the two papers in Figures 23.3 and 23.4 illustrate the use of the fractions *risk* and *odds*. In each case the authors want us to infer a connection between some variable and the subsequent development of a condition.

24

Ratios of Risks and Odds

RISK RATIO (RELATIVE RISK)

You were introduced to the calculation of risks and odds in Chapter 23. The present chapter deals with *ratios* of risks and odds. Researchers in Italy examined evidence that suggested that women with breast cysts might be susceptible to breast cancer (Figure 24.1). They investigated the hypothesis that the chemical composition of the fluid that can be aspirated from a cyst (using a needle and syringe) provides a clue to cancer risk. The women in their study, as part of a breast cancer detection programme, were all followed up for between 2 and 12 years. Using a cohort analytic study design (see Chapter 6), the researchers compared the proportions of women who developed breast cancer among those who had Type I cysts (high concentration of potassium, low concentrations of sodium and chloride) and those shown to have Type II cysts (low concentration of potassium, high concentrations of sodium and chloride).

The researchers here have calculated that the risk of cancer among the women with Type I cysts is $12/417 = 0.029$ (or 2.9%). The risk of cancer among the women with Type II cysts is $2/325 = 0.0062$ (or 0.62%). A popular approach to summarizing these kinds of findings, which the authors have used here, is the *risk ratio* (also known as the *relative risk*). It is a comparison of these two risks – arrived at by dividing one by the other: $2.9/0.62 = 4.7$.

If, for simplicity, we round this risk ratio up to 5, then we might say that the women with Type I cysts have a risk of breast cancer that is about 5 times that seen in women with Type II cysts. Another correct and readily comprehensible way of expressing the finding is to say that breast cancer is 5 times as likely in women with Type I cysts than it is in women with Type II cysts.

By the same logic, if the risks were identical in the two study groups being compared, the risk ratio would be 1. Risk ratios below 1 indicate that the characteristic under scrutiny confers less rather than more risk. Here, the authors could have divided 0.62 by 2.9 (which comes to about 0.2) and thereby reported something like: 'the incidence of breast cancer in women with Type II cysts was lower than in women with Type I cysts (relative risk 0.2)'. Of course 0.2 is the same thing as one-fifth; if the first group has one-fifth the risk of the second group, it is tantamount to saying that the second has 5 times the risk of the first. In other words, it is acceptable for authors to express the risk ratio in either direction as long as they are careful with their wording.

The two terms 'risk ratio' and 'relative risk' are widely used. We prefer *risk ratio* partly because it mirrors what happens with odds in the odds ratio (see below). Chapter 26 describes how confidence intervals are applied to the risk ratio.

ODDS RATIO

In Chapter 23, dealing with risk and odds, we tried to demonstrate that the chance of something happening could reasonably be expressed as a risk or as an odds. No surprise then that the *odds ratio*

Understanding Clinical Papers, Third Edition. David Bowers, Allan House, David Owens and Bridgette Bewick.
© 2014 John Wiley & Sons, Ltd. Published 2014 by John Wiley & Sons, Ltd.

Cohort study of association of risk of breast cancer with cyst type in women with gross cystic disease of the breast

Paolo Bruzzi, Luigi Dogliotti, Carlo Naldoni, Lauro Bucchi, Massimo Costantini, Alessandro Cicognani, Mirella Torta, Gian Franco Buzzi, Alberto Angeli

Abstract

Objective: To assess correlation between type of breast cyst and risk of breast cancer in women with gross cystic disease of the breast.

Design: Cohort study of women with breast cysts aspirated between 1983 and 1993 who were followed up until December 1994 for occurrence of breast cancer.

Setting: Major cancer prevention centre.

Subjects: 802 women with aspirated breast cysts.

Main outcome measures: Type of breast cyst based on cationic content of cyst fluid: type I (potassium:sodium ratio >1.5), type II (potassium:sodium ratio <1.5), or mixed (both types). Subsequent occurrence and type of breast cancer.

Results: After median follow up of six years (range 2–12 years) 15 cases of invasive breast cancer and two ductal carcinomas in situ were diagnosed in the cohort: 12 invasive cancers (and two carcinomas in situ) among the 417 women with type I cysts, two cancers among the 325 women with type II cysts, and one among the 60 women with mixed cysts. The incidence of breast cancer in women with type I cysts was significantly higher than that in women with type II cysts (relative risk 4.62 (95% confidence interval 1.26 to 29.7). These results were confirmed after adjustment for several risk factors for breast cancer (relative risk 4.24 (1.12 to 27.5)).

Conclusions: The increased risk of breast cancer of women with breast cysts seems to be concentrated among women with type I breast cysts.

Design of cohort studies is described in Chapter 6. They commonly report their findings as risk ratios (relative risks).

12 of 417 women with Type I cysts developed cancer (a risk of 2.9%) . . .

. . . while only 2 of 325 women with Type II cysts developed cancer (a risk of 0.62%).

2.9 divided by 0.62 is 4.6, the *risk ratio* (or *relative risk*).

Chapter 26 describes how confidence intervals are applied to the risk ratio.

Chapters 30 and 31 deal with adjusting for confounders.

Table 3 Relative risk of invasive breast cancer among 802 women with gross cystic disease by type of breast cyst and number of cysts aspiration at enrolment

| | No of subjects | No of cases of cancer | Relative risk (95% CI) | |
			Univariate analysis	Multivariate analysis[†]
Type of breast cyst*:				
Type II	325	2	1.00	1.00
Type I	417	12	4.62 (1.26 to 29.7)	4.24 (1.12 to 27.5)
Mixed	60	1	2.57 (0.12 to 26.9)	1.98 (0.07 to 34.4)
No of cysts aspirated:				
Solitary	682	12	1.00	1.00
Multiple	120	3	1.35 (0.31 to 4.24)	1.26 (0.19 to 4.75)

*See text for details of cyst types.
†Adjusted for age, age at menarche, No of births, and family history of breast cancer.

FIGURE 24.1 Summary of a cohort analytic study where the main finding is set out in terms of a risk ratio (relative risk). Reproduced from Bruzzi P, Dogliotti L, Naldoni C, Costantini M, Cicognani A, Torta M, *et al*. Cohort study of association of risk of breast cancer with cyst type in women with gross cystic disease of the breast. *BMJ* 1997, 314: 925–8, © 1997, with permission from BMJ Publishing Group Ltd.

is used to compare two odds in a way that mirrors calculation of the risk ratio for the comparison of two risks.

Back in Italy, but further south in Naples, another research team investigated whether children who experienced a febrile convulsion might be anaemic. The factors that determine why some children suffer convulsions when febrile, while most children do not, are largely unknown. In this case-control study (see Chapter 6) the researchers measured the haemoglobin levels of 146 consecutive children admitted to their hospital as a consequence of a febrile seizure (Figure 24.2). They compared haemoglobin levels for the

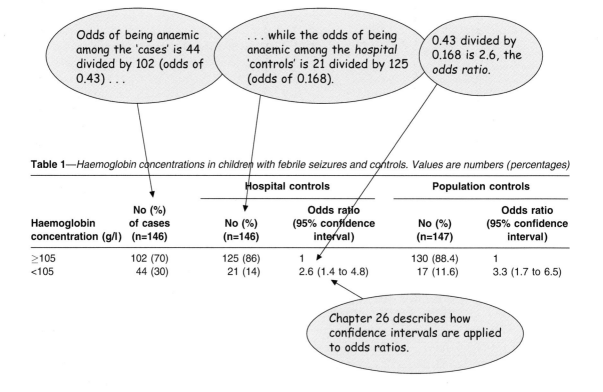

Iron deficiency anaemia and febrile convulsions: case–control study in children under 2 years

Alfredo Pisacane, Renato Sansone, Nicola Impagliazzo, Angelo Coppola, Paolo Rolando, Alfonso D'Apuzzo, Ciro Tregrossi

Case-control studies were described in Chapter 6. They nearly always report their findings as odds ratios.

Odds of being anaemic among the 'cases' is 44 divided by 102 (odds of 0.43) . . .

. . . while the odds of being anaemic among the hospital 'controls' is 21 divided by 125 (odds of 0.168).

0.43 divided by 0.168 is 2.6, the odds ratio.

Table 1—*Haemoglobin concentrations in children with febrile seizures and controls. Values are numbers (percentages)*

Haemoglobin concentration (g/l)	No (%) of cases (n=146)	Hospital controls		Population controls	
		No (%) (n=146)	Odds ratio (95% confidence interval)	No (%) (n=147)	Odds ratio (95% confidence interval)
≥105	102 (70)	125 (86)	1	130 (88.4)	1
<105	44 (30)	21 (14)	2.6 (1.4 to 4.8)	17 (11.6)	3.3 (1.7 to 6.5)

Chapter 26 describes how confidence intervals are applied to odds ratios.

FIGURE 24.2 Table from a case-control study where the main findings are set out in terms of odds ratios. Reproduced from Pisacane A, Sansone R, Impagliazzo N, Coppola A, Rolando P, D'Apuzzo A, *et al*. Iron deficiency anaemia and febrile convulsions: case-control study in children under 2 years. *BMJ* 1996, 313: 343, © 1996, with permission from BMJ Publishing Group Ltd.

children who had seizures with haemoglobin levels for children in two 'control' groups (who had not had seizures): a random sample of 146 children admitted to the same ward but with respiratory or gastrointestinal infections and a random sample of 147 healthy children drawn from the provincial birth register. The table sets out their main findings.

Among the 146 'cases' of children who had seizures, the odds of being anaemic (having a haemoglobin level below 105 g/l) is 44/102 = 0.43. The odds of being anaemic among those in the *hospital* control group is 21/125 = 0.168. The odds ratio comparison of these two odds – arrived at by dividing one by the other – is 0.43/0.168 = 2.6. The odds ratio that compares cases with the *population* control group is worked out in just the same way: odds of anaemia in cases is 44/102 = 0.43; odds of anaemia in population controls is 17/130 = 0.13; odds ratio is 0.43/0.13 = 3.3.

What does the odds ratio tell us? Researchers use the odds ratio not because it conveys meaning to the reader, but because it has mathematical properties that we can only touch on here. As an expression of the comparison between the two kinds of chance it is not easy to interpret. It cannot readily be 'translated' into anything more meaningful; it is purely the fraction formed by dividing the odds of being anaemic in one group by the odds in the other. If you have trouble figuring out what it tells you, do not worry: no one else can do any better than you. The nearest we can get to a common-sense way of expressing this result is to conclude that there is about 3 times the odds of being anaemic if you had a febrile seizure compared with if you did not have a seizure. Just as with the risk ratio, remember that if the odds ratio is 1 then the odds is the same in each group being compared.

One key property of the odds ratio (and one of the reasons why researchers employ such an uninviting measure) can be illustrated from the table in Figure 24.2. Concentrate on the comparison of cases with hospital controls: we are going to rework the calculations in a different direction. In this study, if a child was anaemic then the odds of him or her being in the case group (had a seizure) rather than in the hospital control group (did not have a seizure) is 44/21 = 2.1. Similarly, if a child was not anaemic the odds of her or him being in the case group is 102/125 = 0.82. These odds can be compared in an odds ratio: 2.1/0.82 = 2.6. If you are sharp-eyed you will have spotted that this is the same odds ratio as the one we calculated previously, working the table from a different direction.

We can now draw a new conclusion: that there is about 3 times the odds of getting a febrile convulsion if a child is anaemic rather than not anaemic. This new conclusion is a much more useful one than the conclusion in the previous paragraph. After all, we do not want to conclude after the event that a child who had a convulsion is likely to have been anaemic; rather, we want to conclude that anaemia is a risky state that makes convulsions more likely (so we can do something about anaemic babies and toddlers and thereby prevent seizures).

When a condition is relatively uncommon (and most children do not have a febrile seizure, so it counts as an uncommon condition) the odds ratio is approximately the same as the risk ratio (we are not proving why in this book, but the straightforward proof can be found in most epidemiology books). This transferable property of odds ratios and risk ratios means that, from the present study, we can assert that small children in the catchment area of this Naples hospital have about 3 times the *risk* of getting a febrile convulsion if they are anaemic.

Of course the researchers could have carried out a cohort study instead and calculated the risk ratio directly – without all this jiggery-pokery. However, because febrile convulsions are infrequent, a cohort study would have needed to include many thousands of children in order to come up with a reasonable number of children who had sustained a seizure. The properties of the odds ratio enable researchers to carry out small, quick, cheap case-control studies (rather than large, lengthy, and expensive cohort analytic studies) yet come up with clinically useful findings. Case-control studies pretty well always report their findings in terms of odds ratios.

CLINICAL TRIALS AND 'NUMBERS NEEDED TO TREAT'

Just about everyone finds it easier to comprehend risk ratios than odds ratios. Odds ratios have other properties (not gone into here) that make them valuable in complex mathematics like multivariable analysis (Chapter 31) and meta-analysis (Chapter 33). Unfortunately this seems to have led many researchers to calculate and display their study findings as odds ratios even when they could have given us a risk ratio instead. Consequently some clinicians – concerned that useful research output was being lost in a fog of incomprehensible numbers –came up with what has become a popular way of making sense of some study findings. Where the results of a study come from a clinical trial of treatment or of health-care management, the *number needed to treat* (NNT) is a simple calculation and appeals to many as an intuitively straightforward way to get at the clinical meaning of the finding of a clinical trial.

As an example, researchers across three continents (though mainly in North America) collaborated in a large study to determine what dose of acetylsalicylic acid (aspirin) is the most beneficial to patients undergoing carotid artery surgery (aimed at preventing strokes). They found that fewer patients had a bad outcome (stroke, myocardial infarction, or death) among the low-dose aspirin regimen than among those taking high-dose (Figure 24.3). For the analysis the researchers amalgamated the two lower-dose regimens and the two higher-dose regimens to end up with two (rather than four) comparison groups.

In their table you can see that for the various outcomes, at 30 days and 3 months, they have set out their findings as relative risks (risk ratios) – all falling at around 1.3. But in an attempt to make their findings easier for clinicians to apply in real situations, they have also calculated and displayed the NNT derived from each of their comparisons. Figure 24.3 indicates how they have worked out the NNT. For this calculation, instead of putting the two risks (one for each comparison group) into a ratio, they have subtracted them to generate a difference (sometimes called *absolute difference*) between the risks.

Looking at the top line of their table, notice that the *reduction* in risk due to the better of the two treatments (low-dose aspirin) is $7.0\% - 5.4\% = 1.6\%$. Put another way, a reduction in risk of 1.6% means that of every 100 people treated with low-dose aspirin (rather than high-dose) 1.6 fewer will have a bad outcome (if you do not like 1.6 people in 100, think of 16 people in 1000 – it is the same thing). It is a simple calculation then to say that if 100 treated with low-dose leads to 1.6 fewer bad outcomes, then 100/1.6 (about 61, allowing for some rounding in the arithmetic) people treated with low-dose will result in one less bad outcome. The general formula for the NNT is that it is 100 divided by the percentage absolute risk reduction:

$$\text{Number needed to treat} = 100/\text{percentage absolute risk reduction}$$

This resulting value can be interpreted as follows: 'You would need to treat 61 patients scheduled for carotid endarterectomy with low-dose rather than high-dose aspirin in order to prevent one *extra* patient from experiencing the bad outcome (in this case stroke, heart attack or death)'. Of course, this figure is only an estimate and it might have been displayed together with its confidence interval (not provided in the paper). The NNT is attractive to clinicians who may want to make judgments on the basis of the size of the effect found in a study.

Low-dose and high-dose acetylsalicylic acid for patients undergoing carotid endarterectomy: a randomised controlled trial

D Wayne Taylor, Henry J M Barnett, R Brian Haynes, Gary G Ferguson, David L Sackett, Kevin E Thorpe, Denis Simard, Frank L Silver, Vladimir Hachinski, G Patrick Clagett, R Barnes, J David Spence, for the ASA and Carotid Endarterectomy (ACE) Trial Collaborators*

Summary

Background Endarterectomy benefits certain patients with carotid stenosis, but benefits are lessened by perioperative surgical risk. Acetylsalicylic acid lowers the risk of stroke in patients who have experienced transient ischaemic attack and stroke. We investigated appropriate doses and the role of acetylsalicylic acid in patients undergoing carotid endarterectomy.

Methods In a randomised, double-blind, controlled trial, 2849 patients scheduled for endarterectomy were randomly assigned 81 mg (n=709), 325 mg (n=708), 650 mg (n=715), or 1300 mg (n=717) acetylsalicylic acid daily, started before surgery and continued for 3 months. We recorded occurrences of stroke, myocardial infarction, and death. We compared patients on the two higher doses of acetylsalicylic acid with patients on the two lower doses.

Number needed to treat (NNT) is applied usually to findings from trials and meta-analyses.

The comparison here is between low-dose (81 or 325 mg) and high-dose (650 or 1300 mg).

If you take away the risk of a bad outcome in the low-dose group (5.4%) from the risk in the high-dose group (7.0%) you get the difference in risks (1.6%).

Divide 100 by 1.6 and you find the NNT: around 61.

Event-defining failure	Event rate Low-dose ASA	Event rate High-dose ASA	Relative risk high/low dose (95% CI)	Absolute difference (% [SE])	p	NNT
All patients						
30 days						
Number of patients	1395	1409	. .	. .	. .	. .
Any stroke, MI, or death	75 (5.4%)	99 (7.0%)	1.31 (0.98–1.75)	1.6 (0.9)	0.07	61
Any stroke or death	66 (4.7%)	86 (6.1%)	1.29 (0.94–1.76)	1.4 (0.9)	0.109	72
Ipsilateral stroke or death	58 (4.2%)	81 (5.7%)	1.38 (1.0–1.92)	1.6 (0.8)	0.052	62
3 months						
Number of patients	1395	1409	. .	. .	. .	. .
Any stroke, MI, or death	87 (6.2%)	118 (8.4%)	1.34 (1.03–1.75)	2.1 (1.0)	0.03	46
Any stroke or death	79 (5.7%)	100 (7.1%)	1.25 (0.94–1.67)	1.4 (0.9)	0.12	69
Ipsilateral stroke or death	68 (4.9%)	91 (6.5%)	1.32 (0.98–1.80)	1.6 (0.9)	0.07	63

Figure 4: **Failure rates at 30 days after endarterectomy**

FIGURE 24.3 Table from a clinical trial where the main findings are set out in terms of risk ratios together with numbers needed to treat. Reprinted from *The Lancet* 353: Taylor DW, Barnett HJM, Haynes RB, *et al*. Low-dose and high-dose acetylsalicylic acid for patients undergoing carotid endarterectomy: a randomised controlled trial. 1999; 2179–84, © 1999, with permission from Elsevier.

VI

Analysing the Data:
Estimation and Hypothesis Testing

CHAPTER

25

Confidence Intervals for Means, Proportions, and Medians

Confidence intervals are ubiquitous in clinical papers, so an understanding of them – what they are and how they should be interpreted – will be useful. You will remember from Chapter 10 that clinical researchers inevitably have to use *samples* to study characteristics of 'groups of people' (i.e. *populations*) because it is usually impossible to study populations directly. What is true of the sample is then taken to be also true, *more or less*, of the population (always provided of course that the sample is truly representative of the population). The technical term for this process is *statistical inference*. The 'more or less' bit is taken care of with a confidence interval.

WHAT IS A CONFIDENCE INTERVAL?

Look at Figure 25.1. This is the baseline table taken from a trial which compared annual versus twice-yearly mass azithromycin treatment for the treatment of trachoma (the bacterial infection responsible for so much blindness in the world) among children aged 0–9 in Northern Ethiopia.

You can see that the existing prevalence of trachoma infection in the *sample* of those to be treated annually (sample size was not clearly stated in the original paper, but was probably several hundred) was estimated to be 68.7%. This value is known as the *point estimate* and is the single best guess as to the prevalence of trachoma in the population of children in this part of Northern Ethiopia (many tens, possibly hundreds of thousands of children).

The 95% confidence interval is given as (56.3–81.2)%. How do we interpret this? We can say that there is a 95% chance that the true value for the prevalence of trachoma in this population lies somewhere between 56.3% and 81.2%, and moreover, is more likely to lie around the middle of this interval than towards either end. Statisticians might say that this confidence interval represents *a plausible range of values* for the true (population) prevalence – you need to bear in mind that there is still a 5% chance that the true prevalence lies outside the interval. You can of course also use this interval to see if some predetermined idea of the level of prevalence is supported. For example, say the level of trachoma in Southern Ethiopia is believed to be 50%, then the interval from 56.3% to 81.2% suggests that the percentage of trachoma in the South is not the same in the North. By the way, it is much better practice to write the confidence interval in the form (56.3% to 81.2%), rather than use a hyphen, which can be confusing if there are negative values in the confidence interval. We do not need to be concerned, in this book anyway, with how confidence intervals are calculated – the authors will have derived them using a computer statistics program (SPSS, Minitab, and Stata are among the most common).

Although confidence intervals for single population values such as those in Figure 25.1 are frequently in clinical papers, much more common are those for the *differences* between *two* population values. We will have a look at some common examples of these in the next section.

Understanding Clinical Papers, Third Edition. David Bowers, Allan House, David Owens and Bridgette Bewick.
© 2014 John Wiley & Sons, Ltd. Published 2014 by John Wiley & Sons, Ltd.

Comparison of annual versus twice-yearly mass azithromycin treatment for hyperendemic trachoma in Ethiopia: a cluster-randomised trial

Teshome Gebre, Berhan Ayele, Mulat Zerihun, Asrat Genet, Nicole E Stoller, Zhaoxia Zhou, Jenafir I House, Sun N Yu, Kathryn J Ray, Paul M Emerson, Jeremy D Keenan, Travis C Porco, Thomas M Lietman, Bruce D Gaynor

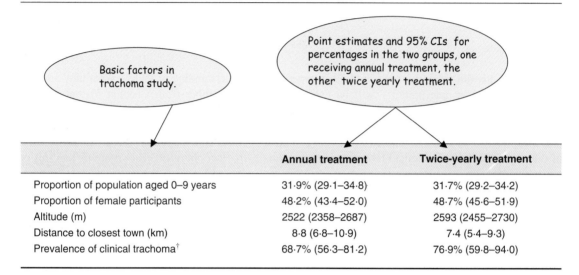

	Annual treatment	Twice-yearly treatment
Proportion of population aged 0–9 years	31·9% (29·1–34·8)	31·7% (29·2–34·2)
Proportion of female participants	48·2% (43·4–52·0)	48·7% (45·6–51·9)
Altitude (m)	2522 (2358–2687)	2593 (2455–2730)
Distance to closest town (km)	8·8 (6·8–10·9)	7·4 (5·4–9·3)
Prevalence of clinical trachoma[†]	68·7% (56·3–81·2)	76·9% (59·8–94·0)

FIGURE 25.1   Confidence intervals from a study comparing annual with twice-yearly treatment with azithromycin for the eradication of trachoma in Ethiopia. Reprinted from *The Lancet* 379: Gebre T, Ayele B, Zerihun M, Genet A, Stoller NE, Zhou Z, *et al.* Comparison of annual versus twice-yearly mass azithromycin treatment for hyperendemic trachoma in Ethiopia: a cluster-randomised trial. 2012; 143–51, © 1999, with permission from Elsevier.

CONFIDENCE INTERVALS FOR DIFFERENCES IN TWO MEANS

Suppose the population mean birthweight of babies born to mothers who smoked during pregnancy is the same as that of babies born to non-smoking mothers. If the means are the same and we subtract one from the other we get 0. As it happens, a random sample of 500 babies produced a point estimate of 33.3 g for the difference in population mean birthweights between the two groups of babies, with a 95% confidence interval for the difference of (−102.9, 169.5) g. Thus we can be 95% confident that the true difference in mean birthweights is somewhere between −102.9 g (babies lighter) and +169.5 g (babies heavier). Since this confidence interval contains 0, we could interpret this result as implying that there was no difference in birthweights. If the confidence interval does not contain 0, the population means are likely to be different. Bear in mind, however, that whether or not the confidence interval contains 0, the most likely difference in both cases is the point estimate of the difference.

As an example of these ideas in practice, Figure 25.2 is from a cohort study into the interactive effects of fitness and statin treatment on mortality risk in veterans with dyslipidaemia. As you can see, the columns in the figure represent the mean total cholesterol levels, the mean triglycerides levels, and the mean high- and low-density lipoprotein (HDL and LDL) cholesterol levels, for patients who had been treated with statins and for those not treated with statins. If we concentrate on total cholesterol levels, you can see that for patients treated with statins, the change in mean total cholesterol level was 1.7 mmol/l, with a 95% confidence interval of (1.6 to 1.7). Since this confidence interval does not include 0, then we can be 95% confident that the difference in mean total cholesterol levels before and after treatment was significantly

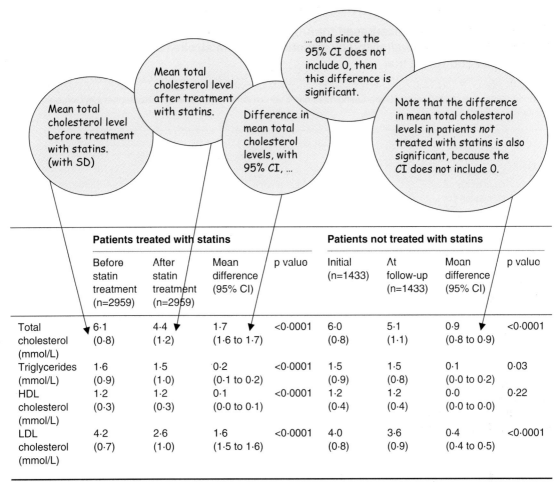

	Patients treated with statins				Patients not treated with statins			
	Before statin treatment (n=2959)	After statin treatment (n=2959)	Mean difference (95% CI)	p value	Initial (n=1433)	At follow-up (n=1433)	Mean difference (95% CI)	p value
Total cholesterol (mmol/L)	6·1 (0·8)	4·4 (1·2)	1·7 (1·6 to 1·7)	<0·0001	6·0 (0·8)	5·1 (1·1)	0·9 (0·8 to 0·9)	<0·0001
Triglycerides (mmol/L)	1·6 (0·9)	1·5 (1·0)	0·2 (0·1 to 0·2)	<0·0001	1·5 (0·9)	1·5 (0·8)	0·1 (0·0 to 0·2)	0·03
HDL cholesterol (mmol/L)	1·2 (0·3)	1·2 (0·3)	0·1 (0·0 to 0·1)	<0·0001	1·2 (0·4)	1·2 (0·4)	0·0 (0·0 to 0·0)	0·22
LDL cholesterol (mmol/L)	4·2 (0·7)	2·6 (1·0)	1·6 (1·5 to 1·6)	<0·0001	4·0 (0·8)	3·6 (0·9)	0·4 (0·4 to 0·5)	<0·0001

Data are mean (SD) unless stated otherwise. p values calculated by paired t test.

FIGURE 25.2 Confidence intervals for differences in lipid and lipoprotein concentrations between patients treated with and without statins. Reprinted from *The Lancet* 381: Kokkinos PF, Faselis C, Myers J, Panagiotakos D, Doumas M. Interactive effects of fitness and statin treatment on mortality risk in veterans with dyslipidaemia: a cohort study. 2013; 394–9, © 2013, with permission from Elsevier.

different. However, this was true also for patients not treated with statins, the difference between mean total cholesterol levels initially and at follow-up was 0.9 mmol/l, with a 95% confidence interval of (0.8 to 0.9). Since this interval did not include 0, this difference was significant.

CONFIDENCE INTERVALS FOR DIFFERENCES IN TWO PERCENTAGES

Figure 25.3 (abbreviated by the present authors) is from a randomised controlled trial to compare outcomes between a multidisciplinary intervention group and a control group, in patients 90 days after admission to hospital following a stroke. The data are shown as proportions and percentages for three outcomes: death and dependency (assessed using a modified Rankin scale, which measures the degree of disability or dependence in the daily activities of people who have suffered a stroke or other causes of neurological disability; the scale runs from 0 (perfect health without symptoms) to 6 (death)), and the

Implementation of evidence-based treatment protocols to manage fever, hyperglycaemia, and swallowing dysfunction in acute stroke (QASC): a cluster randomised controlled trial

Sandy Middleton, Patrick McElduff, Jeanette Ward, Jeremy M Grimshaw, Simeon Dale, Catherine D'Este, Peta Drury, Rhonda Griffiths, N Wah Cheung, Clare Quinn, Malcolm Evans, Dominique Cadilhac, Christopher Levi, on behalf of the QASC Trialists Group

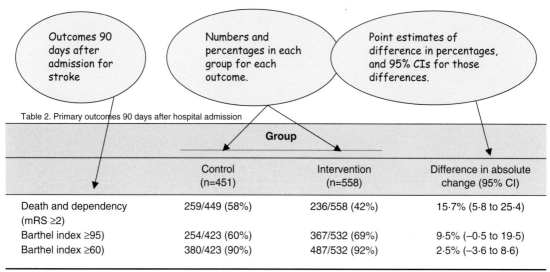

Table 2. Primary outcomes 90 days after hospital admission

	Group		
	Control (n=451)	Intervention (n=558)	Difference in absolute change (95% CI)
Death and dependency (mRS ≥2)	259/449 (58%)	236/558 (42%)	15·7% (5·8 to 25·4)
Barthel index ≥95)	254/423 (60%)	367/532 (69%)	9·5% (−0·5 to 19·5)
Barthel index ≥60)	380/423 (90%)	487/532 (92%)	2·5% (−3·6 to 8·6)

Data are number (%). mRS=modified Rankin scale.

FIGURE 25.3 Comparison of outcomes in patients between a multidisciplinary intervention group and a control group, 90 days after admission to hospital for stroke; from a randomised controlled trial. (Abbreviated by current authors.) Reprinted from *The Lancet* 378: Middleton S, McElduff P, Ward J, Grimshaw JM, Dale S, D'Este C, *et al.*, on behalf of the QASC Trialists Group. Implementation of evidence-based treatment protocols to manage fever, hyperglycaemia, and swallowing dysfunction in acute stroke (QASC): a cluster randomised controlled trial. 2011; 1699–1706, © 2011, with permission from Elsevier.

ability to live independently (measured first by a Barthel Index score ≥ 95 and second by a Barthel Index score ≥ 60; the Barthel Index measures performance in activities of daily living (ADL) – effectively the degree to which the subject can live independently; range is from 0 to 100, higher scores are better).

For the death and dependency outcome (modified Rankin scale ≥ 2) you can see that the percent in the Control group was 58% and in the Intervention group 42%. The 95% confidence interval for the difference in these percentages is (5.8 to 25.4)% with a point estimate of 15.7%. So the most likely value would be 15.7% and we can be 95% confidence that the true difference is between 5.8% and 25.4%. This interval does not include 0, so the difference is significant and definitive. Note that the 95% confidence interval for the difference in both summaries of the Barthel Index scores includes 0, so we must judge these differences not to be significant (i.e. not significantly different from 0). Once again, however, we see that both point estimates are positive, and the upper limit of both confidence intervals also positive. Despite the negative lower confidence interval limits, we cannot exclude the possibility that the difference in the populations are also positive; a larger sample would offer a more definitive answer.

Randomised trial of epidural bupivacaine and morphine in prevention of stump and phantom pain lower-limb amputation

Lone Nikolajsen, Susanne Ilkjaer, Jørgen H Christensen, Karsten Krøner, Troels S Jensen

	Median (IQR) pain		
	Blockade group (n=27)	Control group (n=29)	95% CI for difference (p)
After epidural bolus	0 (0–0)	38 (17–67)	24 to 43 (p<0.0001)
After continuous epidural infusion	0 (0–0)	31 (20–51)	24 to 43 (p<0.0001)
After epidural bolus in operating theatre	0 (0–0)	35 (16–64)	19 to 42 (p<0.0001)

Pain assessed by visual analogue scale (0–100 mm).

Table 2: **Intensity of preamputation pain during treatment with bupivacaine and morphine (blockade group) or saline (control group)**

A plausible range of values for the true difference in median pain levels after the epidural bolus is from 24 to 43 . . .

. . . and there is a significant difference in median pain levels between the two groups at each stage, because none of the CIs includes 0.

FIGURE 25.4 Confidence intervals for differences in median preoperative pain levels in the stump pain study. Reprinted from *The Lancet* 350: Nikolajsen L, Ilkjaer S, Christensen JH, Krøner K, Jensen TS. Randomised trial of epidural bupivacaine and morphine in prevention of stump and phantom pain in lower-limb amputation. 1998; 1353–7, © 1998, with permission from Elsevier.

CONFIDENCE INTERVALS FOR DIFFERENCES IN TWO MEDIANS

Let's return to the study first encountered in Figure 15.2 on the efficacy of bupivacaine given before amputation for the relief of post-amputation stump pain. Patient pre-amputation pain was measured in both the treatment and control groups. The sample median pain levels for each group are shown in Figure 25.4, along with 95% confidence intervals for differences in median pain levels between the two populations.

We can see that the differences in median pain levels between the treatment and control (placebo) groups are significant at all the time points since none of the confidence intervals includes 0. For example, after the epidural bolus (of either bupivacaine or saline), the median pain levels were 0 and 38, respectively. Thus, the difference was 38 and the 95% confidence interval for the population difference was (24 to 43), which does not include 0. So a plausible range for the difference in the population medians is somewhere between 24 and 43.

To sum up. If you are trying to interpret a confidence interval for the true value of the *difference* between two population parameters (such as two means, two medians, or two proportions), then the general rule is as follows:

If the confidence interval for the difference contains 0, you can be 95% confident that there is no statistically significant difference between the populations in terms of the parameter in question. If the interval does not contain 0, then there is a statistically significant difference, and you can also be 95% confident that the confidence interval contains the true value of any difference in the parameters.

Finally, it is worth re-iterating that a confidence interval is a sort of informed guess (based on sample evidence) as to the true value of the corresponding population parameter (or difference in parameters), whose true value *we can never actually know*.

There is another important class of measures for which confidence intervals are commonly quoted, that of *ratios*. In Chapter 26 we will see how the interpretation of the confidence interval for a ratio is shows some important differences.

26

Confidence Intervals for Ratios

You will recall from the discussion in Chapter 24 that risk ratios (often called *relative risks*) are commonly associated with *cohort* studies and odds ratios with *case-control* studies. Clinical researchers need to calculate confidence intervals for the true (population) values of these ratios just as much as they do for the measures (like means and proportions) discussed in Chapter 25. When you read papers which contain the results of such calculations, you still need to be able to understand how to interpret the confidence interval.

However, there is an important difference in the way confidence intervals for ratios are interpreted. In Chapter 25 we saw that if a confidence interval for the *difference* between two population parameters, two means, for example, includes 0, then we can be reasonably confident that there is no statistically significant difference between them. But when we come to the interpretation of confidence intervals for *ratios*, there is a different rule. Why? Well suppose the risk in the population of being born prematurely for those babies whose mothers are clinically obese is 1.25, the *same* as the risk of premature birth for babies whose mothers are not obese, also 1.25. This being so, then if we divide one risk by the other (i.e. determine the risk ratio), the result is 1 (1.25/1.25 = 1).

So if a 95% confidence interval for a risk ratio *contains 1*, then we can be 95% confident that the population risk ratio is *not* significant and the risk factor concerned (obesity in the mother say) is not significant, neither increasing nor decreasing the risk (of premature birth). If the confidence interval *does not contain 1*, we can be 95% confident that the risk factor *does* significantly increase the risk (risk ratio greater than 1) or decrease the risk (risk ratio less than 1). As with the confidence intervals for the differences in population parameters, regardless of whether the confidence interval contains 1 or not, remember that the most likely value (the single best guess) for the population ratio is the point estimate for that ratio.

CONFIDENCE INTERVALS FOR ODDS RATIOS

Let's remind ourselves how ratios, such as odds ratios, are interpreted (see Chapter 23). An example given in Figure 23.4 at the end of that chapter reported an odds ratio of 1.06 for ischaemic heart disease among men with *Helicobacter pylori* compared to men without *H. pylori* (*H. pylori* is the potential *risk factor* in this study). In other words, men with *H. pylori* would appear to have 1.06 times the odds of ischaemic heart disease than men without (6% more if you like).

We use the phrase 'would appear to have' because we still have to decide whether this result is significant – remember that an odds ratio calculated from a sample is only an estimate of the true (population) odds ratio. As we saw above, you need to know whether the interval contains 1 or not.

As it happens, the risk factor *H. pylori* quoted in Chapter 23 is not a statistically significant risk factor for ischaemic heart disease since the 95% confidence interval of (0.86 to 1.31) for the odds ratio includes 1.

Have a look now at Figure 26.1, from a case-control study, which reports odds ratios and their 95% confidence intervals from a study into the possible association between admission to hospital with

Trimethoprim-sulfamethoxazole induced hyperkalaemia in elderly patients receiving spironolactone: nested case-control study

Tony Antoniou, Tara Gomes, Muhammad M Mamdani, Zhan Yao, Chelsea Hellings, Amit X Garg, Matthew A Weir, David N Juurlink,

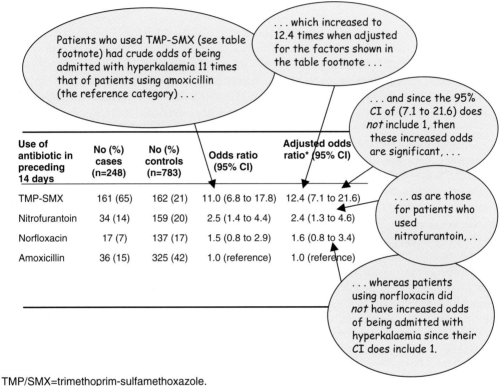

TMP/SMX=trimethoprim-sulfamethoxazole.
*Adjusted for age category, congestive heart failure, chronic liver disease, chronic kidney disease, Charlson co-morbidity index, fifth of income, living in long term care facility, number of prescription drugs in previous year, number of years of spironolactone treatment, and drugs (β adrenergic receptor blockers, potassium sparing diuretics, non-potassium sparing diuretics, non-steroidal anti-inflammatory drugs, potassium supplements, renin-angiotensin-aldosterone inhibitors).

FIGURE 26.1   Crude and adjusted odds ratios for the association between hospital admission involving hyperkalaemia and recent antibiotic use. (See footnote to table for adjustment factors.) Reproduced from Antoniou T, Gomes T, Mamdani MM, Yao Z, Hellings C, Garg AX, *et al.* Trimethoprim-sulfamethoxazole induced hyperkalaemia in elderly patients receiving spironolactone: nested case-control study. *BMJ* 2011, 343: d5228, © 2011, with permission from BMJ Publishing Group Ltd.

hyperkalaemia (high serum potassium) in 248 elderly patients (with 783 controls) using spironolactone, who had then received an antibiotic prescription for either trimethoprim-sulfamethoxazole (TMP-SMX; the potential risk factor), amoxicillin, norfloxacin, or nitrofurantoin. You will notice that the table contains both odds ratios and *adjusted* odds ratios, and we will deal with the idea of adjustment in Chapters 30 and 31, but put simply, it is to discount any factors other than antibiotics which may interfere with the relationship (in fact to control for potential confounders). You will see from the figure that patients who take either TMP-SMX or nitrofurantoin have significantly increased odds of hyperkalaemia compared to patients taking amoxicillin (the reference category, odds ratio = 1) because the 95% confidence intervals do not include 1, whereas patients taking norfloxacin do *not* experience increased odds of hyperkalaemia – their confidence interval *does* include 1.

Notice, by the way, that the value for the odds ratio does not generally sit in the middle of its confidence interval, unlike the case with the confidence intervals for means and proportions.

CONFIDENCE INTERVALS FOR RISK RATIOS

We can interpret a confidence interval for a risk ratio (relative risk) in just the same way as we do an odds ratio. If the confidence interval includes 1, then there is probably no statistically significant risk associated with the factor involved. If the confidence interval does not contain 1, then the risk ratio is significant – if less than 1 the risk is decreased, if greater than 1 the risk is increased.

To illustrate this idea, the table of relative risks (risk ratios) and their 95% confidence intervals shown in Figure 26.2 is taken from a large cohort study (47 000 men and women) into diet and the risk of diverticular disease. The authors compared the risk of diverticular disease between participants with various diets: vegetarians, vegans, meat eaters, and those who ate no meat but some fish. As in Figure 26.1, the authors show both crude and adjusted risk ratios – the factors adjusted for are shown in the table footnote (in this example the adjustment makes no difference to the significance or otherwise of the results, although this will not always be the case). In addition to the confidence intervals the authors also provided *p*-values, which we will consider in Chapter 27. As you can see (looking at the adjusted risks), vegetarians have about two-thirds (the point estimate is 0.70) the risk of diverticular disease compared to non-vegetarians (taken as the referent group, risk ratio = 1), and this is significant because the confidence interval, (0.56 to 0.87), does not contain 1. You will also see that vegans have just over a quarter of the risk (0.28) of diverticular disease as do meat eaters (the referent group) and this too is significant.

CONFIDENCE INTERVALS FOR HAZARD RATIOS

Odds ratios and risk ratios are the ratios frequently seen in the literature, but the *hazard ratio* is also important in the context of survival analysis. We will discuss the hazard ratio in more detail in Chapter 32, but essentially the hazard is a risk, the risk of the specified clinical outcome (for example, death), at any point in time. The interpretation of confidence intervals for hazard ratios is the same as for odds and risk ratios. If the interval contains 1, the risk factor concerned is not a statistically significant hazard. If it does not contain 1, the factor is a statistically significant hazard. Values greater than 1 indicate that the factor increases the hazard, values less than 1 indicate that the hazard is decreased.

In addition to odds, risk, and hazard ratios, clinical research papers will contain references to other ratios and their confidence intervals (e.g. for the ratio of two population means). Whatever the ratio, the rule described in this section, as to whether or not the confidence interval includes 1, still applies.

In Chapters 25 and 26 you have seen how confidence intervals can be helpful in the analysis of research results. In Chapter 27 we will discuss hypothesis testing, which offers an alternative approach, and examine the close relationship between confidence intervals and hypothesis tests.

Diet and risk of diverticular disease in Oxford cohort of European Prospective Investigation into Cancer and Nutrition (EPIC): prospective study of British vegetarians and non-vegetarians

Francesca L Crowe, Paul N Appleby, Naomi E Allen, Timothy J Key

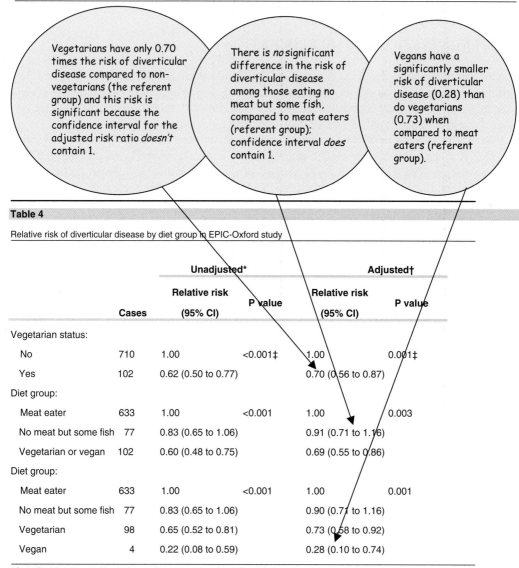

Vegetarians have only 0.70 times the risk of diverticular disease compared to non-vegetarians (the referent group) and this risk is significant because the confidence interval for the adjusted risk ratio *doesn't* contain 1.

There is *no* significant difference in the risk of diverticular disease among those eating no meat but some fish, compared to meat eaters (referent group); confidence interval *does* contain 1.

Vegans have a significantly smaller risk of diverticular disease (0.28) than do vegetarians (0.73) when compared to meat eaters (referent group).

Table 4

Relative risk of diverticular disease by diet group in EPIC-Oxford study

	Cases	Unadjusted* Relative risk (95% CI)	P value	Adjusted† Relative risk (95% CI)	P value
Vegetarian status:					
No	710	1.00	<0.001‡	1.00	0.001‡
Yes	102	0.62 (0.50 to 0.77)		0.70 (0.56 to 0.87)	
Diet group:					
Meat eater	633	1.00	<0.001	1.00	0.003
No meat but some fish	77	0.83 (0.65 to 1.06)		0.91 (0.71 to 1.16)	
Vegetarian or vegan	102	0.60 (0.48 to 0.75)		0.69 (0.55 to 0.86)	
Diet group:					
Meat eater	633	1.00	<0.001	1.00	0.001
No meat but some fish	77	0.83 (0.65 to 1.06)		0.90 (0.71 to 1.16)	
Vegetarian	98	0.65 (0.52 to 0.81)		0.73 (0.58 to 0.92)	
Vegan	4	0.22 (0.08 to 0.59)		0.28 (0.10 to 0.74)	

*Stratified by sex, method of recruitment, and region of residence.
†Stratified by sex, method of recruitment, and region of residence and adjusted for smoking, education level, Townsend deprivation index, self reported hyperlipidaemia, receiving long term medical treatment, ever used oral contraceptives, ever used hormone replacement therapy, and BMI (fully adjusted model).
‡χ^2 test.

FIGURE 26.2   Relative risks (risk ratios) from a large cohort study (47 000 men and women) into diet and the risk of diverticular disease. Reproduced from Crowe FL, Appleby PN, Allen NE, Key TJ. Diet and risk of diverticular disease in Oxford cohort of European Prospective Investigation into Cancer and Nutrition (EPIC): prospective study of British vegetarians and non-vegetarians. *BMJ* 2011, 343: d4131, © 2011, with permission from BMJ Publishing Group Ltd.

27

Testing Hypotheses – the *p*-Value

As you will recall from Chapter 3, researchers usually start with a question, which is often (but not always) formulated as a *hypothesis* (sometimes called a *null hypothesis*) We have seen examples of research questions already. For example: 'Does treatment with statins effect cholesterol levels in patients with hyperlipidemia?', 'Is a telephone helpline effective in promoting smoking cessation?', 'Is there a relationship between diverticular disease and diet?'.

In Chapters 25 and 26 we saw that one way that researchers can deal with such questions is to calculate an appropriate confidence interval (e.g. for the difference in cholesterol levels of the two groups (statins/no statins), or for the risk ratio between vegetarians and non vegetarians). In this present chapter we want to discuss an alternative to confidence intervals, and that is the use of *hypothesis tests*. As an example of this approach, the following is a quote from another study into the benefits of statin therapy:

> It has been suggested that inflammation status, as assessed by C-reactive protein (CRP) concentration, modifies the vascular protective effects of statin therapy. In particular, there have been claims that statins might be more beneficial in people with raised CRP concentrations, and might even be ineffective in people with low concentrations of both CRP and LDL cholesterol. This study aimed to test this hypothesis.
>
> *(Heart Protection Study Collaborative Group, 2011)*

In this chapter we are going to explain the ins and outs of hypothesis testing, and compare the merits of the this approach with that of the confidence interval approach. Conceptually, the hypothesis testing idea is not difficult. You take a representative sample, examine the sample data, decide if the data are consistent with the hypothesis, and then either reject the hypothesis (sample data not consistent with it) or do not reject it (sample data consistent with it). Essentially we are using the sample data as evidence for or against the hypothesis. How then do we decide what constitutes strong enough evidence against the hypothesis? Since the evidence we use is a probability, a few words on probability seem appropriate.

A FEW WORDS ON PROBABILITY

The probability of any event can vary from 0 (meaning it cannot happen, e.g. getting a total of 13 from rolling two dice) to 1 (it is certain to happen, e.g. getting a number from 1 to 6 when one dice is rolled). The closer the probability is to 0, the less likely the event is to happen; the closer to 1 the more likely. If the probability equals 0.5 (i.e. 1 in 2), then the event is as likely to happen as not.

If two events are *independent* then the probability of one event occurring is in no way related to the probability of the other event occurring. So, for example, if we toss a coin twice and get a head with the first toss (the probability of which is 0.5), then the probability of a head on the second toss remains 0.5, because the two events are independent. The probability of two successive heads is $0.5 \times 0.5 = 0.25$. This multiplication rule can be extended to any number of independent events. Probability theory is a huge subject, but that is all we need here.

Understanding Clinical Papers, Third Edition. David Bowers, Allan House, David Owens and Bridgette Bewick.
© 2014 John Wiley & Sons, Ltd. Published 2014 by John Wiley & Sons, Ltd.

ASSESSING THE EVIDENCE AGAINST THE HYPOTHESIS – THE p-VALUE

Let's start by defining the p-value: the p-value is the probability of getting the outcome you found (or one more extreme), when the hypothesis is true.

The idea of the p-value is best illustrated with an example. Imagine you toss a coin 100 times. The hypothesis is that the coin is a fair coin. If you get 92 heads and only eight tails (or 92 tails and only eight heads) you would almost certainly consider this to be strong enough evidence against the hypothesis to enable you to reject it. If you got 60 heads and 40 tails the decision would now be more difficult. How probable is this outcome if your hypothesis were true – that the coin is fair? Does it offer strong enough evidence against the hypothesis – or not? Obviously we need a systematic way of deciding. This is where the p-value comes in.

We compare the probability of the output we obtain with what is known as the *significance level* of the test, denoted alpha (α). (Note that this is different from Cronbach's α related to internal consistency discussed in Chapter 20.) This is conventionally set at 0.05 (sometimes 0.01), but it is important to note that this 0.05 value is completely arbitrary, although firmly established among researchers. So if the probability of getting the outcome that you did get is less than 0.05 (i.e. if $p < 0.05$), this is taken to offer strong evidence against the hypothesis. Such an outcome is so improbable if the hypothesis were true that we are obliged to conclude that the hypothesis is probably not true and we thus reject it.

One of the things you need to be able to tell, therefore, when reading through the results of a hypothesis test is what significance level the authors have used for their tests (although this is almost always 0.05). Furthermore, authors should report p-values clearly and in full (three decimal places is enough). For example, '$p = 0.025$' or 'a p-value of 0.155' or whatever, but not '$p < 0.05$, or $p < 0.01$, or $p > 0.05$', and so on. Even worse than this is the use of asterisks in tables, with a footnote such as '$*p < 0.05$' or '$**p < 0.01$'. The authors should provide the actual p-value. Apart from anything else, it is useful to know how far from 0.05 it is. Note though that some computer programs only give the p-value to three decimal places. So if $p = 0.0006$, some programs will show this as $p = 0.000$ and authors can then only report this as '$p < 0.001$.

MAKING THE WRONG DECISION – TYPES OF ERROR

We need to say a just few words about possible types of error in hypothesis testing because there is a connection to the power of a test (mentioned in Chapter 10). It's worth bearing in mind that when researchers reject or do not reject their null hypothesis on the basis of some *sample* evidence, there is always the possibility that they might, unwittingly, have made the *wrong* decision, either because the sample is not representative enough of the population, or is not big enough to detect an effect. There are two possibilities: Type I and Type II errors.

Type I Errors

Suppose the hypothesis is: 'There is no relationship between diverticular disease and diet'. The researchers may conclude from their sample data that the evidence against this hypothesis is strong enough ($p < 0.05$) for it to be rejected as false when it is in fact true. Statisticians refer to this mistake as a *Type I error*, although the term 'false-positive' means the same thing.

There are three common reasons for researchers to get a false-positive result from a study. First, they may choose a biased sample which is not representative of the study population. Second, they may take too small a sample, so that a false-positive result is obtained by chance. Both these sources of error can be eliminated by careful attention to sampling (see Chapter 10). Third, is the possibility of false-positive results arising from *multiple testing*.

You will remember that the p-value is the probability of a result (or one more extreme) occurring when the hypothesis is true, and conventionally we accept $p < 0.05$ as implying significance. What this means is that there is only a 5% likelihood of a result being due to chance, or 1 in 20. But many studies report the results of multiple significance tests. Bear in mind then, that if authors accept a significance level of $p < 0.05$ and conduct 20 tests, one of them at least may be 'significant' simply by chance.

Researchers can inflate these errors by undertaking lots of subgroup analysis on their data. Subgroups are (by definition) smaller than the original sample, so chance may produce striking findings, and the additional analyses involve more tests so multiple testing becomes a problem. You may see authors reporting methods to overcome this problem. One is to reduce the significance level α from 0.05 to 0.01, thus making the test more rigorous, and to compensate for the number of inferences being made and the need for a stronger level of evidence. Another method is to use the Bonferroni correction, which means dividing the usual significance level α by the number of tests undertaken. With 10 tests this means that the significance level becomes $\alpha/10 = 0.05/10 = 0.005$.

Type II Errors

The second possibility error is when investigators decide that the evidence against the hypothesis is *not* strong enough for it to be rejected as being untrue (*p*-value not less than 0.05), when in fact it *is* untrue and the hypothesis should have been rejected. Again the vagaries of samples might cause this to occur from time to time. Statisticians know this sort of mistake as a *Type II error* (or 'false negative').

False-negative results mainly occur as the result of studies that are too small. For example, suppose we want to know if women are on average shorter than men. If we take a sample of five women and five men we might easily find five tall women and five short men by chance, and conclude (wrongly) that women are not shorter than men. But if we take a sample of 500 in each group we are much less likely to make this mistake (although we might still do so if the sample is biased).

This is where the *power* of a test comes in. The probability of committing a Type II error (i.e. of getting a false negative) is denoted beta (β). Now the power of a test is its ability to detect a true effect if such an effect exists – we want to make sure that we reject the hypothesis of, let us say, no relationship between diverticular disease and diet, when it is not true, and there *is* something going on. Thus, the power of a study equals 1 minus the probability of a Type II error (or $1 - a$ false negative) or $(1 - \beta)$. So the bigger the probability of committing a Type II error, of getting a false negative, the smaller the power of the test. Power is intimately connected with the size of a study – larger studies have more power. If authors are presenting the results of hypothesis tests, they must provide evidence that a calculation, to determine the minimum sample size needed to detect an effect, has been performed. As an example of a sample size calculation, the following extract is from a randomised controlled trial in the management of asthma in pregnancy by measurement of the fraction of exhaled nitric oxide:

> Sample size was calculated with power of 80%, and the type I error rate of 0.05. To detect a 40% reduction in the proportion of participants having an exacerbation from 55% to 33%, 176 women were needed and 210 randomly assigned to allow for a 20% dropout rate.
>
> *(Powell* et al.*, 2011)*

Even if the researchers intend to analyse their data using confidence intervals without performing any tests, the sample size calculation still needs to be done. The problem of too small a sample manifests itself in wide intervals with little precision. These may fail to pick up a significant result (i.e. give a false negative and cause a Type II error).

HYPOTHESIS TESTS AND CONFIDENCE INTERVALS COMPARED

Confidence intervals and hypothesis tests perform a similar function. However, confidence intervals are much to be preferred for a number of reasons. First, because, in addition to indicating whether the hypothesis is to be rejected or not (does the confidence interval include 0 for differences, or 1 for ratios), they also provide a *range of plausible values* for the size of any difference, whereas the hypothesis test only indicates whether any difference is statistically significant, but without any indication of what that difference might be.

Take, for example, the result for the difference in median pain levels of the treatment and control groups, shown in the first row of Figure 25.4. The *p*-value is < 0.0001, which is plenty strong enough for us to reject the hypothesis of equal pain levels in the two populations. But that is all it tells us. However, the 95% confidence interval of (24 to 43) tells us not only that the pain levels are different, because the confidence interval does not include 0, but also that a plausible value for this difference lies somewhere between 24 and 43.

A second reason for preferring to see confidence intervals rather than hypothesis tests is that the plausible range of value provided is in clinically meaningful units, which of course makes interpretation much easier. Far better for you to know that 'the difference in pain levels is most probably between 24 and 43, than just to be told that '$p < 0.0001$'.

Thirdly, in the comparison of two treatments, for example, a confidence interval will give an indication of whether or not the difference in outcomes offers a clinically worthwhile result, *whether or not* the difference in outcomes is significant. For all of these reasons, you will hope to see confidence intervals quoted in papers instead of or in addition to *p*-values. In many circumstances, confidence intervals alone are sufficient.

Two-Tailed Versus One-Tailed Tests

We should mention briefly the difference between two-tailed and one-tailed hypothesis tests (sometimes referred to as two-sided and one-sided, respectively). In the vast majority of published papers the two-tailed test is used, but occasionally you may see a one-tailed test. To illustrate the difference between the two tests with an example, suppose you are investigating a new drug, 'downalol', intended to reduce hypertension. You give one group of hypertensive adults downalol and the other group of similar adults a placebo. Your hypothesis is that there is no difference between the mean diastolic blood pressure in the two groups, and the conventional approach is to assume when you are testing your hypothesis that the difference in the mean diastolic blood pressure may *be either smaller* among the downalol group compared to the placebo group, *or bigger*. In other words you are careful not to pre-judge the outcome, regardless of what you may suspect (or hope for).

Because you are dividing the 0.05 uncertainty into *two* (0.025 for the less than outcome and 0.025 for the more than outcome), this approach is called *two*-tailed hypothesis testing. In recent years papers describing a hypothesis test of *non-inferiority* or equivalence have become more common, which use a one-tailed test. With this approach, the hypothesis would then be that mean diastolic blood pressure in the downalol group was not lower than (i.e. *not inferior* to) or at least equivalent (equal) to, that in the placebo group. In this approach the whole of the 0.05 uncertainty is allocated to the 'not inferior' tail. One criticism of this approach is that if you already know the direction of the difference, why bother doing a hypothesis test at all. A second criticism is that you are more likely to get a favourable outcome because you have the whole of the 0.05 to play with. In the end, of course, the choice of which method to use is up to the researcher.

MATCHED VERSUS INDEPENDENT GROUPS

There are a large number of different statistical tests available to the researcher – we will describe a few of the most common shortly, but you will not perhaps be surprised to discover that the choice of which test is appropriate when two groups are to be compared is governed by the type of data in question and the shape of the distributions (see Chapter 14). In addition, we also need to know whether the groups involved are *independent* or *paired*. For groups to be independent, the selection of the participants in one group must not be influenced by or related to the selection of participants in the other group. However, there are occasions when participants in the groups are not selected independently, but are in fact deliberately matched, such as in some case-control studies (see Chapter 6).

This matching can take two forms. First, matching can be on a person-to-person basis – each individual in the first group is matched with an individual in the second group – same age, same sex, same degree of illness, and so on. Alternatively, the matching can be in proportional terms – the same proportion of males to females in each group, the same proportion of those aged over 60, and so on; this process is often termed *frequency matching*. The choice of an appropriate hypothesis test depends on which type of matching applies. So when the results of any test on two groups appears in a paper, you should be able to tell whether or not the groups were matched. If matched, what is the nature of the matching – individual-to-individual or by proportion? If the latter, then the groups are *not* considered to be matched for the purpose of hypothesis testing. If the groups are supposedly independent you will want evidence that this is true. In either case, you will also want to know exactly how many were in each group.

Now we will briefly describe three hypothesis tests that appear frequently in non-specialist clinical papers: the chi-squared (χ^2) test, the Mann–Whitney test, and the *t*-test.

THREE COMMON TESTS

The χ^2 Test

Suppose you take a sample of 60 male nurses and 140 female nurses working in a large hospital, and record whether or not they smoke. You want to answer the question, 'Is there a relationship between gender and smoking status, or are these two variables independent?'. In other words, are you more (or less) likely to smoke if you are female (say) than if you are male, or does not gender make no difference? Your hypothesis might be that there is no difference in smoking behaviour between the two groups in the population, in other words, the variables are *independent* – gender and smoking are not related. You can express this problem as a 2×2 *contingency* table (a table containing the observed frequencies) like that shown in Figure 27.1.

If the hypothesis is true, if the variables *are* independent, then the proportion of males in each category (smoking and non-smoking), should be approximately the same as the proportion of females in each category. Bear in mind, however, that the *sample* proportions are unlikely to be *exactly* the same even if the hypothesis is true. In this example we can see that the sample proportion of male nurses who smoke is 0.20 (20%) and the sample proportion of female nurses is 0.18 (18%). Are these proportions similar enough for us to assume that they are equal in the population? This is where the χ^2 test comes in – we can use it to determine whether any observed differences in the proportions exceed what we might expect by chance. One condition of the test is that the observations on the two (or more) groups, in this case male nurses and female nurses, *must be independent*. The above example had two categories (smokers and non-smokers) and two groups (males and females), and would be referred to as a 2×2 test, but the test can be used with more than two groups and/or categories, as you will see below.

		Male nurses	Female nurses
Smoke?	No	50	178
	Yes	10	32

FIGURE 27.1 A hypothetical 2×2 contingency table showing sample frequencies of male and female nurses and their smoking habits.

The χ^2 test is used with categorical data (or metric data which has been grouped into categories), provided that the number of categories is not too large – χ^2 is seldom used with more than four or five categories. In fact, the number of categories is limited by the size of the sample. The reasons behind this are a bit technical. As a rough guide, with two groups and three categories, you would need a minimum total sample of 50 or upwards (authors should, of course, give evidence of a power calculation, see Chapter 10). When sample size is small the consequence may be to produce (what are known as) *expected* values which are less than 5. In this case you may see authors using the alternative Fisher's exact test. However, this can only be applied to two-category, two-group, situations. Sample size considerations and the need for the groups to be independent are something to be aware of when you read papers containing χ^2 calculations.

As an example, Figure 27.2 is from a randomised controlled trial of long-term outcomes when using additional catheter-directed thrombolysis versus standard treatment for acute iliofemoral deep vein thrombosis. For each of the two treatments the authors measured three outcomes: post-thrombotic syndrome at 24 months, iliofemoral patency at 6 months, and post-thrombotic syndrome at 6 months. They wanted to know if outcomes and treatments were independent or not and used the χ^2 test to decide. As you can see from Figure 27.2, for the first two outcomes the population proportions are found not to be the same (all $p < 0.05$), so the variables outcome and treatment are not independent, while for the third outcome the p-value is not less than 0.05 so outcome and treatment are independent – it doesn't matter which of the two treatments you get as a patient, you are just as likely to suffer post-thrombotic syndrome at 6 months.

The χ^2 Test with Odds Ratios, Risk Ratios, etc

A second use you will see for the χ^2 test is as a measure of the statistical significance of odds and risk ratios and the like, in the study of potential risk factors for various conditions. If we use the p-value to test hypotheses related to a ratio, for example an odds ratio, then as you saw above, $p < 0.05$ will correspond to a confidence interval for the ratio that does not include 1.

As an example, Figure 27.3 is taken from a randomised controlled trial of the use of aspirin in patients treated with alteplase for acute ischaemic stroke. Patients were randomised into two groups. The first group received aspirin with alteplase, the second group the standard alteplase treatment. Figure 27.3 shows the causes of poor outcomes and the corresponding risk ratios (called here the relative risks), along with 95% confidence intervals, and a p-value derived from the χ^2 test (see figure footnote).

Notice that the p-values are less than 0.05 when the 95% confidence intervals for the risk ratios do not include 1 and *vice versa*.

As another example, take the result for the adjusted relative risk of diverticular disease for vegetarians versus non-vegetarians shown in the first row of Figure 26.2 in Chapter 26. We see that the p-value = 0.001, which is certainly small enough (less than 0.05 for sure!) for us to reject the hypothesis of no difference in risk between the two groups. A similar result can be seen for vegans compared to meat eaters (last row of Figure 26.2), a p = value considerably less than 0.05 – so once again we can reject the hypothesis of no difference in risk between these two groups.

But that is all that these two p-values tell us. However, for the vegetarian versus non-vegetarian groups, the 95% confidence interval of (0.56 to 0.87) tells us not only that the difference in relative risk is significant (because the confidence interval does not contain 1), but that a plausible value for this difference in risk is between 0.56 and 0.87. Similarly, a plausible value for the difference in the vegan versus meat eaters relative risk of diverticular disease lies somewhere between 0.10 to 0.74.

A second reason for preferring to see confidence intervals rather than hypothesis tests is that the plausible range of value provided is in clinically meaningful units, which of course makes interpretation much easier. Far better for you to know that 'the difference in total cholesterol level was most likely between 1.6 and 1.7 mmol/l', than just to be told that '$p < 0.0001$'.

Long-term outcome after additional catheter-directed thrombolysis versus standard treatment for acute iliofemoral deep vein thrombosis (the CaVenT study): a randomised controlled trial

Tone Enden, Ylva Haig, Nils-Einar Kløw, Carl-Erik Slagsvold, Leiv Sandvik, Waleed Ghanima, Geir Hafsahl, Pål Andre Holme, Lars Olaf Holmen, Anne Mette Njaastad, Gunnar Sandbæk, Per Morten Sandset, on behalf of the CaVenT Study Group

	Additional catheter-directed thrombolysis (n=90)		Standard treatment only (n=99)		p value*
	n	% (95% CI)	n	% (95% CI)	
Post-thrombotic syndrome at 24 months[†]	37	41·1% (31·5–51·4)	55	55·6% (45·7–65·0)	0·047
Iliofemoral patency at 6 months[†‡]	58	65·9% (55·5–75·0)	45	47·4% (37·6–57·3)	0·012
Post-thrombotic syndrome at 6 months[§]	27	30·3% (21·8–40·5)	32	32·2% (23·9–42·1)	0·77

Post-thrombotic syndrome defined as Villalta score of 5 points or higher.
* χ^2 test.
† Co-primary outcomes.
‡ Five patients had inconclusive patency assessments and one was lost to follow-up at 6 months.
§ Secondary outcome.

These *p*-value are both less than 0.05, so the proportions (%s) in the populations experiencing either post-thrombotic syndrome at 24 months, or iliopatency at 6 months, when receiving additional catheter-directed thrombolysis versus standard treatment only, are not the same, so treatment and outcome are *not* independent, . . .

. . . whereas this *p*-value is *not* less than 0.05, so the two population proportions are the same, i.e. treatment and outcome might very well be independent.

FIGURE 27.2 Use of the χ^2 test in a comparison of additional catheter-directed thrombolysis versus standard treatment for acute iliofemoral deep vein thrombosis. The question is: are outcome and treatment independent?. Reprinted from *The Lancet* 379: Enden T, Haig Y, Kløw N-E, Slagsvold C-E, Sandvik L, Ghanima W, *et al.*, on behalf of the CaVenT Study Group. Long-term outcome after additional catheter-directed thrombolysis versus standard treatment for acute iliofemoral deep vein thrombosis (the CaVenT study): a randomised controlled trial. 2012, (9810); 31–8, © 2012, with permission from Elsevier.

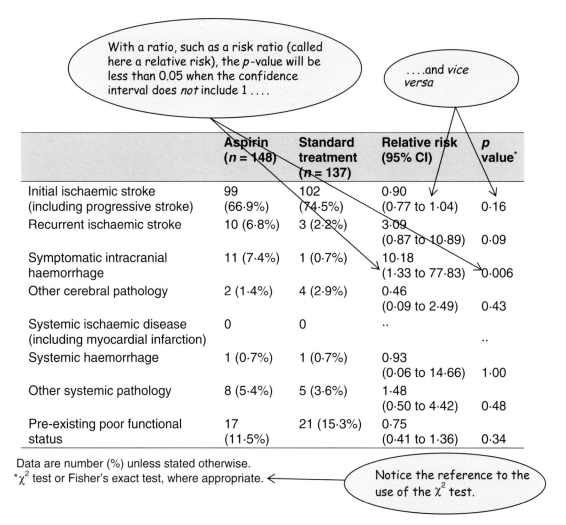

With a ratio, such as a risk ratio (called here a relative risk), the *p*-value will be less than 0.05 when the confidence interval does *not* include 1 ....

....and *vice versa*

	Aspirin (n = 148)	Standard treatment (n = 137)	Relative risk (95% CI)	p value*
Initial ischaemic stroke (including progressive stroke)	99 (66·9%)	102 (74·5%)	0·90 (0·77 to 1·04)	0·16
Recurrent ischaemic stroke	10 (6·8%)	3 (2·2%)	3·09 (0·87 to 10·89)	0·09
Symptomatic intracranial haemorrhage	11 (7·4%)	1 (0·7%)	10·18 (1·33 to 77·83)	0·006
Other cerebral pathology	2 (1·4%)	4 (2·9%)	0·46 (0·09 to 2·49)	0·43
Systemic ischaemic disease (including myocardial infarction)	0	0	..	..
Systemic haemorrhage	1 (0·7%)	1 (0·7%)	0·93 (0·06 to 14·66)	1·00
Other systemic pathology	8 (5·4%)	5 (3·6%)	1·48 (0·50 to 4·42)	0·48
Pre-existing poor functional status	17 (11·5%)	21 (15·3%)	0·75 (0·41 to 1·36)	0·34

Data are number (%) unless stated otherwise.
*χ^2 test or Fisher's exact test, where appropriate. ←

Notice the reference to the use of the χ^2 test.

FIGURE 27.3 Odds ratios for causes of poor outcome in patients with modified Rankin scale score of 3–6 at 3 months. From a study to compare the effects of early addition of intravenous aspirin to alteplase, with standard alteplase without aspirin, in patients with acute ischaemic stroke. (Abbreviated by current authors.) Reprinted from *The Lancet* 380: Zinkstok SM, Roos YB, on behalf of the ARTIS Investigators. Early administration of aspirin in patients treated with alteplase for acute ischaemic stroke: a randomised controlled trial. 2012; 731–7, © 2012, with permission from Elsevier.

The χ^2 Test for Trend

A third and important use for the χ^2 test is as a test for a *trend* in the proportions or percentages across categories, when the categories can be *ordered*. The ordinary χ^2 test is much less powerful than the χ^2 test for trend, which authors should always use in these circumstances. Note that establishing a linear trend across categories implies a relationship between the two variables in question – the hypothesis is that there is no trend (i.e. no relationship). For example, the categories might be the age groups: 0–19, 20–29, and so on, and the two groups might be depressed and not depressed patients. The χ^2 test for trend can then be used to discover if there is a *systematic* trend in the proportion depressed as age group increases. Note that this test is usually applied to 2 × 'something' contingency tables, 2 × 3, 2 × 4, 2 × 5, and so on.

Relation of exposure to airway irritants in infancy to prevalence of bronchial hyper-responsiveness in schoolchildren

Vidar Søyseth, Johny Kongerud, Dagfinn Haarr, Ole Strand, Roald Bolle, Jacob Boe

There is a significant trend across the three age groups (%s of 20, 8 and 4) in the <7 year-exposed children, because the p-value <0.05, . . .

Time spent in Index area	Number (%) in age group (years)			p*
	≤9.0	9.1–11.0	>11.0	
<7 years	16/80 (20%)	4/53 (8%)	2/52 (4%)	0.004
≥7 years	24/118 (20%)	17/118 (14%)	16/108 (15%)	0.27

*χ² test for trend.

Table 3: **Relation between BHR and cumulative exposure**

. . . whereas, there isn't a trend in the %s (20, 14 and 15) for the ≥7 year-exposed children (p-value >0.05).

FIGURE 27.4   An example of the use of the χ^2 test for trend across three age groups among two groups of children. Reprinted from *The Lancet* 345: Søyseth V, Kongerud J, Haarr D, Strand O, Bolle R, Boe J. Relation of exposure to airway irritants in infancy to prevalence of bronchial hyper-responsiveness in schoolchildren. 1995; 217–20, © 1995, with permission from Elsevier.

Figure 27.4 shows the results of a χ^2 test to determine whether there was a trend in the percentages of children exposed to air pollution in two groups across three age groups. One group had been exposed for less than 7 years, the other for 7 years or more.

The χ^2 test is a very versatile procedure and has several other important applications, such as in meta-analysis (see Chapter 33) and in logistic regression (see Chapter 31).

The Mann–Whitney Test

The Mann–Whitney test (also referred to as the Mann–Whitney *U*-test) is a rank-based test of whether two *independent* samples come from the same distribution. This test by itself is not a test of whether the two corresponding population medians are different, but many computer programs (e.g. SPSS, Minitab, and Stata) will produce an associated confidence interval (not *directly* connected to the Mann–Whitney test) for the difference in the medians. This is frequently obtained using what are known as bootstrapping methods. The Mann–Whitney test is a popular but less powerful alternative to the *t*-test (particularly with small samples). The *t*-test is discussed in the next section, but requires the two distributions in question to be both metric and Normally distributed, so the Mann–Whitney test is therefore most appropriately used with either ordinal data or skewed metric data.

As an example of the Mann–Whitney test, Figure 27.5 is taken from a study into the risk factors for depressive symptoms in older people in long-term care in Taiwan. Figure 27.5 shows the median values

Depressive symptoms in long-term care residents in Taiwan

Li-Chan Lin, Tyng-Guey Wang, Miao-Yen Chen, Shiao-Chi Wu and Portwood MJ

Risk factor	Depressed (n=267) Median	Non-depressed (n=246) Median	p-value
Age (y)	78	78	0.585
Time in care (y)	16	14	0.125
Functional status	40	70	< 0.001
Cognitive status	6	8	0.023
Masticatory ability	10	9	0.158

Use of the Mann–Whitney test to identify risk factors for depression. Only two factors are significant with p-values < 0.05.

FIGURE 27.5   Results of a Mann–Whitney test to identify risk factors for depressive symptoms in elderly residents in care. Reproduced from Lin L-C, Wang TG, Chen MY, Wu SC, Portwood MJ (2005)- with permission from John Wiley & Sons.

among depressed and non-depressed groups for five potential risk factors, along with a *p*-value from a Mann–Whitney test. Although the first two factors, age and length of time in care, are metric variables and, distributional requirements permitting, could have been tested using a two-sample *t*-test (see next section), the other three factors are ordinal. In any case, the authors have used the Mann–Whitney test with all five factors. As you can see, only two factors, Functional status and Cognitive status, are significant with $p < 0.001$ and 0.023, respectively.

When the two groups are matched, the Wilcoxon (matched-pairs) signed-rank test can be used, but it appears less frequently in clinical papers and we will not discuss it further.

The *t*-Test

The Two-Sample t-Test

When the sample data are metric, the *t*-test is usually the most appropriate hypothesis test used to determine whether two population means are the same. There are two complementary tests, depending on the way in which the data have been collected. If the groups are matched or paired, the *matched-pairs t*-test is used (see below); if independent, the *two-sample t*-test is used. In order to use the two-sample *t*-test three conditions must be satisfied: the data in both groups must be metric, each should be Normally distributed, and the spreads of the two distributions should be similar (the sample standard deviations can be used to judge whether this is so, although statistics packages usually offer a more formal test).

As it happens, the two-sample *t*-test is fairly tolerant of departures from Normality in the distributions and the need for equal spreads (as a rule-of-thumb, one standard deviation should be no more than twice the other). Authors often don't provide evidence that they have examined the shape of their distributions or the similarity of the spreads before using the two-sample *t*-test, although with large samples the former requirement becomes less crucial. In the event that these requirements for the two-sample *t*-test cannot be satisfied, the Mann–Whitney test (see above) may be used – or the data transformed (see below).

The Matched-Pairs t-Test

With matched or paired data, the matched-pairs *t*-test is used. Both sets of data must be metric, although there is no requirement for either group to have Normally distributed data, but the *differences* between the two sets of data must be Normally distributed, or approximately so. If the Normality of the differences cannot be established, the Wilcoxon (matched-pairs) signed-rank test (see above) is a suitable alternative.

As an example of the decisions that researchers make when choosing an appropriate test, consider the following quote from the authors of Figure 25.1:

> When comparing dichotomous variables in the two treatment groups, we used a two-sided uncorrected χ^2 test. When comparing continuous variables we used a two-sided *t* test, provided that the distributions were sufficiently close to the normal distribution. Otherwise a two-sided Mann–Whitney test was used.
>
> *(Gebre* et al., *2012)*

As an example of the two-sample *t*-test, Figure 27.6 is from a randomised trial comparing laparoscopy-assisted colectomy versus open colectomy for the treatment of non-metastatic colon cancer. The authors used the two-sample *t*-test to compare the differences in means between the two groups for a number of outcomes. Since these outcomes are metric and the groups independent, the two-sample *t*-test is appropriate. The authors do not comment on the shape of any of the distributions in their paper but

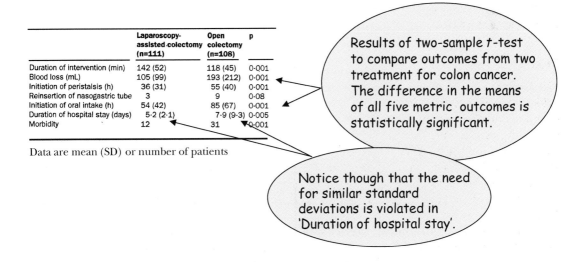

Laparoscopy-assisted colectomy versus open colectomy for treatment of non-metastatic colon cancer: a randomised trial

Antonio M Lacy, Juan C Garcia-Valdecasas, Salvadora Delgado, Antoni Castells, Pilar Taura, Joseph M Pique, Joseph Visa

	Laparoscopy-assisted colectomy (n=111)	Open colectomy (n=108)	p
Duration of intervention (min)	142 (52)	118 (45)	0·001
Blood loss (mL)	105 (99)	193 (212)	0·001
Initiation of peristalsis (h)	36 (31)	55 (40)	0·001
Reinsertion of nasogastric tube	3	9	0·08
Initiation of oral intake (h)	54 (42)	85 (67)	0·001
Duration of hospital stay (days)	5·2 (2·1)	7·9 (9·3)	0·005
Morbidity	12	31	0·001

Data are mean (SD) or number of patients

Results of two-sample *t*-test to compare outcomes from two treatment for colon cancer. The difference in the means of all five metric outcomes is statistically significant.

Notice though that the need for similar standard deviations is violated in 'Duration of hospital stay'.

FIGURE 27.6   Results of two-sample *t*-test to compare outcomes from two treatment for colon cancer. Note that re-insertion of nasogastric tube and morbidity were compared using a χ^2 test. Reprinted from *The Lancet* 359: Lacy AM, Garcia-Valdecasas JC, Delgado S, Castells A, Taura P, Pique JM, *et al.* Laparoscopy-assisted colectomy versus open colectomy for treatment of non-metastatic colon cancer: a randomised trial. 2002; 2224–9, © 2002, with permission from Elsevier.

do provide information on the size of the sample standard deviations. Notice that there is a statistically significant difference for all outcomes shown (all $p < 0.05$).

Transforming Data

Authors can use the Kolmogorov–Smirnov test to examine the hypothesis that a distribution is Normal. If the data turn out not to be Normal (or not Normal-ish), authors can *transform* them to try and achieve approximate Normality before applying the *t*-test. This transformation will often also improve the similarity of the standard deviations. The most common transformation is the $\log_{10}$ transformation, which means that the log to the base 10 of the data is fed into the chosen computer program. The $\log_{10}$ transformation is often more successful in Normalising the data than other possible transformations (such as the square-root transformation), and has the advantage that the back-transformation (by anti-logging) at the end of the analysis can be meaningfully interpreted. It is important to understand that when authors are examining the difference between two means and have log-transformed the data, the back-transformation produces a *ratio*.

For example, imagine we are using the two-sample *t*-test to examine the difference in mean age of male and female trainee nurses in a new intake, and we have had to log-transform the data to make the shape more Normal. Suppose the log results give us a difference in log means (males – females), of 0.078 with a 95% log confidence interval of (0.0715 to 0.0846). When we back-transform by anti-logging we get a

TABLE 27.1   A few of the more common statistical tests

Two-sample *t*-test	Most often used to test for difference in *means* of two *independent* groups. Both sets of data must be metric and Normally distributed, and have similar standard deviations (as a rule of thumb one not more than twice the other).
Matched-pairs *t*-test	Most often used to test for difference in *means* of two *matched* groups. Data must be metric and differences between group scores Normally distributed.
One-way analysis of variance (ANOVA) test	Most often used to test for differences in the means of three or more groups. Data must be metric and Normally distributed in each group, and all standard deviations must be similar.
Mann–Whitney test	Most often used to test whether two independent samples come from the same population distribution. Many computer programs will produce an associated test or confidence interval for the difference in two medians.[a] Data can be either ordinal or metric (any shape distributions but must be similar in each group).
Wilcoxon test	Most often used to test whether the outcome under one condition is no higher, or lower, than the outcome under a second condition. Computer programs will often produce an associated test or confidence interval for the difference in two medians.[b] Data are in matched pairs and can be either ordinal or metric (any shape distribution, but differences in scores must be distributed approximately symmetrically).
Chi-squared (χ^2) test	Most often used to measure whether two variables are *independent* or not; does this by comparing differences in proportions across categories. Data must be categorical and groups independent. When sample size is small, the χ^2 test may not be appropriate. In a two-group, two-category case, Fisher's exact test may be used instead. The same data conditions apply.
Chi-squared (χ^2) test for trend	Most often used to determine whether there is a systematic *trend* in proportions across categories. Data must be categorical and groups independent.
McNemar test	Most often used to measure the difference in *proportions* (or percentages) of two *matched* groups across two categories. Data can be nominal or ordinal.
Kruskal–Wallis test	Most often used to test whether the *medians* of three or more independent groups are the same. Data can be ordinal or metric (any shape distributions but must be similar in each group).

[a]Can be thought of as a test for the difference in medians of two independent groups.
[b]Can be thought of as a test for the difference in medians of two matched groups.

Randomised, controlled trial of efficacy of midwife-managed care

Deborah Turnbull, Ann Holmes, Noreen Shields, Helen Cheyne, Sara Twaddle, W Harper Gilmour, Mary McGinley, Margaret Reid, Irene Johnstone, Ian Geer, Gillian McIlwaine, C Burnett Lunan

Analyses were done for the original groups of allocation (intention to treat). Categorical data were analysed by χ^2 tests. Where appropriate, the χ^2 test for trend was used to test for a linear trend in the relative proportions in each care group. . . 95% CI that do not bracket zero indicate a statistically significant difference at (at least) the 5% level. Mean values were compared by two-sample t tests. p values of less than 0.05 are taken to be statistically significant. All differences are presented as the value of shared care minus that for midwife-managed care.

The authors here provide brief details of the statistical methods used, including confidence intervals, and χ^2 and two-sample t-tests, . . .

. . . and specify a p-value of less than 0.05 for significance.

FIGURE 27.7   Description by authors of types of statistical tests used in a midwife-managed care study. Reprinted from *The Lancet* 348: Turnbull D, Holmes A, Shields N, Cheyne H, Twaddle S, Gilmour WH, *et al*. Randomised, controlled trial of efficacy of midwife-managed care. 1996; 213–8, © 1996, with permission from Elsevier.

difference in means of 1.197 with a 95% confidence interval of (1.179 to 1.215). The correct interpretation of this result is that the mean age of the male nurses is 19.7% *greater* than the mean age of the female nurses, with a 95% confidence interval for the *ratio* of mean ages of from 17.9% older to 21.5% older.

Finally . . .

There are many different statistical tests which you may see in clinical journals. Obviously, we can only discuss a few of the most commonly used. Specialist areas of clinical research will use more specialist tests. The more common tests in the generalist journals are described very briefly in Table 27.1, along with the required data type and distributional (shape) requirements.

Note that the first two tests in Table 27.1 (the two-sample and matched-pairs *t*-tests), are *parametric* tests. That is, they have precise distributional requirements – data needs to be Normally distributed. The remaining tests in the table are *non-parametric* – they have no such precise distributional requirements. In short, the authors should tell you which tests they have used (and why) to get the results they present. With the help of Table 27.1 you should be able to judge whether the chosen test is appropriate.

As an example of authors' description of their choices, Figure 27.7 is from a randomised controlled trial to compare the clinical efficacy of midwife-managed care (midwife only) for pregnant women, with shared care (midwives plus doctors). The Methods section contains a brief summary of the statistical methods employed.

VII

Analysing the Data:
Multivariable Methods

28

Measuring Association

The various types of statistical analysis we have considered so far have involved only a *single* variable, usually measured in two or more groups, such as cholesterol levels in statin and non-statin groups, the degree of stump pain in treatment and placebo groups, diverticular disease in vegetarians and non-vegetarians, and so on. On many occasions, however, researchers want to measure the degree of 'connection' or *association* between *two* or more variables; by 'association' we mean the way that two variables appear to move together, either in the same direction or in opposite directions. For example, weight of baby and weight of mother, or coronary heart disease and hypertension. In this chapter, we will focus on measuring the association between two variables.

In Chapter 29 we will look at ways in which the *agreement* between two variables can be assessed, and in Chapters 30 and 31 we will deal with the inter-relatedness between *more* than two variables. To illustrate the idea the idea of association, suppose a trainee paramedic assesses the Glasgow Coma Scale score of 10 patients. His supervisor simultaneously scores the same patients. Their scores are:

Patient	1	2	3	4	5	6	7	8	9	10
Trainee	5	9	3	7	8	5	4	9	7	5
Supervisor	4	8	2	5	8	4	2	8	6	5

We can see that when the supervisor scores high, the trainee also tends to score high. When the supervisor scores low, the trainee tends to score low. The two sets of scores seem to be positively associated because high scores by one correspond with high scores by the other, and low scores with low scores. (Note though that the degree of actual agreement is poor.)

The opposite situation (high scores with low scores) is called *negative association* (we will come to an example of this shortly). The *strength* of any association between sets of scores will vary from non-existent or weak, through moderate, to strong, and, as above, may be either positive or negative. So how can we measure it?

MEASURING ASSOCIATION

The Scatter Diagram

One simple, but non-quantitative method authors sometimes use for getting an initial feel about the strength and direction (positive or negative) of an association is to plot a *scatter diagram* (or scatterplot) of the data. If we do this for the Glasgow Coma Scale scores, we get the graph shown in Figure 28.1.

For a real example, Figure 28.2 is taken from a study into hospital league tables. The scatter diagram shows the percentage mortality from aortic aneurysm in each of 18 hospitals, plotted against the annual

Understanding Clinical Papers, Third Edition. David Bowers, Allan House, David Owens and Bridgette Bewick.
© 2014 John Wiley & Sons, Ltd. Published 2014 by John Wiley & Sons, Ltd.

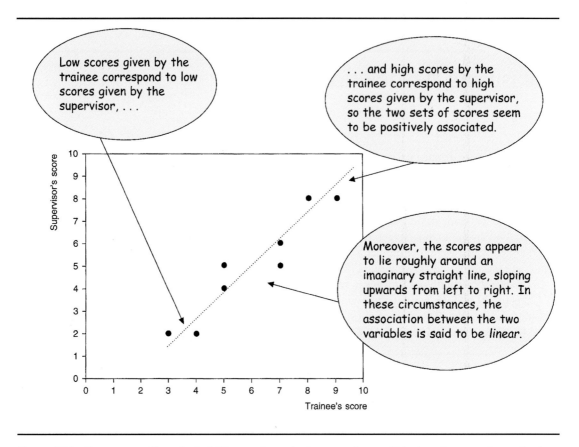

FIGURE 28.1   Scattergram of hypothetical Glasgow Coma Scale scores given to 10 patients by supervisor and trainee paramedic.

number of episodes of this condition treated by each hospital. It is apparent that the two variables are *negatively* associated (negatively, because the scatter slopes down from left to right). In general, hospitals that dealt with low numbers of episodes had high mortality rates, hospitals with high numbers of episodes had low mortality rates (one possible explanation for this is that the more experience the hospital had in dealing with the condition, the better they are at it and *vice versa*).

The *strength* of any association is related to how close the points are to lying on an imaginary straight line drawn through the scatter. The closer they are, the stronger and the more *linear* the association (more on linear relationships in Chapter 30). If all the points fell *exactly* on the line, the association would be described as perfect. Of course, with sample data this never happens. With the aortic aneurysm data (if we disregard the point lying on the horizontal axis, as being a possible anomaly), then we can imagine a straight line drawn through the scatter, which would slope down from left to right, but clearly not all of the points can fall on this line.

This idea may be clearer in Figure 28.3, taken from a study on the usefulness of a general practitioner's documentation of obesity, which compared the patients' own *estimation* of their body mass index (BMI) with an accurate *measurement* taken in a clinic. The two sets of measurements seem to be strongly positively associated, with low estimated body mass indexes associated with low measured BMIs and high with high. The 'best' straight line drawn through the points shows that the majority of them lie close to the line, indicating a *linear* (or straight-line) association.

Mortality league tables: do they inform or mislead?

Martin McKee, Duncan Hunter

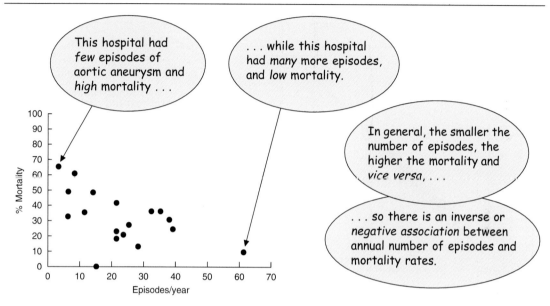

Fig 3   Relation between volume and outcome for aortic aneurysm

---

FIGURE 28.2   Scattergram of percentage mortality from aortic aneurysm in 16 hospitals against number of episodes dealt with per year. Reproduced from McKee M, Hunter D. Mortality league tables: do they inform or mislead? *Quality in Health Care* 1995, 4: 5–12, © 1995, with permission from BMJ Publishing Group Ltd.

However, eyeballing a scatter diagram to judge the strength of an association, although often insightful, suffers limitations (e.g. when we want to judge the *relative* strengths of two or more associations). For this reason, researchers usually employ a *quantitative* measure.

THE CORRELATION COEFFICIENT

The correlation coefficient is the most widely used quantitative measure of association. It is a single numeric measure of the strength of the *linear* association between two variables. (Bear in mind that there may well be a strong association between two variables which is *not* linear – it might be curved for example, but a correlation coefficient of the type discussed here may not detect this as a strong association – or any association at all.) Authors most often use either *Pearson's* correlation coefficient (denoted r) or *Spearman's* correlation coefficient (denoted r_s or rho (ρ)), both of which are similarly interpreted. Both r and r_s can vary between -1 (indicating perfect negative association) and $+1$ (indicating perfect positive association). The further away from 0 the coefficient is (in either direction), the stronger the association.

The choice between r and r_s depends on the type of data and the shape of the distributions. To calculate Pearson's r, and obtain a confidence interval, both sets of data should be metric and (approximately)

GP documentation of obesity: what does it achieve?

PAUL LITTLE

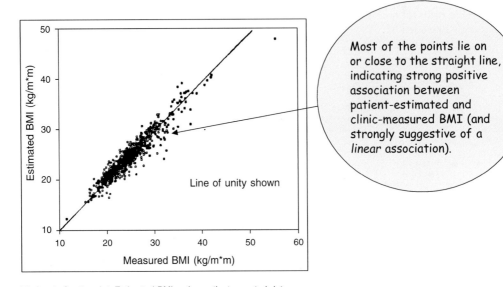

Figure 1. Scatter plot. Estimated BMI: using patient reported data. Measured BMI: using staiometer and scales.

FIGURE 28.3 Scattergram of estimated against measured BMI. Reprinted from Little P. GP documentation of obesity: what does it achieve? *British Journal of General Practice* 1998, 48: 890–4, with permission from the Royal College of General Practitioners.

Normally distributed. If the data are metric but not Normal, or if either variable is ordinal, Spearman's rank-based coefficient r_s should be used. So you need to be told what type of data the authors have used and what shape the distributions have.

The correlation coefficients r and r_s, calculated from sample data, are of course only *estimates* of the true (population) correlation coefficients. To determine whether or not the population correlation coefficients are significant (i.e. not 0), authors can either present confidence intervals or p-values, with the usual rules for significance applying (i.e. confidence intervals not including 0 or $p < 0.05$; see Chapters 25 and 27).

As an example, Figure 28.4 is from an ecological study (see Chapter 6) to investigate how far international variations in infant mortality in the past predict today's adult mortality from stomach cancer, stroke, and other causes. The hypothesis was that *Helicobacter pylori* is a key factor in non-cardiac stomach cancer. *H. pylori* is thought to be acquired in childhood and risk of infection is closely related to living conditions such as hygiene, which can be related to infant mortality. Since infant mortality rates and death rates are both metric, Pearson's r is appropriate, provided that both sets of data are also Normally distributed (unfortunately there is no evidence that the authors have addressed this distributional issue).

In the next (cross-sectional) example (Figure 28.5), the authors were investigating the link between breast size and hormone levels, body constitution, and oral contraceptive use. Although all the variables

Infant mortality, stomach cancer, stroke, and coronary heart disease: ecological analysis

David A Leon, George Davey Smith

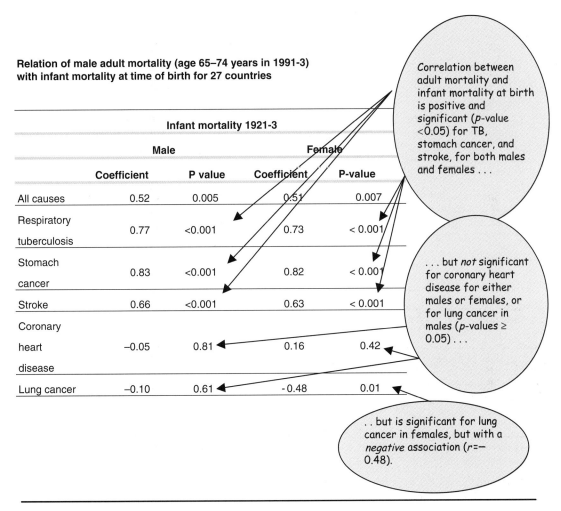

Relation of male adult mortality (age 65–74 years in 1991-3) with infant mortality at time of birth for 27 countries

	Infant mortality 1921-3			
	Male		Female	
	Coefficient	P value	Coefficient	P-value
All causes	0.52	0.005	0.51	0.007
Respiratory tuberculosis	0.77	<0.001	0.73	< 0.001
Stomach cancer	0.83	<0.001	0.82	< 0.001
Stroke	0.66	<0.001	0.63	< 0.001
Coronary heart disease	−0.05	0.81	0.16	0.42
Lung cancer	−0.10	0.61	- 0.48	0.01

Correlation between adult mortality and infant mortality at birth is positive and significant (*p*-value <0.05) for TB, stomach cancer, and stroke, for both males and females . . .

. . . but *not* significant for coronary heart disease for either males or females, or for lung cancer in males (*p*-values ≥ 0.05) . . .

. . but is significant for lung cancer in females, but with a *negative* association (*r*=− 0.48).

FIGURE 28.4 Pearson correlation coefficients (and *p*-values) between adult mortality in 1991–1993 and infant mortality at birth for 27 developed countries. (Abbreviated by current authors.) Reproduced from Leon DA, Smith GD. Infant mortality, stomach cancer, stroke, and coronary heart disease: ecological analysis. *BMJ* 2000, 320: 1705–6, © 2000, with permission from BMJ Publishing Group Ltd.

concerned (except for family history of breast cancer) are metric continuous, they have used Spearman's r_s to measure association, perhaps because of doubts about the Normality of the variables. Their results are shown in Figure 28.5. The authors have chosen to use *p*-values rather than confidence intervals to test the significance of their correlations.

Figure 28.5 shows that, apart from BMI among non-oral contraceptive users, breast size appears to have no connection with most of these physical measurements. It is not surprising that *weight* has an association

Breast Size in Relation to Endogenous Hormone Levels, Body Constitution, and Oral Contraceptive Use in Healthy Nulligravid Women Aged 19–25 Years

Helena Jernström and Håkan Olsson

In 'Never users' of oral contraceptives the Spearman r_S between breast size and body mass index (BMI) is +0.47.

Only BMI and *weight* are significantly associated with breast size among this group (p-values < 0.05).

Breast size is not significantly associated with any of the variables among current oral contraceptive users (all p-values ≥ 0.05).

TABLE 6. Spearman rank correlations (r_S) between breast sizes in healthy Swedish female university students, according to oral contraceptive use and body mass index, height, weight, family history of breast cancer, age at menarche, and age, 1993–1994*

	Oral contraceptive use							
	Never users (n=20)		Former users (n=20)		All nonusers (n=40)		Current users (n=25)	
	r_S	p	r_S	p	r_S	p	r_S	p
Body mass index[†]	0.47	0.038	0.71	<0.001	0.53	<0.001	0.27	0.196
Height	0.25	0.286	0.42	0.068	0.32	0.046	−0.06	0.783
Weight	0.47	0.037	0.55	0.011	0.50	0.001	0.24	0.248
Family history of breast cancer in a first or second degree relative	−0.17	0.473	−0.41	0.071	−0.24	0.131	0.01	0.951
Age at menarche	−0.23	0.329	0.03	0.889	−0.06	0.735	−0.08	0.707
Waist:hip ratio	−0.00	0.985	0.35	0.133	0.18	0.256	0.25	0.226
Age	0.09	0.718	−0.20	0.396	−0.04	0.814	0.15	0.480

* Values from measurements taken during menstrual cycle days 5–10 were used.
[†] Weight (kg)/height (m)^2.

FIGURE 28.5 Spearman correlation coefficients between breast size and a number of factors according to oral contraceptive use. Reproduced from Jernström H, Olsson H. Breast size in relation to endogenous hormone levels, body constitution, and oral contraceptive use in healthy nulligravid women aged 19–25 years. *American Journal of Epidemiology* 1997, 45: 571–80, by permission of Oxford University Press.

if BMI does since the two are linearly related through the formula for BMI (as noted in the table footnote). But again it's not clear which correlation coefficient has been used for the association between breast size and the family history of breast cancer variable, which is dichotomous (yes/no), and for which Spearman's r_s is not suitable. To sum up, whenever you read a paper containing correlation calculations, you should be able to tell which correlation coefficient has been used for which data.

Finally, it is very important to note that correlation implies nothing about *causality* – whether there is a *relationship* (as opposed to simply an association) between any two variables. By 'relationship' we mean do changes in one variable bring about or *cause* subsequent changes in the other variable, and if so, in what way? To answer these questions we need multivariable methods, which we will come to in Chapter 30.

We noted at the beginning of this chapter that association and agreement measure two different things. Association measures the degree to which two sets of values tend to move *together*. Agreement measures the degree to which the values are actually the *same*. However, even if two variables are *associated*, they may not *agree* very well (although if two variables agree they will clearly be associated). Spearman's r_s for the Glasgow Coma Scale scores given in the example at the beginning of this chapter was $+0.962$ with a 95% confidence interval of (0.844 to 0.991). So the association between the scores is strong. However, the percentage of scores which agree is only 20% (2 in 10), so agreement is poor.

We can now turn to the methods used by authors to measure agreement.

29

Measuring Agreement

Health professionals often want to compare two methods of measuring something, such as blood glucose or obesity – they may want to see if a new method (perhaps cheaper and easier) can be used to replace an existing method or if the two methods are perhaps interchangeable. Alternatively, they may want to know how closely two (or more) people (referred to in the literature as 'observers' or 'raters') score some clinical characteristic among a groups of patients. In either case, they will want to know what the level of *agreement* is between the methods, or between the raters. In Chapter 28 we looked at correlation as a means of measuring the level of *association* between two variables, and we noted that association *and* agreement are not the same. In this chapter we are going to examine how clinical papers deal with *agreement* and what you need to look out for. As usual the type of data involved influences the choice of measure. We will start with nominal data.

NOMINAL DATA: COHEN'S KAPPA (κ)

Suppose you ask two nurses to examine separately 10 patients and state, yes or no, whether they need a particular treatment (this is an example of inter-rater agreement). The hypothetical results are:

Patient	1	2	3	4	5	6	7	8	9	10
Nurse A	Y	Y	Y	N	Y	N	N	Y	Y	N
Nurse B	N	Y	Y	Y	Y	N	N	N	Y	Y

The nurses agreed with each other on six patients, but disagreed on four. So their *observed proportional agreement* was 6/10 = 0.6 (or 60%). However, we would have expected them to agree by chance on a few of them anyway, even if they had to take a wild guess without even seeing the patients.

What we need is a measure that adjusts the observed agreement for the number of agreements which are due to chance. This is what *Cohen's κ* does. Cohen's κ measures the proportion of scores that agree (i.e. fall in the same category) *adjusted* for the proportion that could be expected to agree by chance. It is properly known as the *chance-corrected proportional agreement* statistic. (We have already encountered the use of κ to measure agreement by means of test–retest reliability in Chapter 20 in the context of measurement scales.)

Understanding Clinical Papers, Third Edition. David Bowers, Allan House, David Owens and Bridgette Bewick.
© 2014 John Wiley & Sons, Ltd. Published 2014 by John Wiley & Sons, Ltd.

TABLE 29.1   Assessing agreement with κ

κ	Strength of agreement
<0.20	Poor
0.21–0.40	Fair
0.41–0.60	Moderate
0.61–0.80	Good
0.81–1.00	Very good

Interpreting κ

Cohen's κ can vary between 0 (no agreement) and 1 (perfect agreement). Values of κ may be assessed with the help of Table 29.1 (although there is no general agreement on the use of these values and they have no firm analytic foundation). Only values for κ of about 0.60 or more might be considered as indicative of good agreement. In general, variables which are found to be firmly associated will *usually* show good agreement and *vice versa*, although, since this is not invariably the case, the methods are not interchangeable.

One weakness of κ is that it is sensitive to the proportion of subjects in each category, in other words, to prevalence. The consequence of this is that κ values from different studies should not be compared if the prevalences are not the same. Cohen's κ is also inversely sensitive to the number of categories being compared, increasing as the number of categories diminishes. Cohen's κ has many applications, and two typical examples are given below.

Figure 29.1 is taken from a study exploring differences in agreement between Thai couples on their sexual behaviour in the past 12 months, according to their respective HIV status. In one group both partners were HIV-positive, in the other group only one of the partners was. Figure 29.1 shows the levels of both of the couples total percent observed agreement and of their chance-corrected (κ) agreement. As you can see, although total observed percent agreement between the groups was quite similar, overall chance-corrected agreement was quite different.

Figure 29.2 is from a study into the effects of passive smoking on coronary heart disease. The authors used κ to test the *reliability* of data on exposure to risk factors as reported by the subjects in the study. From the original sample of 185, 35 subjects were re-interviewed and their responses were compared with their original responses (this procedure is known as *test–retest*). κ was used to measure the level of agreement between first and second interviews.

ORDINAL DATA: WEIGHTED κ

With ordinal data researchers can calculate a version of κ which is adjusted (or *weighted*) to allow for 'near misses'. This idea is best illustrated with an example. Two experienced trauma doctors were asked to rate 16 patients using the Injury Severity Score (ISS), a scale for assessing the severity of trauma, varying from 0 to 75. The data are shown in Table 29.2 (abbreviated by the present authors). The doctors agree on only five out of 16 cases, so the level of exact agreement is low (Zoltie and de Dombal, 1993).

You can see that some scores are quite different (e.g. Patients 9 and 15). Some scores, although not identical, are close (e.g. Patients 2 and 6). Weighted κ gives credit to these near misses and less credit to those further apart. The frequency with which weighted κ appears in clinical papers does not justify any further discussion here.

Reliability of Self-Reported Sexual Behaviour in Human Immunodeficiency Virus (HIV) Between Concordant and Discordant Heterosexual Couples in Northern Thailand

Melanie A. de Boer, David D. Celentano, Sodsai Tovanabutra, Sungwal Rugpao, Kenrad E. Nelson, and Vinai Suriyanon

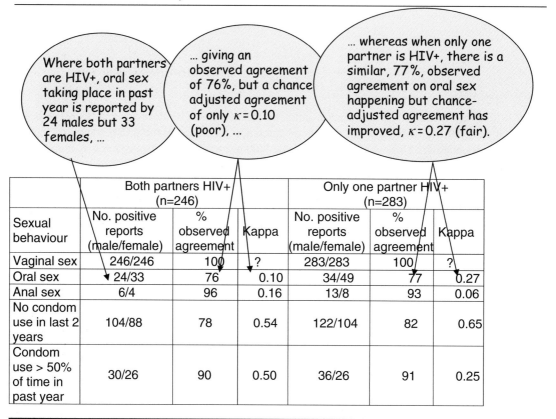

Where both partners are HIV+, oral sex taking place in past year is reported by 24 males but 33 females, ...

... giving an observed agreement of 76%, but a chance adjusted agreement of only $\kappa = 0.10$ (poor), ...

... whereas when only one partner is HIV+, there is a similar, 77%, observed agreement on oral sex happening but chance-adjusted agreement has improved, $\kappa = 0.27$ (fair).

Sexual behaviour	Both partners HIV+ (n=246)			Only one partner HIV+ (n=283)		
	No. positive reports (male/female)	% observed agreement	Kappa	No. positive reports (male/female)	% observed agreement	Kappa
Vaginal sex	246/246	100	?	283/283	100	?
Oral sex	24/33	76	0.10	34/49	77	0.27
Anal sex	6/4	96	0.16	13/8	93	0.06
No condom use in last 2 years	104/88	78	0.54	122/104	82	0.65
Condom use > 50% of time in past year	30/26	90	0.50	36/26	91	0.25

FIGURE 29.1   Agreement between partners of sexual behaviour in the past year by HIV status. Reproduced from de Boer MA, Celentano DD, Tovanabutra S, Rugpao S, Nelson KE Suriyanon V. Reliability of self-reported sexual behaviour in human immunodeficiency virus (HIV) between concordant and discordant heterosexual couples in Northern Thailand. *American Journal of Epidemiology* 1998, 147: 1153–6, by permission of Oxford University Press.

METRIC DATA

Unfortunately there is no single statistic which researchers can use to report agreement between two metric variables. Cohen's κ is of little use since the large number of possible values means that there will be few, if any, pairs of values which are exactly the same. And as we have seen, correlation does not do the same job. One method has been suggested by Bland and Altman (1986). This involves plotting the *differences* between each pair of scores (vertical axis) against their mean (horizontal axis).

Passive smoking at work as a risk factor for coronary heart disease in Chinese women who have never smoked

Y He, T H Lam, L S Li, R Y Du, G L Jia, J Y Huang, J S Zheng

Results on single blind test-re-test by two inter-viewers on 35 hospital subjects (16 cases and 19 controls) showed good agreement, ranging from 75% to 95% for the 10 risk factors tested, with κ values ranging from 0.4 to 0.8 (nine κ values with P<0.01 and one with P<0.05; data not shown).

In this example κ is used to test the reliability of patient-recorded data, by re-interviewing a subsample of the original sample. This is the test–retest procedure.

FIGURE 29.2   Extract from a passive smoking study with the authors' description of using κ for measuring agreement in a test–retest. Reproduced from He Y, Lam TH, Li LS, Du RY, Jia GL, Huang JY, *et al.* Passive smoking at work as a risk factor for coronary heart disease in Chinese women who have never smoked. *BMJ* 1994, 308: 380–4, © 2000, with permission from BMJ Publishing Group Ltd.

In this plot, points showing perfect agreement will lie exactly on the horizontal line drawn through the value 0. The further away the points are from this line, the worse the level of agreement. Moreover, the points should be scattered more or less between horizontal tramlines – an indication that the level of agreement is approximately the same over the whole range of values.

One way of assessing the acceptability of the agreement level is to calculate the standard deviation of the difference scores and then draw two horizontal lines at ± 2 times this standard deviation. If most of the points lie within these tramlines, then agreement between the two measures may be deemed acceptable.

As an example of the Bland–Altman procedure, Figure 29.3 is from a study to assess the accuracy and reliability of two non-invasive thermometers – a chemical thermometer and a tympanic thermometer – by comparing them to the 'gold standard' pulmonary artery catheter (PAC). Temperature data are metric and the authors show two Bland–Altman plots to measure agreement between the PAC and the chemical and tympanic thermometers respectively. The authors have added the ± 2 standard deviation (SD) tramlines.

As you can see, the agreement of the PAC with the chemical thermometer is slightly biased by $+0.2\,°C$ (chemical thermometer measuring $+0.2\,°C$ more than the PAC), but overall agreement is closer, 2

TABLE 29.2   ISS scores given by two observers to 16 trauma patients

Doctor	Patient															
	1	2	3	4	5	6	7	8	9	10	11	12	13	14	15	16
1	9	14	29	17	34	17	38	29	4	29	25	4	16	25	25	45
2	9	13	29	17	22	14	45	10	29	4	25	34	9	25	8	50

Temperature measurement: comparison of non-invasive methods used in adult critical care

Sarah Farnell, Loraine Maxwell, Seok Tan, Andrew Rhodes, and Barbara Philips

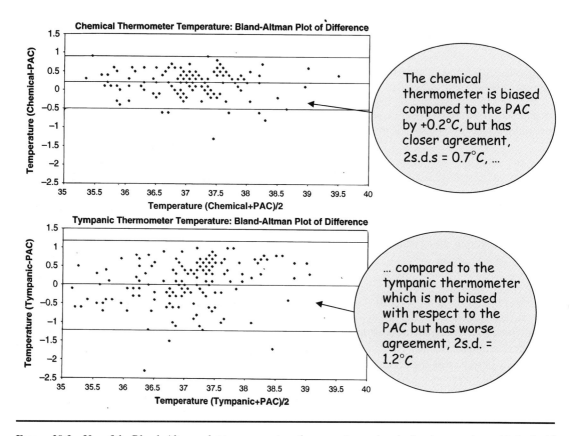

FIGURE 29.3   Use of the Bland–Altman plot to compare two thermometers – chemical and tympanic – with the 'gold standard' pulmonary artery catheter (PAC). Reproduced from Farnell S, Maxwell L, Tan S, Rhodes A, Philips B (2005) with permission from John Wiley & Sons.

SD = 0.7 °C, compared to the tympanic thermometer's 2 SD = 1.2 °C, although the latter is unbiased. There is no evidence that agreement deteriorates over the range of either instrument.

We indicated towards the end of Chapter 28 that we would need to turn to methods which authors can use to investigate causal relationships between variables (rather than associations). That is what we will do in Chapter 30. However, before we leave the subject of agreement, we want to emphasise once again that using correlation to measure agreement is not appropriate. Correlation is a measure of association *not* a measure of agreement.

30

Linear Regression

WHY REGRESSION?

We noted towards the end of Chapter 28 that association does not imply causation. If we were to examine the association between blood pressure and body mass index (BMI), we would most likely find that the two measures were positively correlated; in general, the larger the BMI the greater the blood pressure and *vice versa*. But this association does not *necessarily* mean that it is increased BMI which *causes* increased blood pressure nor that having high blood pressure *causes* high values of body mass index. We can only say that the two are associated.

The χ^2 test is similarly disadvantaged – it will tell us whether two categorical variables are related or not, but it does not indicate anything about the nature of any relationship, the existence or direction of causality, or any size effects. So both correlation and χ^2, although useful procedures, have limitations.

In practice, of course, if researchers suspect a causal relationship between one variable and another, they will also have a belief about the direction of that relationship (e.g. high BMI is a possible *cause* of high blood pressure, but not the other way round).

To investigate such causal relationships they can turn to a powerful family of modelling procedures, collectively known as *multivariable analysis*, which includes *regression analysis*, a procedure which you will come across quite frequently in clinical papers. In these three chapters we want to discuss three different types of regression: *linear* regression (in this chapter), *logistic* regression (in Chapter 31), and *proportional*, or Cox, regression (in Chapter 32, in the context of survival analysis). We must also give a passing mention to *analysis of variance*, related to regression, as you will see, and popular in psychology.

The ideas examined in this chapter are a little more complex than some of the other material in this book. Unfortunately, to understand journal papers which present the results of regression analysis, and to point out what you as a reader need to look out for, we must spend at least a little time discussing some of the basic ideas. We have, as usual, tried to avoid being too technical.

LINEAR REGRESSION

To state the blindingly obvious, regression analysis is done with a *regression model* – a mathematical equation which captures the nature and direction of a causal relationship between one variable and one or more other variables.

To illustrate the general idea, suppose your favourite clinic pastime is to guess each patient's systolic blood pressure (SBP), before you measure it. To your colleagues' surprise, your guesses are quite good, but they do not know that it is all down to a bit of mental arithmetic (but based on having seen a lot of patients). Here's how you do it. For every patient, you always start with the number 4, to which you add

Understanding Clinical Papers, Third Edition. David Bowers, Allan House, David Owens and Bridgette Bewick.
© 2014 John Wiley & Sons, Ltd. Published 2014 by John Wiley & Sons, Ltd.

their age (which you know from their record) multiplied by 1.5; then add their hip girth in centimetres (which you have grown very good at estimating by eye) multiplied by a quarter; then add 10 if they are male; and a further 10 if they are smokers (which you also know from the record). Let us write your mental sum as an equation:

$$SBP \text{ (mmHg)} = 4 + (1.5 \times age) + (0.25 \times hip\ girth) + (10 \times sex) + (10 \times smoker),$$

where *sex* will equal 0 if female and 1 if male, and *smoker* will equal 0 if a non-smoker and 1 if a smoker.

This equation is called a *multivariable linear regression equation* or model. The *model* is said to be *multi*variable because there is more than one variable on the right-hand side of the equation, in this example *age, hip girth, sex*, and *smoker*. These right-hand-side variables are called the *independent*, or *explanatory*, or *predictor* variables, or the *covariates*. These may be metric, ordinal, or nominal. The variable to the left of the 'equals' sign (*SBP* in this example) is called the *outcome, dependent*, or *response* variable and must be metric continuous. The numeric values in front of each variable (e.g. 1.5, 0.25, 10, and 10) are called the *sample regression coefficients*. The value of 4 which stands alone at the beginning of the equation is called the *constant* coefficient and is usually ignored – the only role it plays is to keep an arithmetic balance between the left- and right-hand sides of the regression equation.

Finally, the model is said to be *linear* because we assume here that the effect on systolic blood pressure of an increase in age, say, from 50 to 51, is the same as for age increases from 90 to 91 or 20 to 21, or any other 1-year increase. In other words, the effect of a change in age on systolic blood pressure remains the same right across the age range, and if we were to plot systolic blood pressure against age we would observe that the points were scattered evenly around a straight line, as we saw in Figure 28.1. This linearity property needs also to be true for each of the metric independent variables.

To see how this equation works, if the next patient is a 50-year-old non-smoking male, with a hip girth of 240 cm, then you would estimate his systolic blood pressure to be:

$$SBP = 4 + (1.5 \times 50) + (0.25 \times 240) + (10 \times 1) + (10 \times 0) = 4 + 75 + 60 + 10 + 0 = 149 \text{ mmHg}.$$

In practice, we have to add an uncertainty term (called the *error* or *residual* term, denoted *e*) to the regression equation. However good you are at this guessing game, you can never account for random variations and so you are never likely to be spot on (except coincidentally). So the residual term accounts for the difference between what your model predicts for systolic blood pressure and its true value. If we abbreviate the other variable names, we can summarize the main components of the linear regression model as in Figure 30.1.

The value and sign of each coefficient gives us an *estimate* of the magnitude and direction of the change in the dependent variable if the corresponding independent variable increases by one unit. For example, in our systolic blood pressure model, if age increases by 1 year (age is measured in units of 1 year) then systolic blood pressure will also *increase* (because the sign of the age coefficient is *positive*) by 1.5 mmHg.

In more general terms, the *population* multiple linear regression equation is written as:

$$Y = \beta_0 + \beta_1 \times X_1 + \beta_2 \times X_2 + \ldots + e,$$

where X_1, X_2, and so on, are the independent variables (*age, hip girth*, etc.), and β_1, β_2, and so on, are called the *population regression coefficients*, and we have to estimate their value using sample data, just as we have to estimate the population mean or population proportion. In our blood pressure example, the *sample regression coefficients* 1.5, 0.25, 10, and 10 are our estimates of the population regression coefficients β_1, β_2, β_3, and β_4. In practice, of course, we cannot simply guess these values but have to use some systematic estimation procedure.

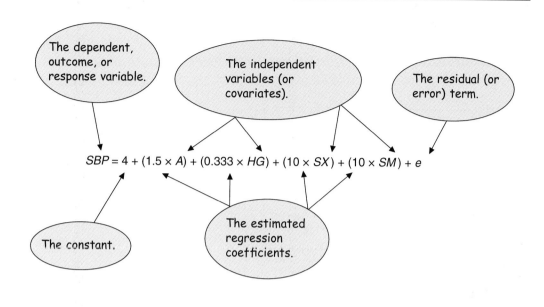

FIGURE 30.1   The main components of a linear regression model.

Estimating the Regression Coefficients – Ordinary Least Squares Estimation

Authors will not usually refer to the estimation process they use, but commonly it will be the method of *ordinary least squares* (OLS). Briefly put, OLS calculates values for the sample regression coefficients which minimizes the sum of all the squared error terms (i.e. minimises $\sum e^2$). The regression equation which is produced by this method gives the 'best' estimates of the population regression coefficients (i.e. at least as close to the true population coefficient values as any other method). The idea is illustrated in Figure 30.2. This shows a regression line drawn through a scatter plot of birthweight against cord serum eicosapentaenoic (EPA) concentration and shows the position of just one of the error terms (there is of course one for each infant).

MEASURING THE STATISTICAL SIGNIFICANCE OF THE REGRESSION PARAMETERS

Since the sample regression coefficients (such as 1.5, 0.333, 10, and 10, in our blood pressure example above) are only *estimates* of the true population parameter coefficients β_1, β_2, and so on, we need to know whether or not each of these parameters is statistically significant. Crucially, are they significantly different from 0? Obviously, if a population regression coefficient is 0, then the independent variable with which it is associated cannot possibly have *any* influence on the dependent variable – it doesn't matter what value this variable takes, once it's multiplied by 0, it drops out. Of course, even if a *population* coefficient is 0, it doesn't mean (samples being what they are) that its sample coefficient will be 0 (and in practice it *never* is). That's why researchers need to assess the statistical significance of each coefficient.

You won't be surprised to learn that they do this either by calculating a confidence interval for each sample coefficient or a p-value. If either the confidence interval does *not* contain 0 or $p < 0.05$, then that

Birthweight in a fishing community: significance of essential fatty acids and marine food contaminants

Philippe Grandjean, Kristian S Bjerve, Pál Weihe and Ulrike Steuerwald

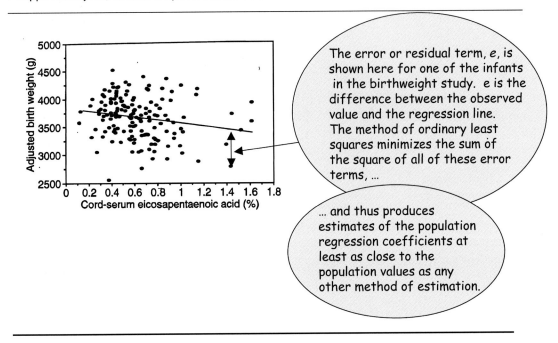

FIGURE 30.2   Scatter plot of birthweight against cord serum EPA acid concentration. EPA concentration is a measure of the availability of polyunsaturated fatty acids to the foetus and is thought to influence foetal growth. Reproduced from Grandjean P, Bjerve KS, Weihe P, Steuerwald U. Birthweight in a fishing community: significance of essential fatty acids and marine food contaminants. *International Journal of Epidemiology* 2000, 30: 1272–7, by permission of Oxford University Press.

variable's population coefficient is probably not 0 and the variable can have a significant influence on the dependent variable.

So when you read a paper which uses linear regression you should be able to find in the table of results either the *p*-value for each coefficient, or better, a confidence interval. By the way, establishing significance in a regression model does not prove causality. The causal nature of a relationship (if any) depends on the inherent nature of the variables and has to be plausibly argued.

MODEL BUILDING AND VARIABLE SELECTION

At the beginning of this chapter we knew which variables were needed to predict the systolic blood pressure of a patient. In practice, researchers will usually have some idea, some working hypothesis, about which independent variables they think will play a role in explaining the variation in their outcome variable. How certain they are about this will influence their variable selection procedure (starting with a list of candidate variables) (i.e. how they build their regression model). Authors should describe their model building procedure so we need to say a few words about the possibilities.

There are two main approaches. First, *automated* variable selection – the computer does it for you. This approach is perhaps more appropriate if you uncertain about which variables are likely to be relevant in the relationship. A second possibility is *manual* selection – you do it! This approach is more appropriate if you have a particular hypothesis to test, so that you have a pretty good idea which independent variable is likely to be the most interesting in explaining your outcome variable. At the same time you may want to adjust for other, potentially confounding, variables (see Chapter 13 for an account of confounding). Being able to take care of potential confounding variables is one of the great strengths (and attractions) of the regression model.

What follows is a very brief description of some of the variable selection procedures, starting with automated methods first. Note that the criteria used by the various computer regression programs to select and de-select variables vary from program to program. Most of these methods start with a series of *univariable* regressions (i.e. each independent variable in turn is regressed separately against the outcome variable and the *p*-value noted). At this stage all variables which have $p \leq 0.2$, or thereabouts, should be identified – using a *p*-value less than this may fail to identify variables which could turn out to be important in the final model.

Automated Variable Selection Methods

- *Forwards selection.* The computer program starts by including on the right-hand side of the model the variable which has the lowest *p*-value (from the univariable regressions). It then adds the other variables one at a time, in lowest *p*-value order, until all variables with $p < 0.05$ are included.
- *Backwards selection.* The reverse of forwards selection! The program starts with all of the candidate variables included in the model, then the variable which has highest $p > 0.05$ is removed. Then the next highest *p*-value variable and so on, until only those variables with $p < 0.05$ are left in the model and all other variables have been discarded.
- *Forward or backward stepwise selection.* After each variable is added (or removed), the variables which were already (or are left) in the model are re-checked for statistical significance; if no longer significant they are removed. The end result is a model where all variables have $p < 0.05$.

These automated procedures have a number of potential disadvantages (including misleadingly narrow confidence intervals and exaggerated coefficient values, and thus their effect size), although they may be useful when researchers have little idea about which variables are likely to be relevant. As an example of this approach the authors of a study into the role of arginase in sickle cell disease, in which the outcome variable was $\log_{10}$ arginase activity (transformed because of distributional shape problems), comment:

> This modeling used a stepwise procedure to add independent variables, beginning with the variables most strongly associated with $\log_{10}$ arginase with $p \leq 0.15$ .... Deletion of variables after initial inclusion in the model was allowed. The procedure continued until all independent variables in the final model had $p \leq 0.05$, adjusted for other independent variables, and no additional variables had $p \leq 0.05$. (Morris *et al.*, 2005)

Manual Variable Selection Methods

These methods are often more appropriate if the investigators are trying to explore the relationship between two variables, say between birthweight (the outcome variable) and mother's weight (the main independent variable), and wish to *adjust* for any possible confounding variables, such as sex of baby, smoking during pregnancy, mother's age, and so on. The identity of potential confounders will have been established by experience, a literature search, discussions with colleagues and users. There are two alternative manual selection procedures:

- *Backward elimination.* The main independent variable plus all of the potentially confounding variables are entered into the model at the start, and the regression analysis performed. The results will then reveal which variables are statistically significant ($p < 0.05$). Non-significant variables can then be dropped from the model, one at a time in decreasing p-value order. However, if the coefficient of any of the remaining included variables changes markedly when a variable is dropped, then the variable should be retained – this may indicate that it is a confounder. (There is no rule about how big a change in a coefficient should be considered noteworthy. A value of 10% has been suggested, but this seems on the small side.)
- *Forward elimination.* The main variable of interest is put in the model, and the other (confounding) variables are added one at a time in order of (lowest) p-value (from the univariable regressions). If statistically significant they are retained, if not, they are dropped, unless any of the coefficients of the existing included variables change noticeably, suggesting that the new variable may be a confounder.

The end result of either manual approach should be a model containing the same variables (although this model may differ from a model derived using one of the automated procedures). In any case, the overall objective is *parsimony* (i.e. having as few independent variables in the model as possible while at the same time explaining the maximum amount of variation in the outcome variable). Parsimony is particularly important when sample size is on the small side; as a rule of thumb, researchers will need at least 20 observations for each independent variable, to obtain reasonable statistical reliability (e.g. narrow-ish confidence intervals).

As an example of the manual backwards selection approach, the authors of the birthweight and cord serum EPA concentration study (Figure 30.2) knew that cord serum EPA was their principal independent variable, and only wanted to add possible confounders to their model. They commented:

> Multiple regression analysis was used to determine the relevant importance of predictors of the outcome (variable). Potential confounders were identified on the basis of previous studies, and included maternal height and weight, smoking during pregnancy, diabetes, parity, gestational length, and sex of the child. Covariates were kept in the final regression equation if statistically significant ($p < 0.01$) after backwards elimination. (Morris *et al.*, 2005)

Incidentally, the main independent variable, cord serum concentration, was found to be statistically significant ($p = 0.037$), as were all of the confounding variables.

Apart from the use of regression models to examine the significance of potential confounding variables, we should mention an additional feature of these models. That is that the value of each coefficient is an *adjusted* value, so that its effect on the dependent variable discounts any possible interactions with the other independent variables in the model. In effect, any possible influence of the other independent variables in the model is *controlled for*. A coefficient thus measures only the '*pure*' effect on the dependent variable of a change by one unit in its own independent variable. This result is hard to achieve using alternative methods of analysis.

Let's now have a look at an example of a regression analysis. Figure 30.3 is from a study into the effect of chronic hypertension in women on the risk of small-for-gestational-age babies. The outcome variable is *birthweight* (g) adjusted for gestational age at delivery. The independent variable of principal focus is chronic hypertension, but a number of other variables are included because the authors believed that they were possible confounders: smoking, and mother's weight, height, age, parity, ethnic origin, and educational level. These additional variables are a mix of metric, ordinal, and nominal types. Figure 30.3 shows, for each independent variable, its estimated coefficient value, denoted β, the standard error (a measure of the preciseness of the estimate – smaller is better), and the p-value.

Effect of Uncomplicated Chronic Hypertension on the Risk of Small-for-Gestational Age Birth

Edwige Haelterman,[1] Gérard Bréart,[2] Josefa Paris-Llado,[2] Michèle Dramaix,[1] and Catherine Tchobroutsky[2,3]

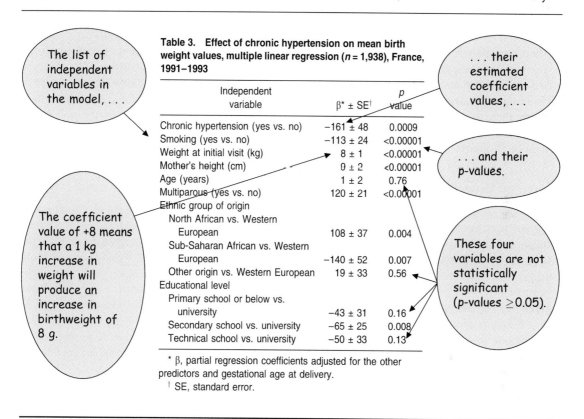

Table 3. Effect of chronic hypertension on mean birth weight values, multiple linear regression ($n = 1,938$), France, 1991–1993

Independent variable	$\beta^* \pm SE^\dagger$	p value
Chronic hypertension (yes vs. no)	−161 ± 48	0.0009
Smoking (yes vs. no)	−113 ± 24	<0.00001
Weight at initial visit (kg)	8 ± 1	<0.00001
Mother's height (cm)	9 ± 2	<0.00001
Age (years)	1 ± 2	0.76
Multiparous (yes vs. no)	120 ± 21	<0.00001
Ethnic group of origin		
North African vs. Western European	108 ± 37	0.004
Sub-Saharan African vs. Western European	−140 ± 52	0.007
Other origin vs. Western European	19 ± 33	0.56
Educational level		
Primary school or below vs. university	−43 ± 31	0.16
Secondary school vs. university	−65 ± 25	0.008
Technical school vs. university	−50 ± 33	0.13

* β, partial regression coefficients adjusted for the other predictors and gestational age at delivery.
† SE, standard error.

Text in surrounding callout bubbles:

The list of independent variables in the model, . . .

. . . their estimated coefficient values, . . .

. . . and their p-values.

The coefficient value of +8 means that a 1 kg increase in weight will produce an increase in birthweight of 8 g.

These four variables are not statistically significant (p-values ≥0.05).

FIGURE 30.3 Results of multiple linear regression analysis of chronic hypertension on risk of small babies. Reproduced from Haelterman E, Bréart G, Paris-Llado J, Dramaix M, Tchobroutsky C. Effect of uncomplicated chronic hypertension on the risk of small-for-gestational age birth. *American Journal of Epidemiology* 1997, 145: 689–95, by permission of Oxford University Press.

You can see that chronic hypertension, the focus of the study, is a statistically significant factor in low-birthweight babies ($p = 0.0009$). In addition, most of the potential confounding variables are in fact significant (*Weight at initial visit, Mother's height, Smoking,* and *Multiparous*; all $p < 0.0001$), the exceptions are: *Age* (p = 0.76), *Other ethnic origin vs. Western European* ($p = 0.56$), and two of the *Educational level* variables ($p = 0.16$ and 0.13).

Interpreting the Regression Coefficients

We explained earlier that the value of the regression coefficient tells us by how much the outcome variable changes if the independent variable increases by 1 unit of measurement. For example, in the hypertensive study, the value of the coefficient of +8 for the variable *Weight at initial visit* means that for every unit

(1 kg) increase in mothers weight, birthweight increases by an average of 8 g. The value for the *Chronic hypertension* coefficient of −161 indicates that when the variable hypertension changes from 0 (no hypertension) to 1 (hypertension), an 'increase', birthweight *decreases* by an average of 161 g. Finally, if a mother has an *Educational level* of primary school or below compared to a university-educated mother, then birthweight will be 43 g lower on average.

Goodness-of-Fit

Authors may also report a *goodness-of-fit statistic*, R^2 (also known as the coefficient of determination), which you may see quoted. R^2, which can vary between 0 and 1, measures the proportion of the observed variation in the outcome variable that is *explained* by the collection of independent variables. The value of R^2 is thus used as an indication of the quality of the model in terms of fitting the data, and can be used to compare alternative models. Note, however, that when an extra variable is added to an existing model, then the goodness-of-fit of the augmented model (compared to the original model) must be assessed using a variant of R^2 known as *adjusted R^2* (usually denoted $\bar{R}^2$).

Dummy (or Design) Variables

As you have seen, linear regression models may contain *nominal* independent variables (e.g. *Ethnic group of origin* as in Figure 30.3). This variable has four categories: European, North African, Sub-Saharan African, and Other. These categories have to be given numerical values before they can be entered into the computer regression program, but they cannot simply be allocated the numbers 1, 2, 3, and 4, since the four categories have no meaningful ordering – why not 3, 4, 1, and 2? Instead, the categories have to be represented by a set of design or *dummy* variables and coded appropriately, and the original variable, ethnicity in our example, replaced by these dummies.

Since authors commonly use dummy variables we need to say a few words about them. As you will see, we need one less dummy variable than there are categories in the original variable. A simple coding scheme, such as that shown in Table 30.1 is commonly used. Here the three dummy variables are labelled *E1*, *E2*, and *E3*, and applied to the Ethnic origin variable in the birthweight example.

So instead of the original single *Ethnic group of origin* variable being entered into the model, the three dummy variables take its place. Thus, an individual whose ethnic origin is Sub-Saharan Africa is given the values: $E1 = 0$, $E2 = 1$, and $E3 = 0$ in the data. Most computer programs will allow you to choose a *reference* or referent category. In this example the authors have chosen European as their reference category, so that, for example, the coefficient on Sub-Saharan African which has a value of −140 (Figure 30.3) is with reference to the birthweight of infants with ethnically European mothers.

TABLE 30.1   A simple coding design for the nominal variable *Ethnic group of origin* in a study of birthweight (Figure 30.3)

Ethnic category	Dummy variable		
	E1	E2	E3
European	0	0	0
North African	0	0	1
Sub-Saharan African	0	1	0
Other	1	0	0

Note the use of three dummy variables to code the four-category *Ethnic group of origin* variable. The European category is the reference category. We will always need one less dummy variable than the number of categories in the variable in question.

Binary nominal variables, the most common example being sex, are also coded with a dummy variable (i.e. the two categories, male and female, are replaced with one dummy variable which can take the value 0 (for a male, say) or 1 (for a female)). We do this without thinking!

If authors include nominal variables with more than two categories in a regression model, they should explain their coding design and indicate clearly their reference category. Ordinal and metric variables can be entered into the model 'as is' (i.e. without the need for coding – unless there is *strong* clinical evidence to suggest that the relationship may be non-linear).

Testing the Assumptions of the Linear Regression Model

We have already seen that the outcome variable must be metric, and that the relationship between the outcome variable and the independent variables must be linear, if we are to use linear regression analysis. There are a few more conditions which must also be met and authors should check that all of these conditions are satisfied (one important condition is that if we plot the error terms they should be Normal). However, since there is scant evidence in clinical papers that authors examine these assumptions, we will skirt gracefully (and gratefully) over this topic.

Effect Modification and Interaction

Suppose we are using a linear regression model to investigate the relationship among a group of individuals between systolic blood pressure (the outcome variable) and age, and we have included gender as a possible confounder. If we discover that systolic blood pressure is related to age, but the relationship is significantly different for men and women, then we would say that systolic blood pressure and gender are *interacting*. We call gender an *effect modifier* because it is acting to modify the effect of age on systolic blood pressure according to whether the individual is a male or female.

If gender was only a confounder and not an effect modifier, it would affect the relationship between age and systolic blood pressure equally for both men and women. So effect modification differs from confounding in that the latter is present for all subgroups and at all levels, whereas an effect modifier acts differentially at different levels and/or with different subgroups.

The presence of effect modification can be tested by including an *interaction* term as an additional independent variable in the model. This term will usually be formed from the product of the two variables in question, in this case (gender × age). If it turns out to have $p < 0.05$, this suggests that effect modification might be present. Authors should only introduce an interaction term in their model if they have made a *strong case* for its inclusion on clinical grounds, and it should not be included if no *main* effect has been found to be statistically significant. The introduction of interaction terms diminishes the model's parsimony (especially if it involves multiple terms in a dummy variable) and may thus lead to problems with sample size.

Summary

The linear regression model is an extremely useful tool for investigating the nature of a possible relationship between some outcome (or dependent) variable and several independent variables, particularly since it allows researchers to examine possible confounders, something difficult to achieve with any other method. When you are reading a clinical paper which reports on the use of a linear regression model, there are, as you have seen, many things to take in. However, at a minimum, the authors should do the following:

- Justify the linear nature of the relationship.
- Provide a list of candidate variables.

- Explain their variable selection procedure (forward, backward, manual, etc.).
- Provide a list of the variables in the final model.
- Explain the coding system for any dummy variables included in the model.
- Present values for the estimated coefficients, preferably with confidence intervals rather than (or as well as) p-values.
- Say something about the goodness-of-fit of their model (i.e. by quoting R^2).
- Offer a reasonably detailed interpretation of their results.

Although the linear regression model frequently appears in clinical papers, the logistic regression model is much more in evidence. We will discuss this procedure in Chapter 31.

ANALYSIS OF VARIANCE

The results of a procedure known as *analysis of variance* (ANOVA) sometimes appears in clinical papers, so needs a brief mention. Linear regression and ANOVA can be shown to be identical facets of what is known to mathematicians as the *generalised linear model*. ANOVA has a history in the social sciences, particularly in psychology and related fields.

However, everything that ANOVA can do, regression can do, and seems to us to be easier to understand. One author in his book on statistics and SPSS, says:

> ANOVA (known as the variance-ratio method) is fine for simple designs, but becomes impossibly cumbersome in more complex situations. The regression model extends very logically to these more complex designs . . . without getting bogged down in mathematics. Finally, . . . the method (ANOVA) becomes extremely unmanageable in some circumstances, such as unequal sample sizes. The regression method makes these situations much easier to deal with. (Field, 2009)

Because ANOVA is not frequently encountered in the principal clinical journals, and because of space limitations, we will not consider it further in this book. Those who want to learn more could do worse than refer to Field (2009) or to Altman (1991).

MULTIVARIATE STATISTICS

There is another powerful class of statistical procedures known collectively as *multivariate statistics*. The multivariate approach is appropriate when there is more than one outcome variable. Included among these methods are factor analysis, discriminant function analysis, and multidimensional scaling. Although these ideas can be very versatile, they are not seen in the main journals with enough frequency to justify any space being devoted to them here.

31

Logistic Regression

In multiple *linear* regression models (considered in Chapter 30), the outcome variable must be metric continuous (e.g. systolic blood pressure, birthweight, blood cholesterol, etc.). However, clinical researchers more often work with *binary* outcome variables (i.e. those which can take only *two* values, such as alive or dead, malignant or benign, has asthma or doesn't, attended hospital or did, etc.), which are usually coded 0 and 1. In these circumstances *logistic regression* models are appropriate. Logistic regression is popular because it provides values for the *odds*, *risk*, and *hazard ratios* for each independent variable. Such independent variables are often potential *risk factors* or confounders. Logistic regression can be used with outcome variables which have more than two possible values, known as *ordinal* logistic regression, although these appear much less often and will not be discussed here.

THE LOGISTIC REGRESSION MODEL

Although you will not see the mathematical form of the binary logistic model appearing in clinical papers, one or two of you (who knows!) might be interested in comparing it with the linear regression model – this is not for the faint-hearted. Let us assume that you have a group of women with a breast lump who are to receive a biopsy which will identify the lump as malignant or benign. We will let this binary diagnosis be our *outcome variable Y*, so $Y = 0$ (benign) or $Y = 1$ (malignant). Let us have just two explanatory variables, $X_1 = $ age and $X_2 = $ whether the woman has ever smoked. The logistic regression equation for this situation can be written as:

$$P(Y = 1) = e^{(\beta_0 + \beta_1 X_1 + \beta_2 X_2 + ...)} / \left[1 + e^{(\beta_0 + \beta_1 X_1 + \beta_2 X_2 + ...)} \right],$$

where the left-hand side of the equals sign is the probability of a malignant diagnosis (i.e. the probability that $Y = 1$, denoted $P(Y = 1)$). As with linear regression, the independent variables X_1, X_2, and so on, can be any mixture of metric, ordinal, or nominal. e is the exponent operator. Notice that the term in brackets is just the same as in the linear regression model. The βs are the population regression parameters which we have to estimate, as in linear regression.

We can't use the linear regression model with a binary outcome variable because there is no guarantee that Y will only take the values between 0 and 1, as required for a probability value. The above logistic equation does the trick nicely.

VARIABLE SELECTION AND MODEL ESTIMATION

The model building situation is much the same as with the linear regression model (see Chapter 30). Either the researcher is uncertain which explanatory variables might be relevant, so the list of candidate variables is long, or a particular hypothesis is to be tested. In other words, the explanatory variable of principal focus is already identified and potential confounders are known from the literature or from experience.

Variable selection procedures are also similar to those used in linear regression, either automated (forward, backwards, or stepwise) or manual. Automated selection has the same limitations previously noted, but may be more appropriate if little is known about which variables might be relevant. Manual selection, as we have seen, offers more control of the model-building process, helps with the identification of potential confounders, and is appropriate if a particular hypothesis is to be examined. There is, however, one change in the criteria used to include or exclude variables. In linear regression we included variables with a $p < 0.05$ (from the univariable regressions) and excluded them otherwise, unless their removal changed any coefficient value by some noticeable amount. In logistic regression we may be more interested in the change in the odds ratio (see next subsection).

As an example of forward selection, the following extract is from a paper examining the risk of adverse perinatal events from vaccination of pregnant women with an MF59 adjuvanted vaccine. The authors used several logistic regression models each with an adverse perinatal outcome as the dependent variable. They describe their model-building procedure thus:

> After assessing the association of several covariates with both the exposure of interest and the outcome, we entered those potential confounders one by one into the model already containing the monovalent MF59 vaccine. We retained variables that changed the crude estimated effect of the vaccine on the outcome by at least 10% in the final model as confounders (number of antenatal visits, maternal age, and smoking). We considered others, such as educational and income level and parity, although the change was between 5% and 10%, on the basis of the bivariate association with both exposure and outcome and their clinical and or epidemiological significance. (Rubinstein *et al.*, 2013)

INTERPRETATION AND STATISTICAL SIGNIFICANCE OF THE REGRESSION COEFFICIENTS

In the linear regression model we use *p*-values and confidence intervals to determine whether the regression coefficients (β_1, β_2, etc.) are statistically significant. The values of these coefficients are also of interest because they tell us by how much the outcome variable will change for each unit change in the associated explanatory variable.

In the logistic regression model we can use the *p*-value of the *Wald* test (related to the χ^2 distribution) to find out whether the coefficients are statistically significant or not. However, in logistic regression we are not nearly as interested in the value of the coefficients as we are in the *value* of the corresponding odds ratio and *its* statistical significance ($p < 0.05$ or confidence interval not including 1). In logistic regression a change of one unit in an independent variable causes a change of β in the log of the odds ratio – so not easy to interpret! However, if we raise e to the power of β, we get the odds ratio! That is, $OR = e^{\beta}$. These odds ratio values are usually provided for us in the computer results, generally with the corresponding confidence interval or *p*-value. It is this ability of logistic regression to produce odds ratios that makes the process so attractive to researchers.

To illustrate these ideas, Figure 31.1 is from a study of the risk factors for depression symptoms in long-term care residents in Taiwan. The outcome variable was, 'Has depressive symptoms (yes or no)'. As you can see, only three risk factors turned out to be statistically significant ($p < 0.05$; confidence intervals not including 1): *Type of institution* (odds ratio = 1.678), *Functional status* (odds ratio = 0.987), and *Impaired swallowing* (odds ratio = 1.686). So a resident with impaired swallowing has nearly 1.7 the odds of having depressive symptoms than does a resident without impaired swallowing.

Notice that the logistic regression coefficient for the risk factor 'impaired swallowing' has a value of 0.522. If you raise e to the power 0.522 (i.e. $e^{0.522}$) on your calculator, the result is 1.686 – which is equal to

Depressive symptoms in long-term care residents in Taiwan

Li-Chan Lin, Tyng-Guey Wang, Miao-Yen Chen, Shiao-Chi Wu and Portwood MJ

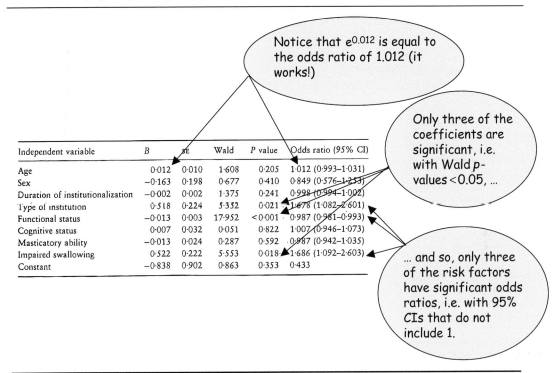

Notice that $e^{0.012}$ is equal to the odds ratio of 1.012 (it works!)

Only three of the coefficients are significant, i.e. with Wald p-values <0.05, ...

... and so, only three of the risk factors have significant odds ratios, i.e. with 95% CIs that do not include 1.

Independent variable	B	SE	Wald	P value	Odds ratio (95% CI)
Age	0·012	0·010	1·608	0·205	1·012 (0·993–1·031)
Sex	−0·163	0·198	0·677	0·410	0·849 (0·576–1·253)
Duration of institutionalization	−0·002	0·002	1·375	0·241	0·998 (0·994–1·002)
Type of institution	0·518	0·224	5·352	0·021	1·678 (1·082–2·601)
Functional status	−0·013	0·003	17·952	<0·001	0·987 (0·981–0·993)
Cognitive status	0·007	0·032	0·051	0·822	1·007 (0·946–1·073)
Masticatory ability	−0·013	0·024	0·287	0·592	0·987 (0·942–1·035)
Impaired swallowing	0·522	0·222	5·553	0·018	1·686 (1·092–2·603)
Constant	−0·838	0·902	0·863	0·353	0·433

FIGURE 31.1 Results of logistic regression analysis of risk factors for depression in long-term care residents in Taiwan. Reproduced from Lin L-C, Wang TG, Chen MY, Wu SC, Portwood MJ. (2005)- with permission from John Wiley & Sons.

the odds ratio for this risk factor seen in the table. A similar result can be demonstrated for all the other regression coefficients and their respective odds ratios.

DUMMY VARIABLES

The treatment of nominal variables also mirrors that in linear regression. Nominal variables must be coded, but ordinal and metric variables can be entered 'as is' (unless there are questions about the linearity of a relationship – see Chapter 30). Authors should provide information about any coding used and identify the reference category.

As an example of the use of dummy variables in logistic regression, Figure 31.2 is from a study of persistent pain in women after treatment for breast cancer, and shows the odds ratios, derived from a logistic regression model, for pain (the outcome variable) and its relationship to five independent variables: one metric (*Age group*) and four nominal (*Breast procedure*, *Axillary procedure*, *Radiotherapy*, and *Chemotherapy*).

The authors have chosen to categorize and code as dummy variables: *Age group* (four categories – reference category is '≥ 70'), *Breast procedure* (two categories), *Axillary procedure* (two categories),

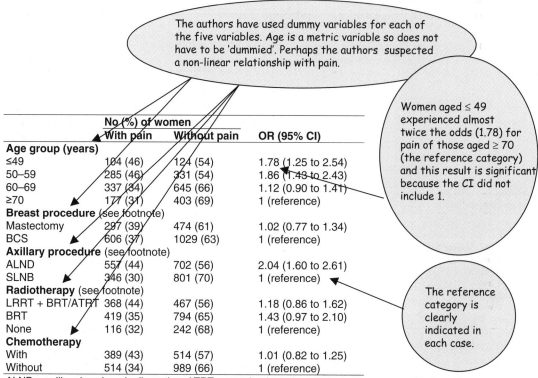

The authors have used dummy variables for each of the five variables. Age is a metric variable so does not have to be 'dummied'. Perhaps the authors suspected a non-linear relationship with pain.

Women aged ≤ 49 experienced almost twice the odds (1.78) for pain of those aged ≥ 70 (the reference category) and this result is significant because the CI did not include 1.

	No (%) of women		OR (95% CI)
	With pain	Without pain	
Age group (years)			
≤49	104 (46)	124 (54)	1.78 (1.25 to 2.54)
50–59	285 (46)	331 (54)	1.86 (1.43 to 2.43)
60–69	337 (34)	645 (66)	1.12 (0.90 to 1.41)
≥70	177 (31)	403 (69)	1 (reference)
Breast procedure (see footnote)			
Mastectomy	297 (39)	474 (61)	1.02 (0.77 to 1.34)
BCS	606 (37)	1029 (63)	1 (reference)
Axillary procedure (see footnote)			
ALND	557 (44)	702 (56)	2.04 (1.60 to 2.61)
SLNB	346 (30)	801 (70)	1 (reference)
Radiotherapy (see footnote)			
LRRT + BRT/ATRT	368 (44)	467 (56)	1.18 (0.86 to 1.62)
BRT	419 (35)	794 (65)	1.43 (0.97 to 2.10)
None	116 (32)	242 (68)	1 (reference)
Chemotherapy			
With	389 (43)	514 (57)	1.01 (0.82 to 1.25)
Without	514 (34)	989 (66)	1 (reference)

The reference category is clearly indicated in each case.

ALND = axillary lymph node dissection; ATRT = anterior thoracic radiotherapy corresponding to anterior thoracic wall; BCS = breast conserving surgery; BRT = breast radiotherapy, corresponding to residual breast tissue; LRRT = locoregional radiotherapy corresponding to periclavicular, axillary level 3, and for right sided breast cancers, internal mammary nodes; SLNB = sentinel lymph node biopsy.
*Adjusted for age, mastectomy/BCS, ALND/SLNB, radiotherapy, and chemotherapy.

FIGURE 31.2 Multivariate logistic regression analysis of effects of method of treatment and age on pain in women after treatment for breast cancer. Of the 2411 women in the study, 903 (37%) reported pain in one or more areas after treatment. Figures are adjusted odds ratios (95% confidence interval). (Abbreviated by current authors.) Reproduced from Mejdahl MK, Andersen KG, Gärtner R, Kroman N, Kehlet H. Persistent pain and sensory disturbances after treatment for breast cancer: six year nationwide follow-up study. *BMJ* 2013, 346: f1865, © 2013, with permission from BMJ Publishing Group Ltd.

Radiotherapy (three categories), and *Chemotherapy* (two categories). The authors do not give reasons for using dummy variables with age (a metric variable), possibly because they suspected non-linear relationships with the outcome variable (pain).

GOODNESS-OF-FIT

We saw that in the linear regression model that the goodness-of-fit of the model is measured by R^2. In the logistic regression model goodness-of-fit is most commonly measured either by the Pearson χ^2 statistic or by the Hosmer–Lemeshow statistic C (Hosmer and Lemeshow, 2013), both of which can be tested using the p-value associated with the χ^2 test (although neither measure is commonly quoted). The hypothesis is that the model is the correct fit. As an example, the following is an extract from a study of severe malnutrition among hospitalised children in rural Kenya (Berkley *et al.*, 2005): 'We evaluated the performance of the resulting models using the Hosmer–Lemeshow goodness-of-fit test' and they later

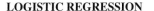

report that the 'Hosmer–Lemeshow goodness-of-fit test $\chi^2 = 8.90$, $p = 0.18$.' Thus, the hypothesis of a good fit is not rejected.

EFFECT MODIFICATION – INTERACTION

The same warnings apply here as in the linear regression model. Interaction terms adversely affect parsimony (particularly with dummy variables) and may lead to problems associated with sample size. Only if they have *strong* clinical justification should authors include interaction terms in their model.

MODEL DIAGNOSTICS

In linear regression not only do we want authors to report a measure of the goodness-of-fit of their model to the data (R^2), we also hope that they will demonstrate the linearity of the relationship and in addition, as a check on some of the basic assumptions of the model, show that they have examined the shape of the error term (it should be Normal), This process is called *model diagnostics*. As we noted though, this does not often happen.

In logistic regression, model diagnostics are much more complex. Because of the binary nature of the outcome variable, the error term is not Normally distributed (it does, in fact, have a binomial distribution – which we have not touched on). See how difficult it soon gets! In addition, the logistic model does not have the set of necessary conditions seen in linear regression, apart from the self-evident – the requirement that the outcome variable is binary. There are model diagnostic procedures available, a lot of them graphical in nature, which are largely concerned with the data patterns in the explanatory variables and the consequences of deleting one or more of these patterns on goodness-of-fit and so on. Because of these problems, it is extremely rare to see any logistic model diagnostics in clinical papers. If you want to know more about the possibilities, try Hosmer and Lemeshow (2013) or Field (2009).

32

Measuring Survival

Clinicians are often interested in questions relating to the survival time of patients following some clinical event, such as 'What is the probability that a patient diagnosed with lung cancer will survive for 12 months?' or 'Which of a number of alternative treatments for breast cancer will offer a patient a longer survival time?'. These are the sorts of questions at which *survival analysis* is aimed. In essence, a sample of patients is regularly monitored from the initial recruitment time point until the study finishes. The time taken by each patient to reach some defined clinical outcome or *end-point* is recorded (an end-point might be death, relapse, repeat of episode, recovery, etc.).

Of course, it is quite possible that some patients may not reach the end-point before the end of the study period. For example, if the end-point is death within 1 year, we might find that 20% of the subjects are still alive after 1 year. The problem is that we do not know for how long these subjects will go on living after the study has concluded nor therefore their true survival time. The data on subjects such as these are said to be *censored*. Censoring can also occur if subjects withdraw from the study before it is completed (e.g. they may relocate or die from a non-related cause).

A second difficulty is that subjects may not all enter a study at the same time, so some of the more recent recruits may be observed for shorter time periods. The problem of censored observations, compounded by unequal observation periods, makes the analysis of such data quite tricky. We can't, for example, calculate the mean survival time, since we don't know all of the survival times. We can, however, often estimate the median survival times, as you will see shortly.

In this chapter we will discuss ways in which these and other problems can be overcome, and at the same time explain some of the ideas and terms which you may encounter with survival studies reported in clinical papers. We start with a commonly used procedure for describing the survival experience of one or more groups of patients, the *Kaplan–Meier* method.

THE KAPLAN–MEIER METHOD – MEDIAN SURVIVAL TIME

The basis of the Kaplan–Meier method is a *life table* which contains the chronological progress of the participants in the study, noting how many experience the end-point of interest every day (or week, month, etc.), how many withdraw prematurely, and what proportion remain. The information in the table is usually presented in the form of the Kaplan–Meier (step-like) curve, which shows the proportion surviving at each successive time period (an example follows shortly).

The method enables researchers to: (i) calculate the survival time for any given proportion of the sample, along with a confidence interval for the survival proportion, (ii) calculate the probability of survival, or (iii) compare the difference in the proportions surviving in two or more groups (along with the appropriate confidence interval).

Figure 32.1 shows two Kaplan–Meier curves from a study into the comparative effectiveness of axitinib (top curve) versus sorafenib for the treatment of patients with advanced renal cell carcinoma. The curves

Understanding Clinical Papers, Third Edition. David Bowers, Allan House, David Owens and Bridgette Bewick.
© 2014 John Wiley & Sons, Ltd. Published 2014 by John Wiley & Sons, Ltd.

Comparative effectiveness of axitinib versus sorafenib in advanced renal cell carcinoma (AXIS): a randomised phase 3 trial

Brian I Rini, Bernard Escudier, Piotr Tomczak, Andrey Kaprin, Cezary Szczylik, Thomas E Hutson, M Dror Michaelson, Vera A Gorbunova, Martin E Gore, Igor G Rusakov, Sylvie Negrier, Yen-Chuan Ou, Daniel Castellano, Ho Yeong Lim, Hirotsugu Uemura, Jamal Tarazi, David Cella, Connie Chen, Brad Rosbrook, Sinil Kim, Robert J Motzer

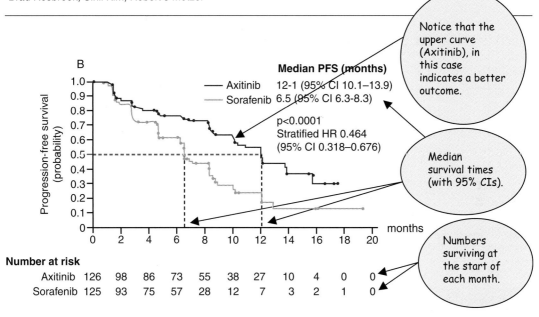

FIGURE 32.1   Kaplan–Meier survival curves from a randomised trial of the effectiveness of axitinib versus sorafenib in advanced renal cell carcinoma among patients previously treated with a cytokine-based regimen. The upper curve represents the axitinib patients, the lower curve the sorafenib patients. The median survival times are 12.1 and 6.5 months, respectively (indicated by the values shown where the horizontal '0.5 progression-free surviving proportion line' intersects each curve). Reprinted from *The Lancet* 378: Rini BI, Escudier B, Tomczak P, Kaprin A, Szczylik C, Hutson TE, *et al.* Comparative effectiveness of axitinib versus sorafenib in advanced renal cell carcinoma (AXIS): a randomised phase 3 trial. 2011; 1931–9, © 2011, with permission from Elsevier.

start with 100% of the patients alive (probability of progression-free survival = 1.0). Each time one of the patients dies, the curve steps down. The numbers still surviving in each treatment group at the start of each month are shown underneath the curves. The median survival times can be found where the horizontal 0.5 (50%) line crosses each curve (12.1 and 6.5 months, respectively). As you can see, the probability of progression-free survival was significantly higher in the axitinib group.

THE LOG-RANK TEST

In the study quoted above, the authors compared the proportions surviving in the two groups by presenting a Kaplan–Meier curve for each group, and determining the median survival times along with their corresponding confidence intervals. Although these values are useful, we are also interested in discriminating between the *complete survival experience* of two (or more) groups. We can do this with the *log-*

Efficacy of azithromycin in prevention of *Pneumocystis carinii* pneumonia: a randomised trial

Michael W Dunne, Samuel Bozzette, J Allen McCutchan, Michael P Dubé, Fred R Sattler, Donald Forthal Carol A Kemper, Diane Havlir, for the California Collaborative Treatment Group

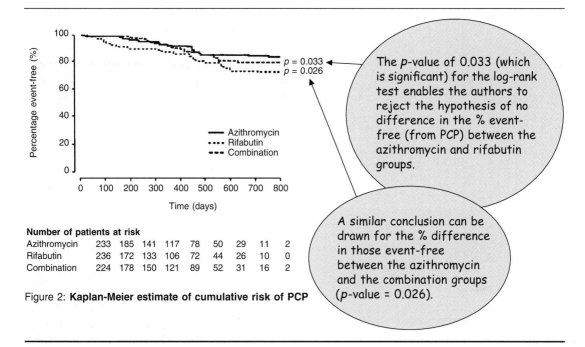

Figure 2: **Kaplan-Meier estimate of cumulative risk of PCP**

FIGURE 32.2 Kaplan–Meier curves showing the percentage of HIV-1-infected patients randomly assigned to three groups (the first group given azithromycin, the second rifabutin, and the third a combination of both drugs), who were event-free (from *P. carinii* pneumonia (PCP)). *p*-values are for the log-rank test of no difference in the percentage event-free (no PCP) between the azithromycin group and the rifabutin and combination groups, respectively. Reprinted from *The Lancet* 354: Dunne MW, Bozzette S, McCutchan JA, Dubé MP, Sattler FR, Forthal D, *et al.*, for the California Collaborative Treatment Group Efficacy of azithromycin in prevention of *Pneumocystis carinii* pneumonia: a randomised trial. 1999; 891–4, © 1999, with permission from Elsevier.

rank test (based on the χ^2 distribution). The working hypothesis is that the different groups are in fact from the same population (i.e. have the same survival experience).

In the study shown in Figure 32.2 the authors wanted to assess the clinical efficacy of azithromycin for prophylaxis of *Pneumocystis carinii* pneumonia in HIV-1-infected patients. Patients were randomly assigned to one of three drug regimens: azithromycin, rifabutin, or a combination of both drugs. The Kaplan–Meier curves show the event-free (no *P. carinii* pneumonia) survival experiences over an 800-day period.

We can use the log-rank test to test the hypothesis of no difference in the percentage event-free between the azithromycin and rifabutin groups (the hypothesis is rejected: $p = 0.033$), and between the azithromycin and the combination groups (the hypothesis is rejected: $p = 0.026$). The authors concluded that azithromycin as prophylaxis for *P. carinii* pneumonia provides additional protection over and above standard *P. carinii* pneumonia prophylaxis. However, these results should be treated with caution because of the very small size of the survivor group towards the end of the study – this can often be a problem.

LOG-RANK TEST FOR TREND

The only difference between the three groups in the example in Figure 32.2 was their drug regimen. However, some groups will be ordered. To see if survival is affected by this ordering we can use the *log-rank test for trend* (again based on the χ^2 distribution). The null hypothesis is that there is no trend in survival across the ordered groups. As an example, in a prospective cohort study to estimate the impact on long-term survival of functional status at 6 months after ischaemic stroke, 7710 patients with ischaemic stroke, registered between 1981 and 2000, were followed up for a maximum of 19 years. Their functional status at 6 months after stroke was assessed with the modified Rankin scale (see Chapter 25). Kaplan–Meier curves, stratified by the Rankin score, were used to monitor mortality during follow-up. The authors comment (our italics):

> There was a significant trend (*log rank test, P < 0.001*) of decreasing survival with increasing Rankin score at six months. . . . Both the separate Rankin scores and level of dependency at six months had a significant effect (P < 0.05) on subsequent survival in the multivariate analyses. The more dependent a patient was at six months, the shorter their subsequent survival.
>
> *(Bruins Slot et al., 2008)*

THE PROPORTIONAL HAZARDS (OR COX'S) REGRESSION MODEL

Although we can use the log-rank test to distinguish survival between groups, the test only provides a *p*-value; it would be more useful to have an estimate of any *difference* in survival, along with the corresponding confidence interval. In addition, the log-rank test does not allow for adjustment for possible confounding variables, which may significantly affect survival. For this reason clinical papers will often contain the results of an approach known as *proportional hazards (or Cox's) regression*. This procedure will provide both estimates and confidence intervals for variables that affect survival and enable researchers to adjust for confounders. To improve your understanding of such material we will discuss briefly the principle underlying the method and the meaning of some of the terms you may encounter.

The focus of proportional hazards regression is the *hazard* (first introduced in Chapter 26). The hazard is akin to a failure rate. If the end-point is death, for example, then the hazard is the rate at which individuals die at some point during the course of a study. The hazard can go up or down over time, and the distribution of hazards over the length of a study is known as the *hazard function*. You won't see authors quote the hazard regression function or equation, but for those interested it looks like this:

$$\text{Hazard} = h_0 + e^{(\beta_1 X_1 + \beta_2 X_2 + ...)},$$

where h_0 is the baseline hazard and is of little importance. As with linear and logistic regression, the explanatory or independent variables X_1, X_2, and so on, can be any mixture of nominal, ordinal, or metric, and nominal variables can be 'dummied', as described previously (Chapters 30 and 31). The same variable selection procedures (i.e. automated or by hand) can also be used.

The most interesting property of this model is that e^{β_1}, e^{β_2}, and so on, give us the *hazard ratios* for the variables X_1, X_2, and so on (notice the obvious similarity with the odds ratios in logistic regression). The hazard ratios are effectively *risk ratios*, but usually (although not always) referred to as hazard ratios in the context of survival studies. So if X_1 is, for example, the 'Presence of

Laparoscopy-assisted colectomy versus open colectomy for treatment of non-metastatic colon cancer: a randomised trial

Antonio M Lacy, Juan C Garcia-Valdecasas, Salvadora Delgado, Antoni Castells, Pilar Taura, Joseph M Pique, Joseph Visa

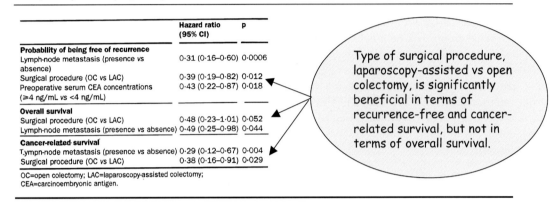

	Hazard ratio (95% CI)	p
Probability of being free of recurrence		
Lymph-node metastasis (presence vs absence)	0·31 (0·16–0·60)	0·0006
Surgical procedure (OC vs LAC)	0·39 (0·19–0·82)	0·012
Preoperative serum CEA concentrations (≥4 ng/mL vs <4 ng/mL)	0·43 (0·22–0·87)	0·018
Overall survival		
Surgical procedure (OC vs LAC)	0·48 (0·23–1·01)	0·052
Lymph-node metastasis (presence vs absence)	0·49 (0·25–0·98)	0·044
Cancer-related survival		
Lympn-node metastasis (presence vs absence)	0·29 (0·12–0·67)	0·004
Surgical procedure (OC vs LAC)	0·38 (0·16–0·91)	0·029

OC=open colectomy; LAC=laparoscopy-assisted colectomy; CEA=carcinoembryonic antigen.

Type of surgical procedure, laparoscopy-assisted vs open colectomy, is significantly beneficial in terms of recurrence-free and cancer-related survival, but not in terms of overall survival.

FIGURE 32.3 Results of a Cox proportional hazards regression analysis comparing the survival of patients with laparoscopy-assisted colectomy versus open colectomy for the treatment of non-metastatic colon cancer. Reprinted from *The Lancet* 359: Lacy AM, Garcia-Valdecasas JC, Delgado S, Castells A, Taura P, Pique JM, *et al.* Laparoscopy-assisted colectomy versus open colectomy for treatment of non-metastatic colon cancer: a randomised trial. 2002; 2224–9, © 2002, with permission from Elsevier.

micrometastases, Yes/No', then HR1 is the hazard, or risk, of death for a patient when micrometastases are present compared to when they are absent. All of this is true only if the relative effect (essentially the *ratio*) of the hazard on the two groups (e.g. the relative effect of micrometastases on the survival of each group) remains constant over the whole course of the study. Authors should show that they have checked the assumption of *proportional* hazard for each variable in the model, but don't always do so (although an exception is given below).

As an example of proportional hazards regression, Figure 32.3 is taken from a study into the relative survival of two groups of patients with non-metastatic colon cancer – one group having laparoscopy-assisted colectomy, the other open colectomy (we also looked at this study in Chapter 27 in the context of the two-sample *t*-test, see Figure 27.6). Figure 32.3 shows the hazard ratios and confidence intervals for the probability of being free of recurrence, of overall survival, and of cancer-related survival, after the patients were stratified according to tumour stage.

So, for example, patients with lymph node metastasis do only about a third as well in terms of being recurrence-free over the course of the study compared to patients without lymph node metastasis (hazard ratio = 0.31) and this difference is statistically significant since the confidence interval does not include 1 (and the *p*-value of 0.0006 is less than 0.05). Patients with lymph node metastasis also compare badly with non-metastasis patients in terms of both overall survival (only about a half as well, hazard ratio = 0.49) and cancer-related survival (just over a quarter as well, hazard ratio = 0.29), respectively. Both these results are statistically significant. Note that type of surgery, laparoscopy-assisted versus open colectomy, is not statistically significant in terms of overall survival – the confidence interval, (0.23–1.01), includes 1. However, laparoscopy-assisted colectomy has significantly greater benefit than open colectomy for being recurrence-free and for cancer-related survival; 61% less chance of reoccurrence and 62% less chance of cancer-related death, respectively.

Checking the Proportional Hazards Assumption

The proportional hazards assumption can be checked graphically using what is known as the *log-log* plot. You will sometimes find authors mentioning that they have carried out this check. For example, in a study of prostate cancer survival after radical prostatectomy, the authors state that:

> The proportional hazards assumption of the Cox model was tested through the graphical examination of the log-log plots of the variables used in the model. These plots formed approximate paralleled lines as required.
>
> *(Freedland* et al., *2005)*

Unfortunately, we do not have the space to discuss this or other procedures any further; interested readers should refer to Hosmer and Lemeshow (1999).

33

Systematic Review and Meta-Analysis

If you diagnose a patient as having sciatica, you will want to know (if you do not already) the current consensus on the most appropriate treatment. You will consult colleagues and look through all the relevant journals that you can get your hands on, to identify those studies that deal with treatments for this condition. If you had easy access to one or more clinical databases – such as PubMed, MEDLINE, Embase, or CINAHL (Cumulative Index to Nursing & Allied Health Literature) – your job would be that much easier. Because your interest is in treatments, it would make sense to concentrate on the findings from well-conducted clinical trials (Chapter 7) because they generally offer the best protection against confounding bias (Chapter 13). Even so, you may well encounter three problems with the studies you uncover:

- Many trials will be based on participants who are highly selected and probably unrepresentative of typical patients – so it may be tricky to generalise the findings to your practice.
- Many trials will be based on smallish samples which, as we have seen earlier, lead to imprecise and unreliable findings.
- Partly as a consequence of the above problems, many of the trials come to differing and conflicting conclusions.

One possible response to these three difficulties is to identify all relevant trials and then somehow combine them into one big study to produce a single overall finding which, based as it is on a much larger aggregated sample, is likely to be more precise. This combination of many separate studies will generally get closer to representing the real-world population of patients – the highly selected patient groups in one trial are likely to be dissimilar to the highly selected patients in another trial, so a wide range of study populations will have been sampled by a wide range of researchers. This combination procedure is known as a *meta-analysis*, of which more later.

In practice, clinicians do not usually do any of the above themselves, relying instead on others who are more expert in this work, and who have in recent years been compiling and disseminating reviews of the effectiveness of a whole array of treatments. These reviews often incorporate critical appraisal of the quality of the individual studies and will sometimes make recommendations or issue guidelines that carry the seal of approval of health departments or others who fund patient care. This book does not tackle this literature, often deemed part of *evidence-based practice* – there are many books and websites available that do. But we do regard the explanation of these *systematic reviews* of trials as important for an understanding of clinical papers and the rest of this chapter is a guide to some of the procedures used by systematic reviewers. In particular, we deal with the amalgamation of individual trials – with meta-analysis.

SYSTEMATIC REVIEW

A written review of treatments for a condition can amount to the opinion of its authors, backed up by findings that support that opinion. Of course, where the author is an acknowledged expert, the message

Understanding Clinical Papers, Third Edition. David Bowers, Allan House, David Owens and Bridgette Bewick.
© 2014 John Wiley & Sons, Ltd. Published 2014 by John Wiley & Sons, Ltd.

emerging from the review might be supported by his or her own research, together with that of his or her chums; research from the wider world might be cited when it agrees with the author's view, but ignored when it does not. Plainly, such a review would not be a satisfactory guide to treatment. Instead, it would be better if the review had followed a strict protocol that set out how the reviewer could ensure that as much of the relevant literature as possible has been searched, and that the applicable findings had all been appraised for quality, before synthesis into the final conclusion. In short, this kind of systematic review mimics a primary research study: it has a specific question to answer and its methods are made clear (including the steps taken to minimize bias), such that the work could be replicated by another reviewer.

In the extract from a systematic review (Figure 33.1) there is a clearly stated question, ' . . . to identify all unconfounded randomised trials of dietary advice to lower cholesterol concentration'. The primary research studies that were to be included are described in a few words, but with great clarity: they have to

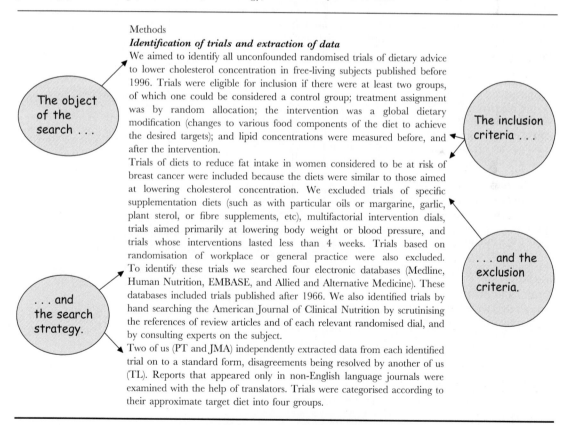

Systematic review of dietary intervention trials to lower blood total cholesterol in free-living subjects

J L Tang, J M Armitage, T Lancaster, C A Silagy, G H Fowler, H A W Neil

Methods
Identification of trials and extraction of data
We aimed to identify all unconfounded randomised trials of dietary advice to lower cholesterol concentration in free-living subjects published before 1996. Trials were eligible for inclusion if there were at least two groups, of which one could be considered a control group; treatment assignment was by random allocation; the intervention was a global dietary modification (changes to various food components of the diet to achieve the desired targets); and lipid concentrations were measured before, and after the intervention.

Trials of diets to reduce fat intake in women considered to be at risk of breast cancer were included because the diets were similar to those aimed at lowering cholesterol concentration. We excluded trials of specific supplementation diets (such as with particular oils or margarine, garlic, plant sterol, or fibre supplements, etc), multifactorial intervention dials, trials aimed primarily at lowering body weight or blood pressure, and trials whose interventions lasted less than 4 weeks. Trials based on randomisation of workplace or general practice were also excluded. To identify these trials we searched four electronic databases (Medline, Human Nutrition, EMBASE, and Allied and Alternative Medicine). These databases included trials published after 1966. We also identified trials by hand searching the American Journal of Clinical Nutrition by scrutinising the references of review articles and of each relevant randomised dial, and by consulting experts on the subject.

Two of us (PT and JMA) independently extracted data from each identified trial on to a standard form, disagreements being resolved by another of us (TL). Reports that appeared only in non-English language journals were examined with the help of translators. Trials were categorised according to their approximate target diet into four groups.

The object of the search . . .

The inclusion criteria . . .

. . . and the search strategy.

. . . and the exclusion criteria.

FIGURE 33.1 Authors' description of their search strategy and the inclusion and exclusion criteria in a study into dietary intervention and blood cholesterol. Reproduced from Tang JL, Armitage JM, Lancaster T, Silagy CA, Fowler GH, Neil HAW. Systematic review of dietary intervention trials to lower blood total cholesterol in free-living subjects. *BMJ* 1998, 316: 1213–9, © 1998, with permission from BMJ Publishing Group Ltd.

have a certain kind of design, certain standards for the allocation of the treatments have to be met, the intervention has to be of a narrowly defined type, and benefit has to be measured in a certain way. There are also some sensible and explicit exclusions. The reader is told how the authors searched the biomedical literature (and the literature on alternative health treatments) and something about how the findings are extracted.

Figure 33.1 doesn't state that the quality of the studies was appraised by the authors. Figure 33.2, on the other hand, shows part of the Abstract for a systematic review (for the treatment of cutaneous warts) that does refer to this process of appraising methodological quality. The main text (not shown) describes in

Local treatments for cutaneous warts

Gibbs, S; Harvey, I; Sterling, JC; Stark, R
Cochrane Database of Systematic Reviews

Background:
Viral warts caused by the human papilloma virus represent one of the most common diseases of the skin. Any area of skin can be affected although the hands and feet are by far the commonest sites. A very wide range of local treatments are available.

Objectives:
To assess the effects of different local treatments for cutaneous, non-genital warts in healthy people.

Search strategy:
We searched the Cochrane Controlled Trials Register (January 2003), the Skin Group trials register (January 2003), MEDLINE (1966 to January 2003), EMBASE (1980 to January 2003) and a number of other key biomedical and health economics databases. In addition the cited references of all trials identified and key review articles were searched. Pharmaceutical companies involved in local treatments for warts and experts in the field were contacted. The most recent searches were carried

Selection criteria:
Randomised controlled trials of local treatments for cutaneous non-genital viral warts in immunocompetent human hosts were included.

Data collection and analysis:
Study selection and assessment of methodological quality were carried out by two independent reviewers.

Main results:
Fifty-two trials were identified which fulfilled the criteria for inclusion in the review. The evidence provided by these studies was generally weak because of poor methodology and reporting. In 17 trials with placebo groups that used participants as the unit of analysis the average cure rate of placebo preparations was 30% (range 0 to 73%) after an average period of 10 weeks (range 4 to 24 weeks). . . . .

> The Cochrane Library contains thousands of systematic reviews and has information about hundreds of thousands of randomised trials

> In this Review, the reviewers assessed the quality of each trial that was included. The main text of the Review gives details of how they did it.

FIGURE 33.2 Cochrane Review of local treatments for skin warts showing that the included studies were assessed for their quality. Reproduced from Gibbs S, Harvey I, Sterling JC, Stark R (2005) with permission from John Wiley & Sons.

more detail how the reviewers used three criteria to judge the quality (concealment of allocation, blinding of outcome assessment, and handling of withdrawals and dropouts) – together with the overall quality of reporting and handling of data in the trials. You might notice that these three criteria are ones that we have paid attention to earlier in this book, when dealing with trials (in Chapter 7).

The example in Figure 33.2 is taken from the Cochrane Library – an electronic database largely dedicated to the publication of systematic reviews. It is a tremendously rich source of reviewed and appraised evidence about health-care interventions of all kinds, and it sets very high standards for the reviews that it publishes. It also contains many useful sources of guidance concerning searching, reviewing, combining, and appraising research.

PUBLICATION AND OTHER BIASES

The success of any systematic review depends critically on how thorough and wide-ranging the search for relevant studies is. One frequently quoted difficulty is that of *publication bias*, which can arise from a number of sources:

- There is a tendency for journals to favour the acceptance of studies showing positive outcomes at the expense of those with negative outcomes.
- There is a tendency for authors to favour the submission to journals of studies showing positive outcomes at the expense of those with negative outcomes.
- Studies with positive results are more likely to be published in English language journals, giving them a better chance of capture in the search process.
- Studies with positive results are more likely to be cited, giving them a better chance of capture in the search process.
- Studies with positive results are more likely to be published in more than one journal, giving them a better chance of capture in the search process.
- Some studies are never submitted for publication. For example, those which fail to show a positive result, those by pharmaceutical companies (particularly if the results are unfavourable), graduate dissertations, and so on.

There are a number of other sources of potential bias. *Inclusion bias*, for example, arises from the possibility that inclusion and exclusion criteria will be set to favour the admission of studies with particular outcomes over less 'helpful' studies. A further potential problem is that smaller studies tend to be less methodologically sound, with wider variability in outcomes, and are consequently less reliable. Moreover, lower-quality studies tend to show larger effects. In the light of all this, it is important that the paper should contain clear evidence that the authors have addressed these issues. One possibility is for them to provide a *funnel plot*.

THE FUNNEL PLOT

In a funnel plot the size of the study is represented on the vertical axis and the size of the treatment's effect (which in the example that follows is represented by the odds ratio on the horizontal axis). In the absence of bias, the funnel plot should have the shape of a *symmetric* upturned cone or funnel. Larger studies shown at the top of the funnel will be more precise (their results will not be so spread out), smaller studies, shown towards the bottom, less precise, and therefore more spread out. These differences produce the funnel shape. However, if the funnel is asymmetrical (e.g. if parts of the funnel are missing or poorly represented), then this is suggestive of bias of one form or another.

A large clinical trial tends to be published whatever it finds because lots of people and a lot of money will have been needed to carry it out, so its very existence will be known to many; failure to publish a large trial because the results disappoint some of those involved will lead to adverse scrutiny and comment. Small studies, on the other hand, are often not published and few people know (or care) about the consequent loss to the literature. Publication bias therefore arises especially with smaller studies and, as described above, would usually be expected to lead to the preferential publication of trials showing effects that favour active or new treatments (rather than placebos or treatment-as-usual). The clever characteristic of the funnel plot is that its design locates the missing blobs – due to publication bias – down near the base of the funnel (where the small studies are plotted) and towards the side that represents benefit for the placebo or treatment-as-usual.

For example, authors reporting the results of a meta-analysis into the use of beta-blockers as a secondary prevention after myocardial infarction produced the resulting funnel plot shown in Figure 33.3.

Each point in Figure 33.3 represents one of the studies. Values to the left of the value 1 on the horizontal axis show reductions in mortality, values to the right show increases. The congregation of values around

Bias in location and selection of studies

Mathias Egger, George Davey Smith

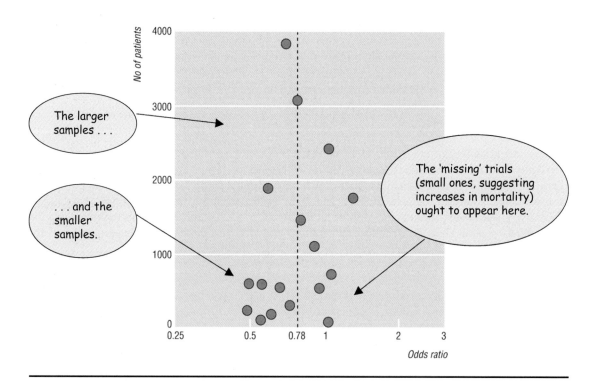

FIGURE 33.3 Funnel plot used to check for publication bias in a meta-analysis of beta-blockers to prevent secondary myocardial infarction. Reproduced from Egger M, Smith GD. Bias in location and selection of studies. *BMJ* 1998, 316: 61–6, © 1998, with permission from BMJ Publishing Group Ltd.

0.78 (about 80%) indicates an overall 20% reduction in the odds of mortality. The authors comment as follows:

> The funnel plot is shown in [Figure 33.3]. Visual assessment shows some asymmetry, which indicates that there was selective non-publication of smaller trials with less sizeable benefit. However, in formal statistical analysis the degree of asymmetry is found to be small and non-significant (P > 0.1). Furthermore, exclusion of the smaller studies had little effect on the overall estimate. Bias does not therefore seem to have distorted the findings from this meta-analysis. (Egger and Smith, 1998, footnotes removed)

HETEROGENEITY

Even when a set of potentially similar studies has been identified, authors have to make sure they are similar *enough* to be combined. For example, they should have similar participants, the same type and level of intervention, the same output measure, the same treatment effect, and so on. The underlying assumption (i.e. the null hypothesis) of meta-analysis is that all the studies measure the same effect in the same population and that any difference between them is due to chance alone. When the results are combined, the chance element cancels out. Only if studies are homogenous in this way can they be properly combined.

You might find the comments on heterogeneity (the opposite state to homogeneity where studies are dissimilar) by the authors of the diet and cholesterol study quoted earlier (Figure 33.1) illuminating:

> The design and results of these dietary studies differed greatly. They were conducted over 30 years and varied in their aims, in the intensity and type of intervention, and in the different baseline characteristics of the subjects included. Completeness and duration of follow up also differed. Unsurprisingly, the heterogeneity between their effects on blood cholesterol concentration was also significant. Among the longer trials some, but not all, of the heterogeneity between the effects on blood cholesterol concentration seemed to be due to the type of diet recommended. Deciding which trials should be included in which groups is open to different interpretation and, although we tried to be consistent, for some trials the target diets either were not clearly stated or did not fit neatly into recognised categories such as the step 1 and 2 diets. It is important to be cautious in interpreting meta-analysis when there is evidence of significant heterogeneity; although there was no evidence that the overall results were influenced by trials with outlying values. (Tang *et al.*, 1998)

Authors should present some evidence that the homogeneity assumption has been tested – one possibility is for them to provide readers with a *L'Abbé plot* (see Figure 33.4, from a study into the use of non-steroidal anti-inflammatory drugs (NSAIDs) for pain relief). The L'Abbé plot displays *outcomes* from a number of studies, with the percentage of successes (or the event rate, reduction in risk, etc.) with the treatment group on the vertical axis and the same measure for the control/placebo group on the horizontal axis. The 45° line is thus the boundary between effective and non-effective treatment. Values above the line show beneficial results. If possible, authors should use varying sized plotting points proportional to sample size (not done in this example). The compactness of the plot is a measure of the degree of homogeneity across the studies; the more compact, the more homogenous the studies. The *overall* meta-analytic result can also be shown on the same plot (but is not shown in Figure 33.4).

Two more commonly used alternatives which you will see in clinical papers dealing with meta-analysis are the *Cochrane Q test for heterogeneity*, which uses the χ^2 distribution (see Chapter 27), and the I^2 statistic, also based on χ^2 (Higgins and Thompson, 2002). The problem with the Q test is that it is not powerful enough to detect actual heterogeneity when the number of studies is small (the usual case) and too powerful in detecting negligible heterogeneity when the number of studies is large. The I^2 statistic, which has the advantage of not depending on study size, is a measure of the percentage of the variation in effect sizes between studies due to heterogeneity rather than chance.

Quantitive systematic review of topically applied non-steroidal anti-inflammatory drugs

R A Moore, M R Tramèr, D Carroll, P J Wiffen, H J McQuay

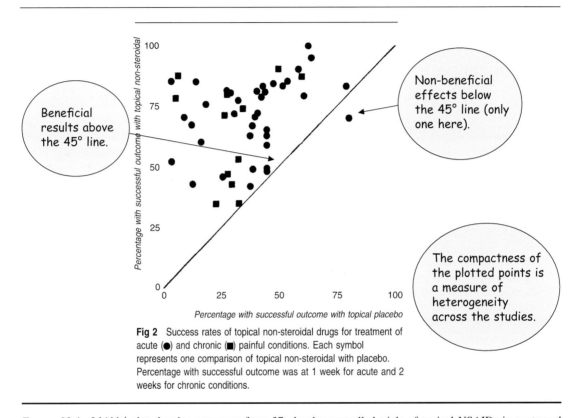

Fig 2 Success rates of topical non-steroidal drugs for treatment of acute (●) and chronic (■) painful conditions. Each symbol represents one comparison of topical non-steroidal with placebo. Percentage with successful outcome was at 1 week for acute and 2 weeks for chronic conditions.

FIGURE 33.4   L'Abbé plot showing outcomes from 37 placebo-controlled trials of topical NSAIDs in acute and chronic pain conditions. Reproduced from Moore RA, Tramèr MR, Carroll D, Wiffen PJ, McQuay HJ. Quantitative systematic review of topically applied non-steroidal anti-inflammatory drugs. *BMJ* 1998, 316: 333–8, © 1998, with permission from BMJ Publishing Group Ltd.

An example of the Q statistic is given in Figure 33.5, taken from a study which 'aimed to identify and evaluate all published randomised trials of hospital versus general practice care for people with diabetes'. The author's Table 2 presents a summary of the weighted (by sample size) mean differences for a number of different outcomes. Table 3 presents similar information for different outcomes in terms of the odds ratio. The p-values for the Q statistic are given in the last column. Only one set of studies displays evidence of heterogeneity – chiropody (with $p < 0.05$).

COMBINING THE STUDIES: THE MANTEL–HAENSZEL PROCEDURE

Providing that the question of effect-size heterogeneity between studies has been resolved, the final step in a meta-analysis is to *combine* the studies often using the Mantel–Haenszel procedure (which we do not

Diabetes care in general practice: meta-analysis of randomised control trials

Simon Griffin

p-values for tests of heterogeneity across studies for a number of different outcomes.

Table 2   Summary weighted differences comparing prompted general practice care with hospital care

Outcome	Weighted difference in mean values (95% CI)		χ^2 test of between trial heterogeneity	P value
	Favours prompted GP care	Favours hospital care		
Glycated haemoglobin (%) (3 trials, n=535)	−0.28 (−0.59 to 0.03)		3.90	>0.10
Systolic blood pressure (mm Hg) (2 trials, n=369)		1.62 (−3.30 to 6.53)	2.56	>0.10
Diastolic blood pressure (mm Hg) (2 trials, n=369)		0.56 (−1.69 to 2.80)	0.10	>0.75
Frequency of review (per patient per year) (2 trials, n=402)	0.27 (0.07 to 0.47)		0.59	>0.30
Frequency of glycated haemoglobin test (per patient per year) (2 trials, n=402)	1.60 (1.45 to 1.75)		0.05	>0.80

Table 3   Summary odds ratios comparing prompted general practice care with hospital care

Outcome	Odds ratios (95% CI)		χ^2 test of between trial heterogeneity	P value
	Favours prompted GP care	Favours hospital care		
Mortality (2 trials, n=456)		1.06 (0.53 to 2.11)	0.0	1.0
Losses to follow up (3 trials, n=589)	0.37 (0.22 to 0.61)		1.63	>0.30
Referral to chiropody (2 trials, n=399)	2.51 (1.59 to 3.97)		9.77	<0.005
Referral to dietitian (2 trials, n=399)		0.61 (0.40 to 0.92)	0.56	>0.30

The only heterogeneity is across the chiropody studies (but there are only two of these!).

FIGURE 33.5   The Mantel–Haenszel test for heterogeneity in studies with differing outcomes in a diabetes care study. The null hypothesis is that the studies are homogenous. Only one outcome (chiropody) has significant heterogeneity. Reproduced from Griffin S. Diabetes care in general practice: meta-analysis of randomised control trials. *BMJ* 1998, 317: 390–6, © 1998, with permission from BMJ Publishing Group Ltd.

describe) to produce a single-value overall summary of the net effect across all studies, as in the next example. Figure 33.6 is known as a forest plot, and is a graph of study outcome often arranged vertically and in order of effect size (although not this example, which is arranged by publication date – also done quite frequently) versus outcome measure on the horizontal axis. Figure 33.6 is taken from a meta-analysis of randomised controlled trials and observational studies to evaluate the association of chocolate consumption with the risk of developing cardiovascular disorders. The outcome measure might be

Chocolate consumption and cardiometabolic disorders: systematic review and meta-analysis

Adriana Buitrago-Lopez, Jean Sanderson, Laura Johnson, Samantha Warnakula, Angela Wood, Emanuele Di Angelantonio, Oscar H Franco

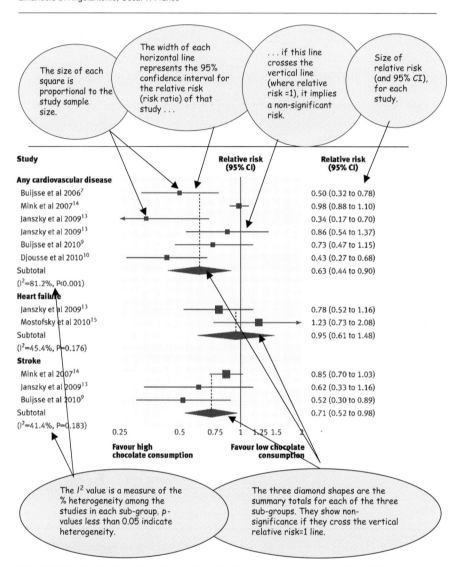

FIGURE 33.6 Forest plot from a study of the relative risks for cardiovascular disease, heart failure, and stroke, comparing adults with higher and lower levels of chocolate consumption, respectively. The individual studies are listed to the left of the forest plot, the associated relative risks (risk ratios) for each study to the right of the plot. Reproduced from Buitrago-Lopez A, Sanderson J, Johnson L, Warnakula S, Wood A, Di Angelantonio E, *et al.* Chocolate consumption and cardiometabolic disorders: systematic review and meta-analysis. *BMJ* 2011, 343: d4488, © 2011, with permission from BMJ Publishing Group Ltd.

odds or risk ratios, means or proportions or their differences, event rates, and so on – in this study the outcome measure is the relative risk (or risk ratio). Each study is represented by a box with a horizontal line through it, which represents the width of the 95% confidence interval. The area of each box should be proportional to its sample size. In this example, the authors have split the studies into three groups: any cardiovascular disease (six studies), heart failure (two studies), and stroke (three studies). The overall net outcome effect for each subgroup is shown with a diamond shape. The area of the diamond is proportional to the total number of studies represented and its width to the 95% confidence interval.

Values to the left of a relative risk of 1 (bottom axis) show reductions in cardiovascular disease (favouring high levels of chocolate consumption), those to the right an increase. The Mantel–Haenszel procedure was used to produce the final subgroups results shown in Figure 33.6. The aggregate relative risks in each of the three groups are 0.63, 0.95 (not significant because the confidence interval includes 0), and 0.71.

The I^2 statistic (percentage heterogeneity) is given for each subgroup – as a rule of thumb, values of 0–25% indicate low heterogeneity, 50% moderate heterogeneity, and 75% high heterogeneity. Heterogeneity is high and significant ($p < 0.05$) in the 'Any cardiovascular disease' subgroup, but not significant either of the other two subgroups.

The number of meta-analytic studies in the journals has increased steadily over the past few years. With the increasing favour of evidence-based practice, this trend is likely to be maintained. However, not all researchers are unreservedly enthusiastic about this procedure and worry about various shortcomings (due to bias and other problems). Unfortunately, we do not have the space to devote to these reservations in what is still an emerging method.

34

Analysing Qualitative Data

The process of analysing qualitative data enables the researcher to move from the raw data to a *meaningful interpretation* of the information obtained. This process includes a number of steps. How these steps are implemented differs, depending on the approach taken but analysis generally includes:

- A process of *familiarisation* with the data. Usually by reviewing material collected (e.g. reading interview transcripts; looking over images collected; reading field notes).
- *Description of reoccurring meaning* present in the data (e.g. by coding for reoccurring themes) (e.g. Figure 34.1).
- *Grouping of description of meanings* that share commonalities to form categories (Figure 34.2).
- Putting together, or *synthesizing*, categories to develop explanations (Figures 34.3 and 34.4)

The different approaches to qualitative analysis use a variety of labels for each step. The order of the steps and the number of iterations also differs between approaches. Within their writing authors should explain how they move from interacting with the raw data to developing explanations of the meanings assigned to the data collected. The explanation of how meanings were assigned helps the reader to understand the level of abstraction within the analysis strategy.

For example, some approaches seek to minimise the researchers' interpretation of participant accounts, while others maximise interpretation of material, seeking to understand the unspoken meaning within the data. The explanation also helps the reader to understand whether the analysis was driven by the data (perhaps by identifying reoccurring themes as they emerge) or if instead the themes were driven by another source (maybe the framework developed to address existing policies; coding developed using a theoretical model). Whatever the approach taken, the material presented in the published paper should enable the reader to understand the process of analysis, including how meaning was assigned.

Researchers often use computer software to assist with management of data and data analysis. It is worth emphasising that the software is a tool for managing the analysis process, the software cannot take over the identification of themes nor can software independently generate codes. The identification of reoccurring meaning, the grouping of description of meanings, and synthesis of categories is done by the researcher as he or she uses the software to keep track of the process.

Qualitative analysis can be viewed as a process of segmentation followed by a process of reconstruction. It is the process of reconstruction that enables new ways of thinking about the topic of interest to be discovered. The process of synthesizing pulls the segmented meaning back together to enable the telling of a coherent story that furthers our understanding of the topic of interest. We have noticed that people new to qualitative analysis sometimes present the segmentation findings, for example, by describing individual themes identified in the data, without presenting an explanation of how the segmented pieces fit together.

Understanding Clinical Papers, Third Edition. David Bowers, Allan House, David Owens and Bridgette Bewick.
© 2014 John Wiley & Sons, Ltd. Published 2014 by John Wiley & Sons, Ltd.

Waiting for a Liver Transplant

Jill Brown, James H. Sorrell, Jason McClaren, and John W. Creswell

Invariant Structure	Meaning Unit
I miss working so much it upsets me	The inability to work is experienced as a feeling ofloss
I feel just incredibly blessed	Patients feel gratitude and privilege of being listed
The only time I feel like I'm waiting is the time I feel they are intruding on my life	Waiting is felt when interferes with goals
I know that a transplant opens up a whole other group of problems . . .	Questioning rationality of surgery
I can't get into the negative—I don't like it—I don't like personally being there and sometimes it's a lot of work	Resisting negative outlook
In the beginning, it was a good feeling, like something is going to finally happen	Initial excitement/elation with being listed
When frustrated, I can't do anything—when frustrated I can' control going down	Frustration from waiting renders people impotent and out of control

Clear illustration of the link between raw data (what these authors call invariant structure) and the meaning assigned (meaning unit).

FIGURE 34.1 Exploring what meaning people ascribe to the experience of invariant structures and their corresponding meaning units. From a study of feelings among those waiting for a liver transplant. (Abbreviated by current authors.) Reproduced from Brown J, Sorrell JH, McClaren J, Creswell JW. Waiting for a liver transplant. *Qualitative Health Research* 2006, 16: 129–36, © SAGE Publications. Reprinted by permission of SAGE Publications.

Waiting for a Liver Transplant

Jill Brown, James H. Sorrell, Jason Mc Claren and John W. Creswell

Theme	Meaning Units
Loss	The inability to work is experienced as a feeling of loss The rules of the waiting list interfere with other life goals The feeling of waiting is worse when it interferes with goals There is a lack of control over one's own life Awareness of disease renders one undependable . . . . . .
Transformations	There is a change in perspective through the transformative experience of illness New self-identity during waiting Illness makes one face own mortality New understanding of what is sacred Refusal to see illness as part of identity . . . . . .
Searching	Blame attributed to one's self Patients want justice and fairness in the transpla nt process . . . . . .

Authors provide evidence of how meaning units were grouped together (shared meaning).

In the text the authors explain how the analysis was driven by participant data.

FIGURE 34.2 Sample of three themes and corresponding meaning units. From a study of feelings among those waiting for a liver transplant. Reproduced from Brown J, Sorrell JH, McClaren J, Creswell JW. Waiting for a liver transplant. *Qualitative Health Research* 2006, 16: 129–36, © SAGE Publications. Reprinted by permission of SAGE Publications.

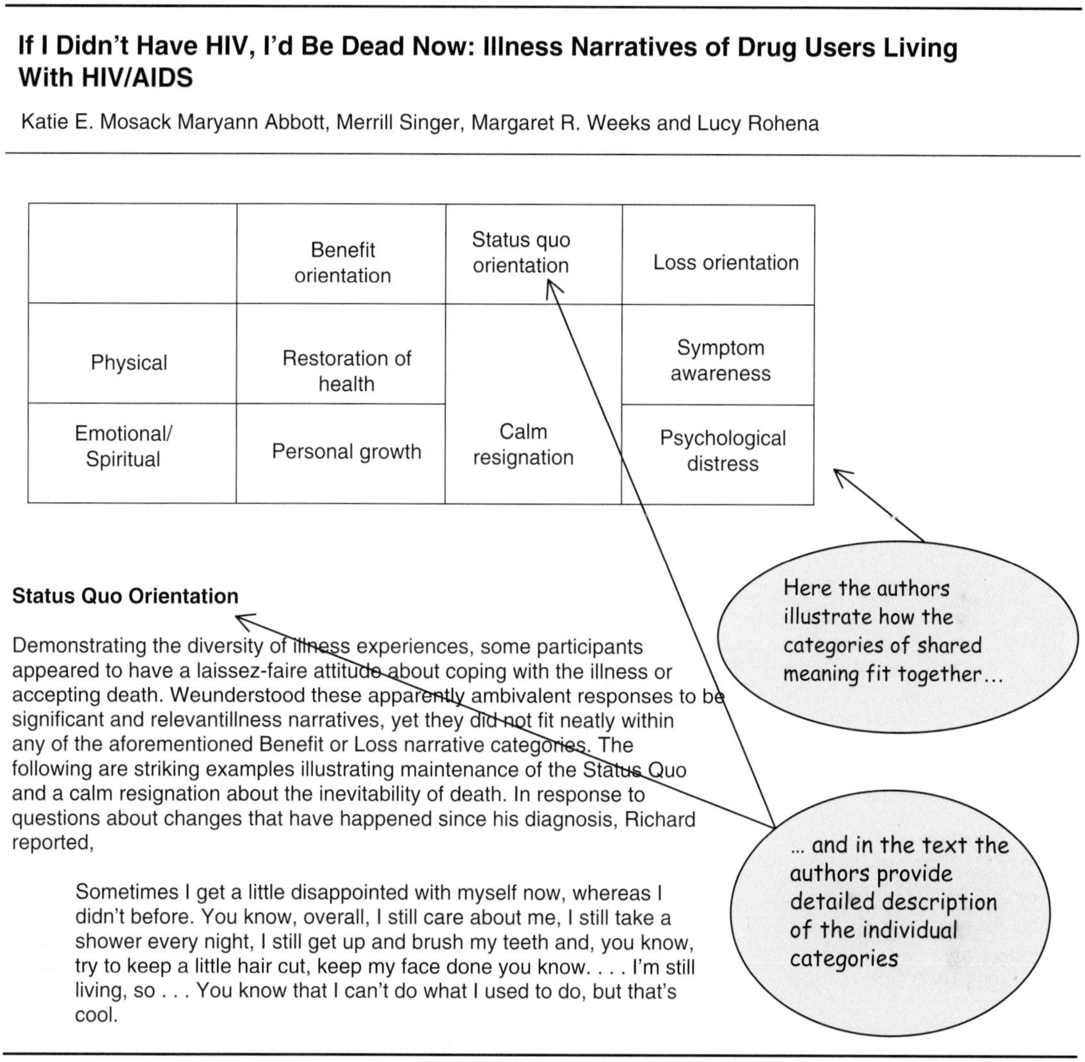

If I Didn't Have HIV, I'd Be Dead Now: Illness Narratives of Drug Users Living With HIV/AIDS

Katie E. Mosack Maryann Abbott, Merrill Singer, Margaret R. Weeks and Lucy Rohena

	Benefit orientation	Status quo orientation	Loss orientation
Physical	Restoration of health		Symptom awareness
Emotional/ Spiritual	Personal growth	Calm resignation	Psychological distress

Status Quo Orientation

Demonstrating the diversity of illness experiences, some participants appeared to have a laissez-faire attitude about coping with the illness or accepting death. We understood these apparently ambivalent responses to be significant and relevant illness narratives, yet they did not fit neatly within any of the aforementioned Benefit or Loss narrative categories. The following are striking examples illustrating maintenance of the Status Quo and a calm resignation about the inevitability of death. In response to questions about changes that have happened since his diagnosis, Richard reported,

> Sometimes I get a little disappointed with myself now, whereas I didn't before. You know, overall, I still care about me, I still take a shower every night, I still get up and brush my teeth and, you know, try to keep a little hair cut, keep my face done you know. . . . I'm still living, so . . . You know that I can't do what I used to do, but that's cool.

Here the authors illustrate how the categories of shared meaning fit together...

... and in the text the authors provide detailed description of the individual categories

FIGURE 34.3   Illness narratives among drug users living with HIV/AIDS. Reproduced from Mosack KE, Abbott M, Singer M, Weeks MR, Rohena L. If I didn't have HIV, I'd be dead now: illness narratives of drug users living with HIV/AIDS. *Qualitative Health Research* 2005, 15: 586–605, © SAGE Publications. Reprinted by permission of SAGE Publications.

Reconciling Incompatibilities: A Grounded Theory of HIV Medication Adherence and Symptom Management

Holly Skodol Wilson, Sally A. Hutchinson and William L. Holzemer

The explanatory schema generated from interview data reveals that adherence or nonadherence is significantly more complex than a matter of medications' being too costly and inaccessible or people's being too busy or forgetting (Gifford, 1999). Adherence choices occur in a particular context and in the face of conditions, which appeared repeatedly as themes in this study's data. The context and conditions contribute to a state of mind that can result in postponing taking medications until symptoms and or disease markers are considerably more dire, or in making adherence choices to comply, not comply, or self-tailor patients' participation in their medication regimen. It is important to note that choices can change on a day-to-day, if not dose-by-dose, basis and that adherence or nonadherence is a fluctuating phenomenon and not a fixed or static one (see Figure1).

The authors provide a description of the model generated from their analysis . . .

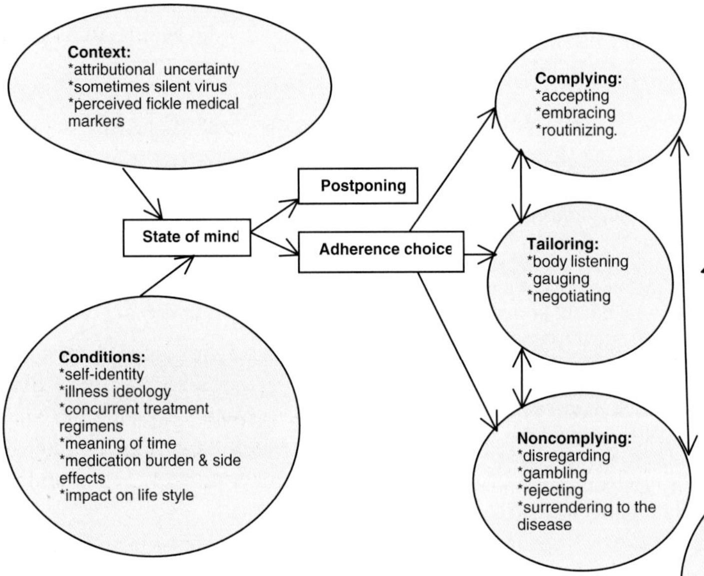

.. and a figure is used to show how the components of the model fit together. The arrows show the direction of influence.

In the text the authors provide a description of each component of this model. Their description is evidenced with participant quotes.

Illness ideology represented the body of doctrine and belief systems people held about the nature of HIV and its treatment. Some of the study participants were fully convinced of the truth of medico-science theories of their condition, and some departed dramatically from this in the direction of alternative beliefs and practices. In the words of one patient in the first category, "I just keep my faith in the doctors and trust that the medication will work and keep my viral load down and keep me from getting opportunistic infections. By contrast, another participant shared a . . .

FIGURE 34.4 A theory of reconciling incompatibilities. Reproduced from Wilson HS, Hutchinson SA, Holzemer WL. Reconciling incompatibilities: a grounded theory of HIV medication adherence and symptom management. *Qualitative Health Research* 2002, 12: 1309, © SAGE Publications. Reprinted by permission of SAGE Publications.

35

Results in Text and Tables

RAW RESULTS AND COOKED FINDINGS

Study results are often set out in three stages: (i) the raw *results*, (ii) the selection and summary of results into *findings*, and (iii) the interpretation of these findings to produce *conclusions* (conclusions are dealt with in Chapter 37). Often some raw results and the consequent findings are presented in the text. Another strategy is to present raw results in tables, with the text extracting the findings that the authors reckon to be the key points (Figure 35.1).

Equally often, raw results are displayed in tables but analysed further before being written out again in the text as summarised findings. In the example in Figure 35.2, from a study of bleeding from the upper gastrointestinal tract, the text and table set out raw results in some detail, but the text goes on to make selected key points after applying further calculations.

INTERESTING FINDINGS

Many of the most interesting findings from research investigations are those arising from comparisons between two (or more) groups of subjects. Notice in the text of Figure 35.2 that the authors have calculated and drawn our attention to higher incidences of bleeding and greater mortality among older people, and in men compared with women. In setting out these kinds of comparisons researchers often employ two technical devices. First, they tell us the findings, accompanied by the statistical estimates of confidence intervals or hypothesis tests (described in Chapters 25–27).

Second (although not applied to the data in Figure 35.2), they may express their comparisons in terms of the kinds of fractions and ratios described in Chapters 22–24. To comprehend the findings of many papers you will need to be comfortable with risk ratios (relative risk) and odds ratios (Chapter 24), and the confidence intervals for each (Chapter 26). Risk ratios are typically used to describe the findings of cohort studies and clinical trials, while odds ratios are applied to case-control studies. There is an unfortunate tendency for authors to use odds ratios to report the results of clinical trials; it is not incorrect to summarize trial findings as odds ratios, but it is difficult to interpret their meaning. Almost everyone finds risk ratios easier to translate into the everyday parlance of chance, such as 'twice the chance of recovery in one group compared with the other'. Figures 35.3 and 35.4 are illustrations of typical reporting of risk ratios (here called relative risk) (Figure 35.3) and odds ratios (Figure 35.4).

Prevalence of serious eye disease and visual impairment in a north London population: population based, cross sectional study

A Reidy, D C Minassian, G Vafidis, J Joseph, S Farrow, J Wu, P Desai, A Connolly

Results

The survey was carried out from April 1995 to October 1996, and 1547 people were examined and included in the sample. Of these, 1459 (94.3%) were white. Age and sex distribution in the sample was similar to that of the population of the area sampled (figure on website).

Response rate

The overall response rate was 1547/1840 (84% of those invited to participate). This was achieved after up to three rounds of invitation to attend. Non-responders were similar to respondents in terms of age, sex, and attending hospital clinics or opticians. Not having access to a telephone at home was more common in non-responders and in those who had to be re-invited for the third time.

Population prevalence of eye disorders

Table 1 shows that the population prevalence of visual impairment caused by cataract was 30%, that caused by age related macular degeneration was 8%, and that caused by refractive error was 9%. The prevalence of chronic open angle glaucoma was 3%, and a further 7% of subjects were suspected of having glaucoma. Table 2 shows that impaired vision in one or both eyes, present in more than half of the sample (815/1547), was potentially remediable in 69% of cases.

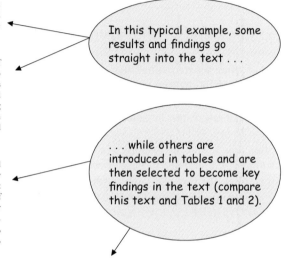

In this typical example, some results and findings go straight into the text . . .

. . . while others are introduced in tables and are then selected to become key findings in the text (compare this text and Tables 1 and 2).

Notice how the precision of the results is estimated using confidence intervals.

Table 1 Population prevalence (%) of main eye disorders

Eye disorders	No of cases in sample	Estimated population prevalence (95% CI)*	Estimated No of cases in population of 13 371 (95% CI)*
Cataract (lens opacity; one or both eyes; visual acuity <6/12)	451	30 (25.1 to 35.3)	4037 (3351 to 4723)
Had cataract surgery (one or both eyes)	162	10 (8.5 to 12.4)	1399 (1141 to 1657)
Age related macular degeneration (visual acuity <6/12)	133	8 (5.8 to 10.8)	1108 (776 to 1440)
Glaucoma (chronic open angle)	47	3 (2.3 to 3.6)	395 (306 to 485)
Suspected glaucoma	109	7 (5.4 to 8.4)	924 (719 to 1128)
Refractive error causing visual impairment one or both eyes; visual acuity <6/12	136	9 (7.0 to 11.4)	1228 (935 to 1521)

*Weighted average of cluster specific prevalence measures; calculations take into account the two stage cluster random sampling design.

Table 2 Visual impairment in the population and the proportion likely to be remediable through surgery or refraction and dispensing of spectacles

Visual impairment or blindness (visual acuity <6/12)	Estimated population prevalence (%) (95% CI)*	No of cases in sample†	Proportion (%) potentially remediable
One eye only	23.6 (20.9 to 26.3)	367	65
Both eyes	30.2 (24.8 to 35.5)	448	72
Total	53.8 (48.4 to 59.2)	815	69

*Weighted average of cluster specific prevalence measures; calculations take into account the two stage cluster random sampling design. †Eye disorders causing visual impairment: cataract, corneal opacity, posterior subcapsular opacity, and refractive error (including uncorrected aphakia or pseudophakia).

FIGURE 35.1 Extract from a Results section to illustrate the interplay of text and tables. Reproduced from Reidy A, Minassian DC, Vafidis G, Joseph J, Farrow S, Wu J, *et al.* Prevalence of serious eye disease and visual impairment in a north London population: population based, cross sectional study. *BMJ* 1998, 316: 1643–6, © 1998, with permission from BMJ Publishing Group Ltd.

Acute upper gastrointestinal haemorrhage in west of Scotland: case ascertainment study

Oliver Blatchford, Lindsay A Davidson, William R Murray, Mary Blatchford, Jill Pell

Results

A total of 1882 adult cases were coded. This includes 61 patients whose acute upper gastrointestinal haemorrhage occurred while they were inpatients for other reasons and 61 patients who were transferred from other hospitals. Table 1 shows summary details of the patients' ages, sex distribution, and diagnoses.

In eight cases the final outcome of the episode was not recorded owing to incompleteness of the clinical record. No postcode could be traced in 24 cases, and the recorded postcodes were not valid in 52.

Incidence

The adult population of the area from which these patients were admitted was 2 184 285 at the 1991 census, giving an overall incidence of 172 per 100 000 people aged 15 and over per annum (95% confidence interval 165 to 180).

The incidence rose sharply with age, being 5.7 times higher among those over 75 than among those aged 15 to 29; P<0.00001), and it was twice as high among men as among women (P<0.00001). Table 1 also shows that the incidence of acute upper gastro-intestinal haemorrhage also rose with increasing Carstairs deprivation score, being 2.2 times greater in the most deprived quarter than in the most affluent quarter (P<0.00001).

Mortality

There were 153 deaths among the 1882 patients, resulting in an overall population mortality of 14.0 per 100 000 per annum (11.9 to 16.4). The population mortality increased sharply with increasing age (113 times greater among those over 75 than among those aged 15 to 29; P<0.00001) (table 1), and mortality among men was 1.6 times greater than among women (P−0.005). The population mortality in the most deprived quarter was double that in the least deprived quarter (P<0.0002).

This section of the text shows raw results – details of sample size, inclusions and exclusions.

This section of the text summarizes findings drawn from the preceding results in text and table – first applying additional calculations.

Notice that the text: (i) condenses raw table results (on age and deprivation) into clear statements about the findings and (ii) describes further analysis of table results on incidence.

Table 1 Patient characteristics by incidence of and mortality and case fatality from acute upper gastrointestinal haemorrhage

	No of patients	Incidence (95% CI) (per 100 000 per year)	No of deaths	Mortality (95% CI) (per 100 000 per year)	Case fatality (%)
All cases	1882	172 (165 to 180)	153	14.0 (11.9 to 16.4)	8.1 (6.9 to 9.6)
Sex:					
Male	1208	236	89	17.4	7.4
Female	674	116	64	11	9.6
Statistics:					
Relative risk (95% CI) for women		0.49 (0.45 to 0.54)		0.63 (0.46 to 0.87)	1.29 (0.95 to 1.76)
χ^2 for trend (p value)		229 (<0.00001)		7.96 (0.005)	2.67 (0.1)
Age group (years):					
15–29	251	84	2	0.7	0.8
30–44	316	111	5	1.8	1.6
45–59	410	176	23	9.9	5.6
60–74	500	260	56	29.2	11.2
≥75	405	480	67	79.3	16.6
χ^2 for trend (p value)		635 (<0.00001)		261 (0.00001)	80 (<0.00001)
Deprivation score (quarters):*					
1 (most affluent)	316	114	27	9.7	9.4
2	389	144	20	7.4	5.4
3	433	159	45	16.5	11.6
4 (least affluent)	668	247	52	19.2	8.5
χ^2 for trend (p value)		141 (<0.00001)		14.6 (<0.0002)	0.24 (0.6)

*Excludes 76 cases in which deprivation score was missing.

FIGURE 35.2 Extract from another Results section to illustrate more complex interplay between text and tables. Reproduced from Blatchford O, Davidson LA, Murray WR, Blatchford M, Pell J. Acute upper gastrointestinal haemorrhage in west of Scotland: case ascertainment study. *BMJ* 1997, 315: 510–4, © 1997, with permission from BMJ Publishing Group Ltd.

Mortality associated with oral contraceptive use: 25 year follow up of cohort of 46 000 women from Royal College of General Practitioners' oral contraception study

Valerie Beral, Carol Hermon, Clifford Kay, Philip Hannaford, Sarah Darby, Gillian Reeves

Abstract

Objective To describe the long term effects of the use of oral contraceptives on mortality.

Design Cohort study with 25 year follow up. Details of oral contraceptive use and of morbidity and mortality were reported six monthly by general practitioners. 75% of the original cohort was "flagged" on the NHS central registers.

Setting 1400 general practices throughout Britain.

Subjects 46 000 women, half of whom were using oral contraceptives at recruitment in 1968–9. Median age at end of follow up was 49 years.

Main outcome measures Relative risks of death adjusted for age, parity, social class, and smoking.

Results Over the 25 year follow up 1599 deaths were reported. Over the entire period of follow up the risk of death from all causes was similar in ever users and never users of oral contraceptives (relative risk=1.0, 95% confidence interval 0.9 to 1.1; P=0.7) and the risk of death for most specific causes did not differ significantly in the two groups. However, among current and recent (within 10 years) users the relative risk of death from ovarian cancer was 0.2 (0.1 to 0.8; P=0.01), from cervical cancer 2.5 (1.1 to 6.1; P=0.04), and from cerebrovascular disease 1.9 (1.2 to 3.1, P=0.009). By contrast, for women who had stopped use ≥10 years previously there were no significant excesses or deficits either overall or for any specific cause of death.

> Remember that a relative risk (risk ratio) of 1 indicates the same risk in each group; hence, the statement here that death from all causes was as likely among users and non-users (see Chapter 24).

> The way these findings are worded, a relative risk below 1 suggests less risk of ovarian cancer among pill users.
>
> A relative risk above 1 suggests greater risk of cervical cancer among pill users.

FIGURE 35.3 The display of risk ratios (relative risk) to summarize findings from a cohort study. Reproduced from Beral V, Hermon C, Kay C, Hannaford P, Darby S, Reeves G. Mortality associated with oral contraceptive use: 25 year follow up of cohort of 46 000 women from Royal College of General Practitioners' oral contraception study. *BMJ* 1999, 318: 96–100, © 1999, with permission from BMJ Publishing Group Ltd.

LEGENDS AND BRACKETS

Tables can be difficult to follow – not surprising when many contain a great deal of information. But even simple tables are hard to understand if they are not set out well and labelled with care. A table should bear a clear description of what it contains, together with a guide to its components – often called its *legend* (or heading). We find the legend of Table 1 in Figure 35.5 a model of clarity. It is taken from a randomised controlled trial that compared routine general practitioner care with the effect of putting the patient in

Risk factors for erysipelas of the leg (cellulitis): case-control study

Alain Dupuy, Hakima Benchikhi, Jean-Claude Roujeau, Philippe Bernard, Loïc Vaillant, Oliver Chosidow, Bruno Sassolas, Jean-Claude Guillaume, Jean-Jacques Grob, Sylvie Bastuji-Garin

Abstract

Objective To assess risk factors for erysipelas of the leg (cellulitis).

Design Case-control study.

Setting 7 hospital centres in France.

Subjects 167 patients admitted to hospital for erysipelas of the leg and 294 controls.

Results In multivariate analysis, a disruption of the cutaneous barrier (leg ulcer, wound, fissurated toe-web intertrigo, pressure ulcer, or leg dermatosis) (odds ratio 23.8, 95% confidence interval 10.7 to 52.5), lymphoedema (71.2, 5.6 to 908), venous insufficiency (2.0, 1.0 to 8.7), leg oedema (2.5, 1.2 to 5.1) and being overweight (2.0, 1.1 to 3.7) were independently associated with erysipelas of the leg. No association was observed with diabetes, alcohol, or smoking. Population attributable risk for toe-web intertrigo was 61%.

Conclusion This first case-control study highlights the major role of local risk factors (mainly lymphoedema and site of entry) in erysipelas of the leg. From a public health perspective, detecting and treating toe-web intertrigo should be evaluated in the secondary prevention of erysipelas of the leg.

Just as with the risk ratio, when the odds ratio is 1, it signifies that odds are the same in each group (see Chapter 24).

All the odds ratios here are greater than 1, suggesting greater risk of cellulitis in those with each characteristic. In particular, it looks like broken skin or lymphoedema are especially prevalent among cellulitis sufferers.

FIGURE 35.4 The display of odds ratios to summarize findings from a case-control study. Reproduced from Dupuy A, Benchikhi H, Roujeau J-C, Bernard P, Vaillant L, Chosidow O, *et al*. Risk factors for erysipelas of the leg (cellulitis): case-control study. *BMJ* 1999, 318: 1591–4, © 1999, with permission from BMJ Publishing Group Ltd.

touch with a facilitator (from the 'Amalthea Project') whose task was to facilitate contact with relevant voluntary organisations. Study subjects were patients whose general practitioner thought they had psychosocial problems well suited to voluntary sector assistance. The table legend sets out first what the table contains – baseline characteristics of the subjects at the start of the study. Second, it tells us what the numerical values indicate – in this case, numbers of subjects unless stated otherwise. Third, it tells the reader what the brackets contain (percentages).

DASHES

Brackets cause confusion when the legend doesn't tell you what is in them. Dashes are even more hazardous: the problem is that we use the same device – a dash – to indicate range and as a minus sign. Figure 35.6 presents extracts from two further tables from the same study as Figure 35.5. It is self-evident that the dashes in their Table 5 are being used to indicate range. You may find it less obvious that the dashes

A randomised controlled trial and economic evaluation of a referrals facilitator between primary care and the voluntary sector

Clare Grant, Trudy Goodenough, Ian Harvey, Chris Hine

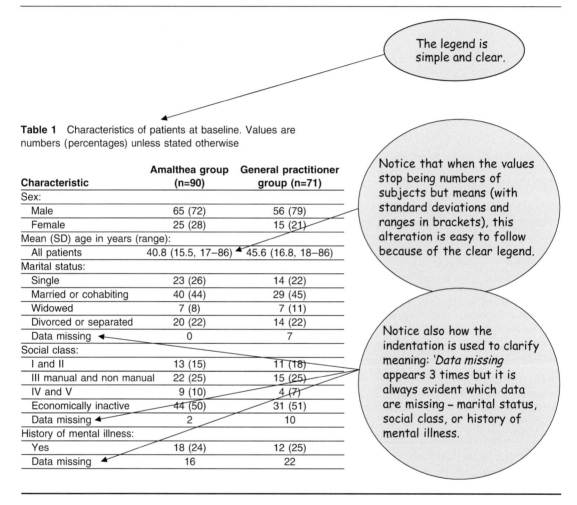

The legend is simple and clear.

Table 1 Characteristics of patients at baseline. Values are numbers (percentages) unless stated otherwise

Characteristic	Amalthea group (n=90)	General practitioner group (n=71)
Sex:		
Male	65 (72)	56 (79)
Female	25 (28)	15 (21)
Mean (SD) age in years (range):		
All patients	40.8 (15.5, 17–86)	45.6 (16.8, 18–86)
Marital status:		
Single	23 (26)	14 (22)
Married or cohabiting	40 (44)	29 (45)
Widowed	7 (8)	7 (11)
Divorced or separated	20 (22)	14 (22)
Data missing	0	7
Social class:		
I and II	13 (15)	11 (18)
III manual and non manual	22 (25)	15 (25)
IV and V	9 (10)	4 (7)
Economically inactive	44 (50)	31 (51)
Data missing	2	10
History of mental illness:		
Yes	18 (24)	12 (25)
Data missing	16	22

Notice that when the values stop being numbers of subjects but means (with standard deviations and ranges in brackets), this alteration is easy to follow because of the clear legend.

Notice also how the indentation is used to clarify meaning: 'Data missing appears 3 times but it is always evident which data are missing – marital status, social class, or history of mental illness.

FIGURE 35.5 How the clarity of a table depends on its layout and the legend. Reproduced from Grant C, Goodenough T, Harvey I, Hine C. A randomised controlled trial and economic evaluation of a referrals facilitator between primary care and the voluntary sector. *BMJ* 2000, 320: 419–23, © 2000, with permission from BMJ Publishing Group Ltd.

in their Table 4 indicate minus signs. The legend for Table 4 tells us that the first column of values refers to *differences* in various measures before and after the study interventions. A minus difference on the scales shown here indicates improvement (for example less anxiety).

Displaying confidence intervals requires particular care (see Chapter 25). The interval might reasonably be written, for example, as (4–9). But you may recall that when confidence intervals

A randomised controlled trial and economic evaluation of a referrals facilitator between primary care and the voluntary sector

Clare Grant, Trudy Goodenough, Ian Harvey, Chris Hine

Table 4 Difference between outcome measure scores of patients in two arms of trial from repeated measures analysis of covariance after adjustment for baseline score

In all the values here, the dash is a minus sign, so the word 'to' is used to indicate range.

Outcome measure	Differences for combined follow up period (95% CI)	P value
Hospital anxiety and depression scale		
Anxiety	−1.9 (−3.0 to −0.7)	0.002
Depression	−0.9 (−1.9 to 0.2)	0.116
DUKE-UNC functional social support scale		
Confidant support	−0.9 (−2.4 to 0.6)	0.221
Affective support	−0.3 (−1.2 to 0.7)	0.594

Table 5 Mean and range of resource utilisation for patients in two arms of trial

Outcome measure	Amalthea group (n=89)*	General practitioner group (n=68)[†]
No of contacts with primary healthcare team	4.4 (1–13)	4.4 (1–13)
Cost of contacts with primary healthcare team (£)	61 (14–188)	69 (9–202)
No of prescriptions	3.2 (0–30)	2.9 (0–16)
No of mental health prescriptions	1.9 (0–30)	0.9 (0–8)
Cost of prescriptions (£)	25 (0–169)	22 (0–209)
No of referrals	0.3 (0–2)	0.5 (0–4)
No of mental health referrals	0.2 (0–2)	0.3 (0–2)
Cost of referrals (£)	21 (0–146)	42 (0–322)
Total cost of primary healthcare team contacts, prescribing, and referrals (£)	107 (14–340)	133 (10–452)

(1–13) obviously indicates a range between 1 and 13.

FIGURE 35.6 How the clarity of a table depends on its layout and the legend. Reproduced from Grant C, Goodenough T, Harvey I, Hine C. A randomised controlled trial and economic evaluation of a referrals facilitator between primary care and the voluntary sector. *BMJ* 2000, 320: 419–23, © 2000, with permission from BMJ Publishing Group Ltd.

express the plausible range around a difference between two proportions or between two means, then one or both of the confidence limits often has a minus sign. No wonder then that it is sensible always to write the interval as something like (4 to 9) or (−4 to 9) to prevent ambiguity. In Table 5 in Figure 35.6 there are lots of minus signs, so it is a mercy that the intervals are consistently written as one value *to* another. Not all authors or journals are as careful about this simple safeguard as in the examples here, so watch out for dashes.

The last table in this section (Figure 35.7) has been included to show how authors and journal editorial staff, by liberal but careful use of brackets, dashes and 'to', can successfully and economically display a lot of different kinds of results yet avoid confusing the reader. Despite their efforts they don't always achieve final products as clear as this one and the earlier tables shown in this section.

Patient satisfaction with outpatient hysteroscopy versus day care hysteroscopy: randomised controlled trial

Christian Kremer, Sean Duffy, Michelle Moroney

> The legend is very brief because the variables keep changing so each variable and its brackets is defined in turn.

> Brackets, 'to', and two kinds of dashes – yet always clear.

Table 3 Main outcomes

Variable	Outpatient group (n=49)	Day case group (n=48)	Difference (95% CI)	P value
No (%) of patients satisfied	41 (84)	37 (77)	4.0 (−9 to 22)	0.42
No (%) of patients who needed analgesia at end of hysteroscopy	6 (12)	7 (14)	1.0 (−10 to 17)	0.74
Pain score at 30 minutes (scale 0–10)	0.4 (0–1.2)	0.3 (0–2.2)		0.34
Minutes to recovery of full mobility (interquartile range)	0 (0–5)	105 (80–120)		<0.001
No (%) of patients needing pain relief D0*	15 (30)	16 (33)	−1.0 (−13 to 24)	0.77
No (%) of patients needing pain relief D1†	11 (22)	11 (23)	0 (−14 to 19)	0.93
Median No (range) of days of analgesia	0 (0–2)	0 (0–4)		0.27
Full recovery on day (interquartile range)	2 (1–2.7)	3 (2–4)		<0.05
Days away from work (interquartile range)	1 (0–1.6)	3 (2–4)		<0.0001
Minutes away from home (interquartile range)	120 (110–170)	480 (450–525)		<0.0001

*Patients who need some form of oral or injectable analgesia on day of procedure (immediately after procedure or at home).
†Patients who need some form of oral or injectable analgesia on day after procedure.

FIGURE 35.7 A table that successfully uses brackets, dashes and the word 'to'. Reproduced from Kremer C, Duffy S, Moroney M. Patient satisfaction with outpatient hysteroscopy versus day case hysteroscopy: randomised controlled trial. *BMJ* 2000, 320: 279–82, © 2000, with permission from BMJ Publishing Group Ltd.

36

Results in Pictures

WHY USE CHARTS AND FIGURES?

Research authors and journal publishers generally do their best to make sure that the display of figures is informative and economical of space, so that '*A picture paints a thousand words*'. There are two ways that figures can achieve these aims: either by displaying data graphically when they cannot readily be shown another way or by using the figure to create a striking impact – even when the findings might effectively have been placed within text or tables. In practice these aims are not consistently met, and sometimes the publisher's main aim in printing charts and figures may be to break up large blocks of unattractive text and tables.

Figure 36.1 is an example of a chart that shows how the study data, in two groups of subjects, are derived from all the people who might possibly have been subjects. It's hard to imagine how the information here could be presented as clearly and concisely as text or in a table

The next example in Figure 36.2 is one where the data might readily have been placed in either text or table, but the impact of the pie charts is intended to demonstrate how study samples are divided into proportions according to some variable (in this case cause of death); it works well enough. Pie charts show the parts of a whole, so comparisons between two or more groups can be displayed only by placing multiple pies side by side. Bar charts, on the other hand, lend themselves to the comparison of two or more groups, all in one figure. The apparently simple chart in Figure 36.3 has considerable impact, displaying a striking reduction in the tropical eye disease trachoma after fly control in villages in The Gambia. On closer inspection, though, it is surprisingly complex – comparing villages that were sprayed with those that were not, in two seasons of the year, in each case measuring trachoma prevalence twice. You will need to concentrate to comprehend the whole story behind the data; we think that neither text nor table could readily present the findings as clearly or economically.

There are a great many possible additions and refinements to the basic bar chart. One extra feature you will often encounter is a line, often known as an *error bar*, sticking out of and penetrating into the main bar, as in Figure 36.4. The authors are using the error bars to illustrate how precisely the main bars estimate the population values (see Chapter 25). In general, authors use either the standard error or the 95% confidence interval; they should tell you which one (although often they forget to). Neither is particularly to be preferred to the other. Less often the error bar may be a standard deviation (see Chapter 15), which is rarely if ever helpful on a bar chart.

Sometimes you will see a line graph instead of a bar chart – particularly when the horizontal axis is time. When there are two or more samples being compared, the effect of joining up the points for each sample shows the pattern over time rather better than would a comparable bar chart (Figure 36.5). Error bars are often included with line graphs and fulfil much the same function as they do with bars.

Understanding Clinical Papers, Third Edition. David Bowers, Allan House, David Owens and Bridgette Bewick.
© 2014 John Wiley & Sons, Ltd. Published 2014 by John Wiley & Sons, Ltd.

Intensity of leg and arm training after primary middle-cerebral-artery stroke: a randomised trial

Gert Kwakkel, Robert C Wagenaar, Jos W R Twisk, Gustaaf J Lankhorst, Johan C Koetsier

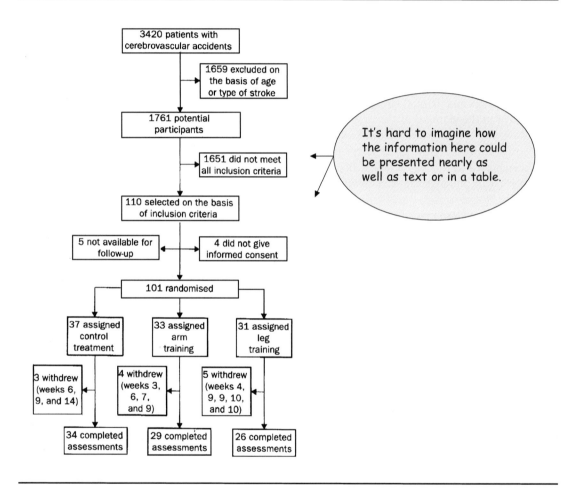

FIGURE 36.1   Trial profile: showing what happened to all potentially eligible subjects. Reprinted from *The Lancet* 354: Kwakkel G, Wagenaar RC, Twisk JWR, Lankhorst GJ, Koetsier JC. Intensity of leg and arm training after primary middle-cerebral-artery stroke: a randomised trial. 1999; 191–6, © 1999, with permission from Elsevier.

Another trimming sometimes added to the bar chart is the splitting of the bars into subdivisions, giving the feel of bars stacked on top of one another. The advantage of economy of information is countered by a problem with visual interpretation because only the lowest part of the bar has a fixed baseline, so the pattern of the higher parts of the bars can easily be missed. In the fairly typical example shown here as Figure 36.6 the patterns evident in the lowest part of the bars are the easiest to grasp.

Effect of metoprolol CR/XL in chronic heart failure: Metoprolol CR/XL Randomised Intervention Trial in Congestive Heart Failure (MERIT-HF)

MERIT-HF Study Group

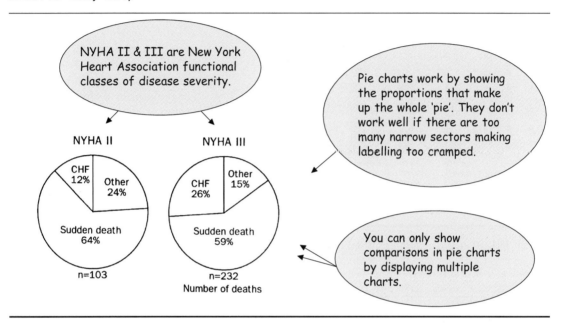

FIGURE 36.2   Pie charts showing severity of heart failure and mode of death. Reprinted from *The Lancet* 353: MERIT-HF Study Group. Effect of metoprolol CR/XL in chronic heart failure: Metoprolol CR/XL Randomised Intervention Trial in Congestive Heart Failure (MERIT-HF). 1999; 2001–7, © 1999, with permission from Elsevier.

The layout of a bar chart suggests some content to the area of each bar – between the baseline and the limit of the bar – often used to display values for proportions or means. When the value to be displayed is an odds ratio or a risk ratio, then there is no baseline and consequently no substance to any of the space. Consequently, values for risk ratios or odds ratios are often, as in Figure 36.7, marked on the chart with no bar to be seen.

SHAPE OF DISTRIBUTIONS

Histograms show a distributed, metric variable chopped up into equal sized bands – such that the shape of the accumulated bars accurately displays the *shape* of the data (see Chapter 14). In the example in Figure 36.8, the graph shape shows that there was over-representation of older people among the sample of patients who had experienced pulmonary emboli. Although bar charts are drawn with gaps between bars, histograms keep the whole data set together without gaps.

When data are skewed or when the data are of the ordinal categorical type (see Chapter 14) researchers may choose to present the distribution graphically using a box plot (or box-and-whisker chart). The example in Figure 36.9 explains how these pictures are constructed. They use the measures of spread based on rank order that were set out in Chapter 15.

Effect of fly control on trachoma and diarrhoea

Paul M Emerson, Steve W Lindsay, Gijs EL Walraven, Hannah Faal, Claus Bøgh, Kebba Lowe, Robin L Bailey

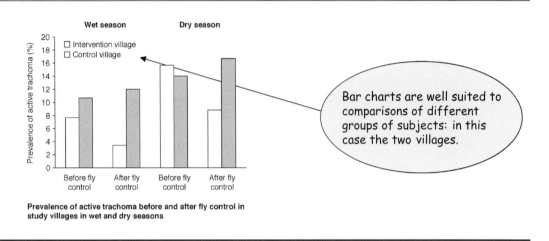

Prevalence of active trachoma before and after fly control in study villages in wet and dry seasons

FIGURE 36.3 Bar chart comparing disease prevalence before and after fly control in control and intervention study villages in wet and dry seasons. Reprinted from *The Lancet* 353: Emerson PM, Lindsay SW, Walraven GE, Faal H, Bøgh C, Lowe K, *et al.* Effect of fly control on trachoma and diarrhoea. 1999; 1401–3, © 1999, with permission from Elsevier.

Quantitative assessment of cervical spondylotic myelopathy by a simple walking test

Anoushka Singh, H Alan Crockard

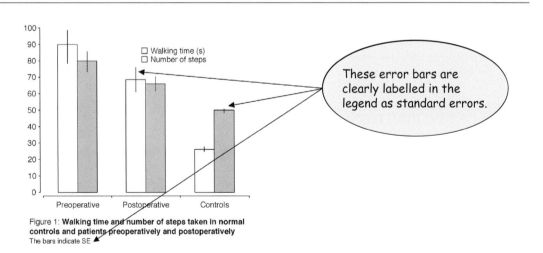

Figure 1: **Walking time and number of steps taken in normal controls and patients preoperatively and postoperatively** The bars indicate SE

FIGURE 36.4 Bar chart with error bars. Reprinted from *The Lancet* 354: Singh A, Crockard HA. Quantitative assessment of cervical spondylotic myelopathy by a simple walking test. 1999; 370–3, © 1999, with permission from Elsevier.

Comparison of combination therapy with single-drug therapy in early rheumatoid arthritis: a randomised trial

Timo Möttönen, Pekka Hannonen, Marjatta Leirisalo-Repo, Martti Nissilä, Hannu Kautianinen, Markku Korpela, Leena Laasonen, Heikki Julkunen, Raijo Luukkainen, Kaisa Vuori, Leena Paimela, Harri Bläfield, Markku Hakala, Kirsti Ilva, Urpo Yli-Kerttula, Kari Puolakka, Pentti Järvinen, Mikko Hakola, Heikki Piirainen, Jari Ahonen, Ilppo Pälvimäki, Sinikka Forsberg, Kalevi Koota, Claes Friman, for the FIN-RACo trial group

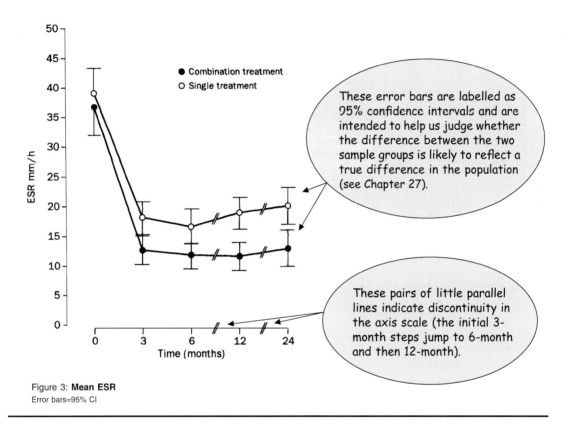

Figure 3: **Mean ESR**
Error bars=95% CI

FIGURE 36.5 Line graph with error bar, showing mean erythrocyte sedimentation rate (ESR) over 2 years of follow-up showing ESR for single and combination treatment groups. Reprinted from *The Lancet* 353: Möttönen T, Hannonen P, Leirisalo-Repo M, Nissilä M, Kautiainen H, Korpela M, *et al.* Comparison of combination therapy with single-drug therapy in early rheumatoid arthritis: a randomised trial. 1999; 1568–73, © 1999, with permission from Elsevier.

Clinical progression and virological failure on highly active antiretroviral therapy in HIV-1 patients: a prospective cohort study

Bruno Ledergerber, Matthias Egger, Milos Opravil, Amalio Telenti, Bernard Hirschel, Manuel Battegay, Pietro Vernazza, Philippe Sudre, Markus Flepp, Hansjakob Furrer, Patrick Francioli, Rainer Weber, for the Swiss HIV Cohort Study*

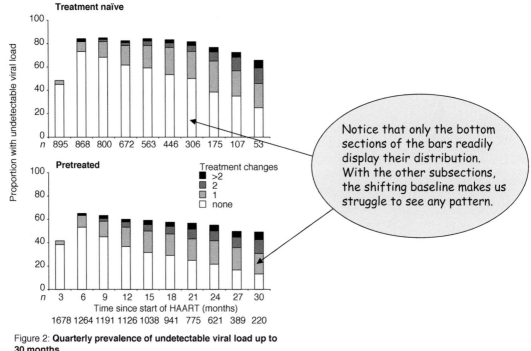

Figure 2: **Quarterly prevalence of undetectable viral load up to 30 months**
Shaded bars=number of changes made to initial regimen.

FIGURE 36.6 Stacked bar charts displaying time pattern of undetectable viral load for four subdivisions of the sample according to number of treatment changes. Reprinted from *The Lancet* 353: Ledergerber B, Egger M, Opravil M, Telenti A, Hirschel B, Battegay M, *et al.* Clinical progression and virological failure on highly active antiretroviral therapy in HIV-1 patients: a prospective cohort study. 1999; 863–8, © 1999, with permission from Elsevier.

Factors influencing the effect of age on prognosis in breast cancer: population based study

Niels Kroman, Maj-Britt Jensen, Jan Wohlfahrt, Henning T Mouridsen, Per Kragh Andersen, Mads Melbye

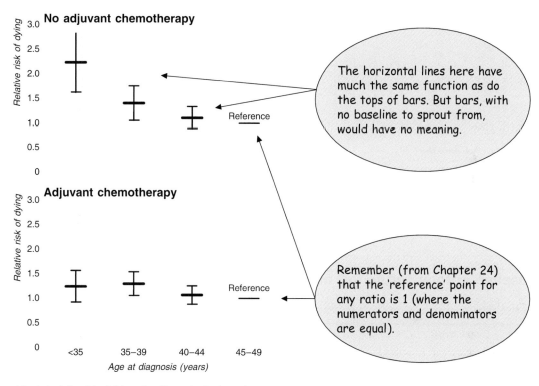

Adjusted relative risk of dying after diagnosis of primary breast cancer according to age at diagnosis among 4329 low risk patients who received no adjuvant treatment (top) and 2824 high risk patients who received adjuvant cytotoxic treatment (bottom). Women aged 45–49 at diagnosis were used as reference. Bars indicate 95% confidence intervals. Relative risk was adjusted for tumour size, nodal status, histological grading, year of diagnosis, and expected mortality

FIGURE 36.7   Chart using horizontal marks (with error bars) to indicate relative risks for four age groups in two cohorts who received or did not receive adjuvant chemotherapy for the treatment of breast cancer. Reproduced from Kroman N, Jensen M-B, Wohlfahrt J, Mouridsen HT, Andersen PK, Melbye M. Factors influencing the effect of age on prognosis in breast cancer: population based study. *BMJ* 2000, 320: 474–9, © 2000, with permission from BMJ Publishing Group Ltd.

Acute pulmonary embolism: clinical outcomes in the International Cooperative Pulmonary Embolism Registry (ICOPER)

Samuel Z Goldhaber, Luigi Visani, Marisa De Rosa, for ICOPER*

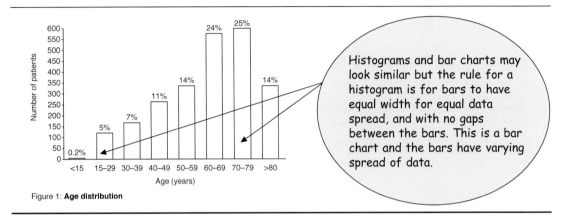

Figure 1: **Age distribution**

FIGURE 36.8　Bar chart of age distribution of 2454 consecutive patients with acute pulmonary embolism drawn from 52 hospitals in seven countries. Reprinted from *The Lancet* 353: Goldhaber SZ, Visani L, De Rosa M. Acute pulmonary embolism: clinical outcomes in the International Cooperative Pulmonary Embolism Registry (ICOPER). 1999; 1386–9, © 1999, with permission from Elsevier.

Decline in total serum IgE after treatment for tuberculosis

J F A Adams, E H Schölvinck, R P Gie, P C Potter, N Beyers, A D Beyers

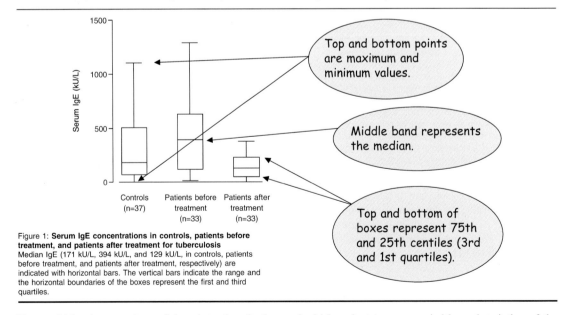

Figure 1: **Serum IgE concentrations in controls, patients before treatment, and patients after treatment for tuberculosis**
Median IgE (171 kU/L, 394 kU/L, and 129 kU/L, in controls, patients before treatment, and patients after treatment, respectively) are indicated with horizontal bars. The vertical bars indicate the range and the horizontal boundaries of the boxes represent the first and third quartiles.

FIGURE 36.9　A comparison of three box plots (or box-and-whisker charts) accompanied by a description of the conventional layout of the box plot. Reprinted from the *The Lancet* 353: Adams JFA *et al*. Decline in total serum IgE after treatment for tuberculosis. 1999; 353:2030–2, © with permission for Elsevier.

37

The Discussion and Conclusions

The Discussion section of a paper usually comes at the end, after the presentation of Results, and is meant to put those results in context for the reader – indicating the authors' beliefs about the meaning of their findings and their implications for the future.

The Discussion varies considerably in content and length, according to the style of the journal, but it is likely to contain some or all of the following elements. Discussions often start with a brief summary of the main findings of the study, as in Figure 37.1. This summary will usually contain little or no data or statistics – its purpose is to 'remind' you of the main message the authors would like you to take from their paper. It should certainly contain no new data, which always belong in the results section.

The findings may then be compared with those from other similar work, to point out whether they broadly agree with previous research or whether they disagree. This business of comparing findings with others can be difficult, mainly because it is so hard to get an accurate, unbiased view of the previous research in an area. We tend to know certain papers well – especially if we have enjoyed them or they support our own views – and yet be unaware of other equally important work. The best approach would be to refer to a *systematic review* of the literature (see Chapter 33), but one may not exist. If one doesn't (or if it isn't quoted by the authors) then be cautious about the possibilities of bias from selective quotation in this mini-review.

Good Discussions include a brief *critical appraisal* of the work that is presented: pointing out the main strengths *and weaknesses* of the study, and considering whether the results could have been due to some flaw in its design or conduct. A typical example is shown in Figure 37.2.

So far in the Discussion, the authors should have reminded you of what their findings are and where they fit in to the total picture, and they should have indicated the likelihood that their results are believable and not due to problems with the study. Next you may find a suggestion as to the meaning of the findings: is there a plausible explanation for them? Any reader of crime or thriller novels knows that a plausible story may not turn out to be a true one, but nonetheless this is a useful exercise. If results fly in the face of everything we know, they may present an exciting challenge to our theories, but we are more likely to think twice about whether they are reliable. Journals (and authors) vary considerably in how much they like to explore this side of the work – 'getting away from the data' – and some Discussions can seem too much like reviews in their own right.

Another way to examine the meaning of results is to ask what their implications are for future practice. In clinical practice, the question is: 'If we believe these results, should it change how we work, and if so how?' Incidentally, this is a very good question to ask of yourself: to decide whether you really *do* believe the results and whether you really base your practice on evidence! Of course, answers are rarely clear-cut and the other question to ask of the future is: 'What research do we need to do to build on the findings from this study or to answer questions raised by it?'

A few papers finish with a Conclusions or Summary section, but for most the Abstract and Discussion serve those purposes. Journals often have boxes (Figure 37.3) or bullet-point lists, to tell you about a paper. They can offer you a quick summary of what a paper is about and they tell you what the authors conclude from their study.

Understanding Clinical Papers, Third Edition. David Bowers, Allan House, David Owens and Bridgette Bewick.
© 2014 John Wiley & Sons, Ltd. Published 2014 by John Wiley & Sons, Ltd.

The equity impact of participatory women's groups to reduce neonatal mortality in India: secondary analysis of a cluster randomised trial

Tanja AJ Houwelling, Prasanta Tripathy, Nirmala Nair, Shibanand Rath, Suchitra Rath, Rajkumar Gope, Rajesh Shina, Casper W Looman, Anthony Costello and Audrey Prost

Discussion

Our study shows that the women's group intervention strongly reduced the NMR among lower socio-economic groups in the areas of India in which the study was conducted. The effects were substantially stronger among the most socio-economically marginalised groups. This is remarkable, given that interventions often lead to increasing, rather than declining socio-economic inequalities in mortality. [7, 12,14,43,44.] Our findings are important in view of the paucity of evidence for specifically effective means for reducing socio-economic inequalities in mortality. We show that a low cost[45] participatory community intervention can contribute to an equitable achievement of MDG4.

The authors start with a brief summary of their main finding.

Evaluation of data and methods

Measurement bias is unlikely to explain our findings. Neonatal mortality rate was the primary outcome measure of the original trial, and stringent measures were taken to ensure completeness and reliability of the data relating to this measure.[41] Birth and newborn death data in the trial were collected through prospective surveillance ,[41] which constitutes an important advance over often-used retrospective surveys, which rely on mothers' recall.[46-47] More generally, because the study used a randomised design, potential confounders are expected to be evenly distributed between the study arms...

They go on to consider whether methodological weakness might explain the results.

...Mechanisms

Two complementary mechanisms may explain the stronger intervention effect among the most marginalised groups in the study. First, the uptake of the intervention (women's group attendance, behavioural improvements) was similar among the most and less marginalised groups, whereas interventions normally.

Having decided not, the authors outline possible mechanisms for the effect they observed.

FIGURE 37.1 A Discussion that starts with a résumé of the study findings before considering possible explanations. Reproduced from Houwelling TAJ, Prasanta T, Nirmala N, Shibanand R, Suchitra R, Rajkumar G, *et al*. The equity impact of participatory women's groups to reduce neonatal mortality in India: secondary analysis of a cluster-randomised trial. *International Journal of Epidemiology* 2013, 42: 520–32 by permission of Oxford University Press.

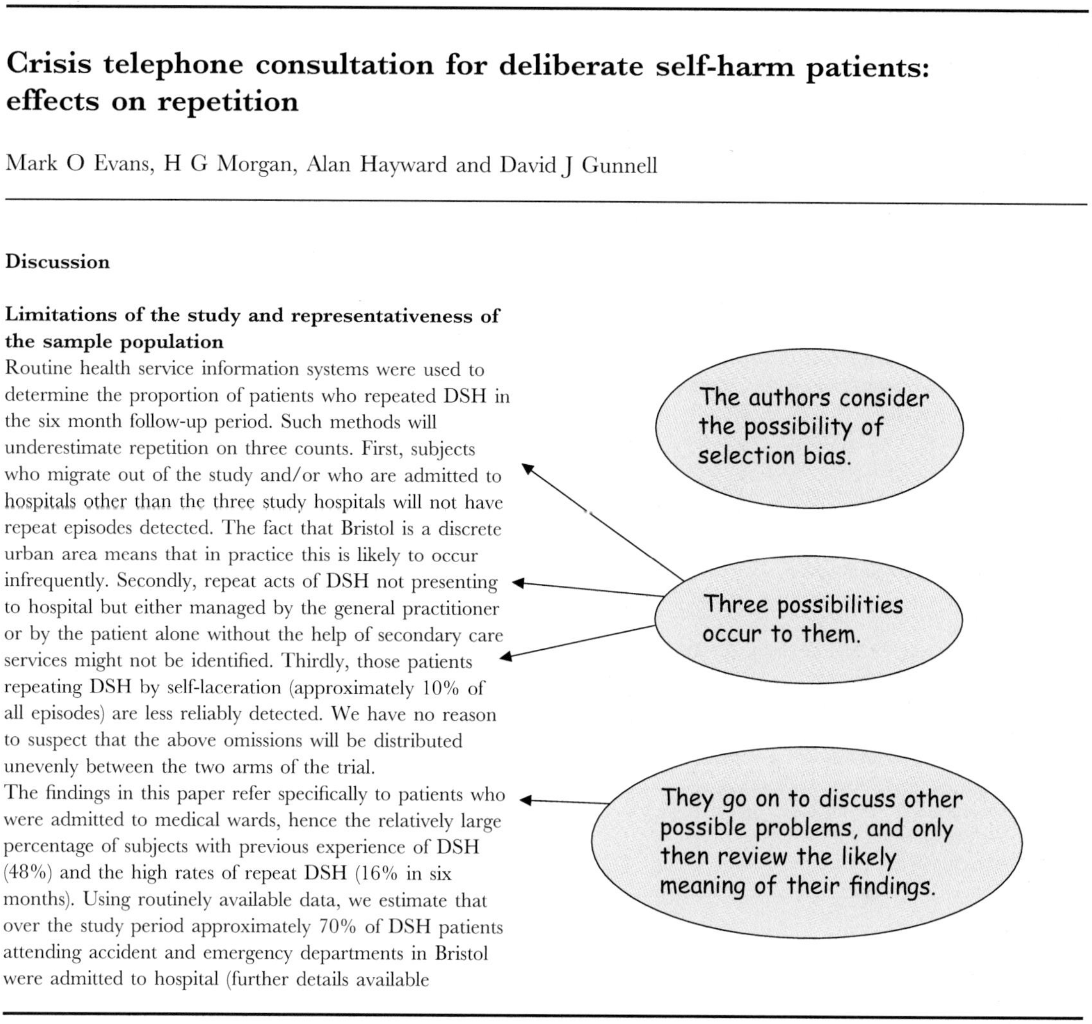

Crisis telephone consultation for deliberate self-harm patients: effects on repetition

Mark O Evans, H G Morgan, Alan Hayward and David J Gunnell

Discussion

Limitations of the study and representativeness of the sample population

Routine health service information systems were used to determine the proportion of patients who repeated DSH in the six month follow-up period. Such methods will underestimate repetition on three counts. First, subjects who migrate out of the study and/or who are admitted to hospitals other than the three study hospitals will not have repeat episodes detected. The fact that Bristol is a discrete urban area means that in practice this is likely to occur infrequently. Secondly, repeat acts of DSH not presenting to hospital but either managed by the general practitioner or by the patient alone without the help of secondary care services might not be identified. Thirdly, those patients repeating DSH by self-laceration (approximately 10% of all episodes) are less reliably detected. We have no reason to suspect that the above omissions will be distributed unevenly between the two arms of the trial.

The findings in this paper refer specifically to patients who were admitted to medical wards, hence the relatively large percentage of subjects with previous experience of DSH (48%) and the high rates of repeat DSH (16% in six months). Using routinely available data, we estimate that over the study period approximately 70% of DSH patients attending accident and emergency departments in Bristol were admitted to hospital (further details available

The authors consider the possibility of selection bias.

Three possibilities occur to them.

They go on to discuss other possible problems, and only then review the likely meaning of their findings.

FIGURE 37.2   Critical appraisal of a study's results. Reproduced from Evans MO, Morgan HG, Hayward A, Gunnell DJ. Crisis telephone consultation for deliberate self-harm patients: effects on repetition. *British Journal of Psychiatry* 1999, 175: 23–7, © 1999, with permission from the Royal College of Psychiatrists.

Risk of subarachnoid haemorrhage in first degree relatives of patients with subarachnoid haemorrhage: follow up study based on national registries in Denmark

Favid Gaist, Michael Vaeth, Ioannis Tsiropoulos, Kaare Christensen, Elisabeth Corder, Jørn Olsen, Henrik Toft Sørensen

What is known on this topic

Several observational studies have indicated that first degree relatives of patients with subarachnoid haemorrhage are at increased risk of having this disorder. However, the validity of the risk estimates could be questioned owing to potential problems of selection and recall bias.

What this paper adds

This follow up study overcame some of these problems by using national registries in Denmark to create pedigrees and to identify incident cases of subarachnoid haemorrhage.

The study confirmed that first degree relatives of patients with subarachnoid haemorrhage are at a threefold to fivefold increased risk of experiencing a subarachnoid haemorrhage compared with the general population but the incidence rate of subarachnoid haemorrhage is low.

Summary boxes like this will often appear near the end of a paper. They may help you decide whether the paper is likely to interest you, but you should never believe what they say without checking out the study for yourself.

FIGURE 37.3   A summary box which outlines a study's importance and main findings. Reproduced from Gaist F, Vaeth M, Tsiropoulos I, Christensen K, Corder E, Olsen J, *et al*. Risk of subarachnoid haemorrhage in first degree relatives of patients with subarachnoid haemorrhage: follow up study based on national registries in Denmark. *BMJ* 2000, 320: 141–5, © 2000, with permission from BMJ Publishing Group Ltd.

References

Adams JFA, Schölvinck EH, Gie RP, Potter PC, Beyers N, Beyers AD. Decline in total serum IgE after treatment for tuberculosis. *Lancet* 1999, 353: 2030–2.

Adish AA, Esrey SA, Gyorkos TW, Jean-Baptiste J, Rojhani A. Effect of consumption of food cooked in iron pots on iron status and growth of young children: a randomised trial. *Lancet* 1999, 353: 712–6.

Alderson SL, Foy R, Glidewell L, McLintock K, House A. How patients understand depression associated with chronic physical disease – a systematic review. *BMC Family Practice* 2012, 13: 41.

Altman D. *Practical Statistics for Medical Research*. London: Chapman & Hall, 1991.

Anderson EH, Spencer MH. Cognitive representations of AIDS: a phenomenological study. *Qualitative Health Research* 2002, 12: 1338–52.

Antoniou T, Gomes T, Mamdani MM, Yao Z, Hellings C, Garg AX, *et al.* Trimethoprim-sulfamethoxazole induced hyperkalaemia in elderly patients receiving spironolactone: nested case-control study. *BMJ* 2011, 343: d5228.

Appleby L, Shaw J, Amos T, McDonnell R, Harris C, McCann K, *et al.* Suicide within 12 months of contact with mental health services; national clinical survey. *BMJ* 1999, 318: 1235–9.

Appleby L, Warner R, Whitton A, Faragher B. A controlled study of fluoxetine and cognitive-behavioural counselling in the treatment of postnatal depression. *BMJ* 1997, 314: 932–5.

Arolker M, Epstein M, Seale C. A critical appraisal of ethical sedative use for dying patients: comparative ethnographic study of three palliative care units. *BMJ Supportive & Palliative Care* 2012, 2: A34.

Baker JA, Richards DA, Campbell MG. Nursing attitudes towards acute mental health care: development of a measurement tool. *Journal of Advanced Nursing* 2005, 49: 522–9.

Basso O, Olsen J, Johansen AMT, Christensen K. Change in social status and risk of low birthweight in Denmark: population based cohort study. *BMJ* 1997, 315: 1498–502.

Bebbington-Hatcher M, Fallowfield LJ. A qualitative study looking at the psychosocial implications of bilateral prophylactic mastectomy. *The Breast* 2003, 12: 1–9.

Bennett B, Goldstein D, Lloyd A, Davenport T, Hickie I. Fatigue and psychological distress – exploring the relationship in women treated for breast cancer. *European Journal of Cancer* 2004, 40: 1689–95.

Beral V, Hermon C, Kay C, Hannaford P, Darby S, Reeves G. Mortality associated with oral contraceptive use: 25 year follow up of cohort of 46 000 women from Royal College of General Practitioners' oral contraception study. *BMJ* 1999, 318: 96–100.

Berkley J, Mwangi I, Griffiths K, Ahmed I, Mithwani S, English M, *et al.* Assessment of severe malnutrition among hospitalised children in rural Kenya. *Journal of the American Medical Association* 2005, 294: 591–5.

Bhagwanjee S, Muckart DJJ, Jeena PM, Moodley P. Does HIV status influence the outcome of patients admitted to a surgical intensive care unit? A prospective double blind study. *BMJ* 1997, 314: 1077.

Bland JM, Altman DG. Statistical methods for assessing agreement between two clinical measurements. *Lancet* 1986, i: 307–10.

Blatchford O, Davidson LA, Murray WR, Blatchford M, Pell J. Acute upper gastrointestinal haemorrhage in west of Scotland: case ascertainment study. *BMJ* 1997, 315: 510–4.

Blazeby JM, Soulsby M, Winstone K, King PM, Bulley S, Kennedy RH. A qualitative evaluation of patients' experiences of an enhanced recovery programme for colorectal cancer. *Colorectal Disease* 2010, 12 (10 Online): e236–42.

Bowers D. *Statistics from Scratch: An Introduction for Health Professionals*, 2nd edn. Chichester: John Wiley, 2008.

Boyles CM, Bailey PH, Mossey S. Chronic obstructive pulmonary disease as disability: dilemma stories. *Qualitative Health Research* 2011, 21: 187–98.

Brandon S, Cowley P, McDonald C, Neville P, Palmer R, Wellstood-Eason S. Electroconvulsive therapy: results in depressive illness from the Leicestershire trial. *BMJ* 1984, 288: 23–6.

Brown J, Sorrell JH, McClaren J, Creswell JW. Waiting for a liver transplant. *Qualitative Health Research* 2006, 16: 129–36.

Bruins Slot K, Berge E, Dorman P, Lewis S, Dennis M, Sandercock P, on behalf of the Oxfordshire Community Stroke Project, the International Stroke Trial (UK), and the Lothian Stroke Register. Impact of functional status at six months on long term survival in patients with ischaemic stroke: prospective cohort studies. *BMJ* 2008, 336: 376.

Bruzzi P, Dogliotti L, Naldoni C, Bucchi L, Costantini M, Cicognani A, *et al.* Cohort study of association of risk of breast cancer with cyst type in women with gross cystic disease of the breast. *BMJ* 1997, 314: 925–8.

Buitrago-Lopez A, Sanderson J, Johnson L, Warnakula S, Wood A, Di Angelantonio E, *et al.* Chocolate consumption and cardiometabolic disorders: systematic review and meta-analysis. *BMJ* 2011, 343: d4488.

Burden SR, Hill J, Shaffer JL, Campbell M, Todd C. An unblinded randomised controlled trial in preoperative oral supplements in colorectal cancer patients. *Journal of Human Nutrition and Dietetics* 2011, 24: 441–8.

Burns E, Schmied V, Fenwick J, Sheehan A. Liquid gold from the milk bar: constructions of breastmilk and breastfeeding women in the language and practices of midwives. *Social Science & Medicine* 2012, 75: 1737–45.

Buston KM. Experiences of, and attitudes towards, pregnancy and fatherhood amongst incarcerated young male offenders: findings from a qualitative study. *Social Science & Medicine* 2010, 71: 2212–8.

Chapple A, Ziebland S, Hewitson P, McPherson A. What affects the uptake of screening for bowel cancer using a faecal occult blood test (FOBt): a qualitative study. *Social Science & Medicine* 2008, 66: 2425–35.

Chosidow O, Chastang C, Brue C, Bouvet E, Izri M, Monteny N, *et al.* Controlled study of malathion and *d*-phenothrin lotions for *Pediculus humanus* var *capitis*-infected schoolchildren. *Lancet* 1994, 344: 1724–9.

Cooper KG, Bain C, Parkin DE. Comparison of microwave endometrial ablation and transcervical resection of the endometrium for treatment of heavy menstrual loss: a randomised trial. *Lancet* 1999, 354: 1859–63.

Corcoran P, Arensman E, Perry IJ. The area-level association between hospital treated deliberate self-harm, deprivation and social fragmentation in Ireland. *Journal of Epidemiology & Community Health* 2007, 61: 1050–5.

Coste J, Delecoeuillerie G, Cohen de Lara A, Le Parc JM, Paolaggi JB. Clinical course and prognostic factors in acute low back pain: an inception cohort study in primary care practice. *BMJ* 1994, 308: 577–80.

Cousens SN, Zeidler M, Esmonde TF, De Silva R, Wilesmith JW, Smith PG, *et al.* Sporadic Creutzfeldt-Jakob disease in the United Kingdom: analysis of epidemiological surveillance data for 1970–96. *BMJ* 1997, 315: 389–95.

Crooks VA. Exploring the altered daily geographies and lifeworlds of women living with fibromyalgia syndrome: a mixed method approach. *Social Science & Medicine* 2007, 64: 577–88.

Crowe FL, Appleby PN, Allen NE, Key TJ. Diet and risk of diverticular disease in Oxford cohort of European Prospective Investigation into Cancer and Nutrition (EPIC): prospective study of British vegetarians and non-vegetarians. *BMJ* 2011, 343: d4131.

Culbertson DS, Griggs M, Hudson S. Ear and hearing status in multilevel retirement facility. *Geriatric Nursing* 2004, 25: 93–6.

de Boer MA, Celentano DD, Tovanabutra S, Rugpao S, Nelson KE, Suriyanon V. Reliability of self-reported sexual behaviour is human immunodeficiency virus (HIV) between concordant and discordant heterosexual couples in Northern Thailand. *American Journal of Epidemiology* 1998, 147: 1153–61.

Diekman ST, Ballesteros MF, Berger LR, Carabello RS, Kegler SR. Ecological level analysis of the relationship between smoking and residential-fire mortality. *Injury Prevention* 2008, 14: 228–31.

Drach-Zahavy A, Goldblatt H, Granot M, Hirschmann S, Kostintski H. Control: patients' aggression in psychiatric settings. *Qualitative Health Research* 2012, 22: 43–53.

Dunne MW, Bozzette S, McCutchan JA, Dubé MP, Sattler FR, Forthal D, *et al.*, for the California Collaborative Treatment Group. Efficacy of azithromycin in prevention of Pneumocystis carinii pneumonia: a randomised trial. *Lancet* 1999, 354: 891–4.

Dupuy A, Benchikhi H, Roujeau J-C, Bernard P, Vaillant L, Chosidow O, *et al.* Risk factors for erysipelas of the leg (cellulitis): case-control study. *BMJ* 1999, 318: 1591–4.

Dyson SM, Atkin K, Culley LA, Dyson SE, Evans H, Rowley DT. Disclosure and sickle cell disorder: a mixed methods study of the young person with sickle cell at school. *Social Science & Medicine* 2010, 70: 2036–44.

Egger M, Smith GD. Bias in location and selection of studies. *BMJ* 1998, 316: 61–6.

Ellenbecker CH, Frazier SC, Verney S. Nurses' observations and experiences of problems and adverse effects of medication management in home care. *Geriatric Nursing* 2004, 26: 164–70.

Emerson PM, Lindsay SW, Walraven GE, Faal H, Bøgh C, Lowe K, *et al*. Effect of fly control on trachoma and diarrhoea. *Lancet* 1999, 353: 1401–3.

Enden T, Haig Y, Kløw N-E, Slagsvold C-E, Sandvik L, Ghanima W, *et al.*, on behalf of the CaVenT Study Group. Long-term outcome after additional catheter-directed thrombolysis versus standard treatment for acute iliofemoral deep vein thrombosis (the CaVenT study): a randomised controlled trial. *Lancet* 2012, 379(9810): 31–8.

Evans MO, Morgan HG, Hayward A, Gunnell DJ. Crisis telephone consultation for deliberate self-harm patients: effects on repetition. *British Journal of Psychiatry* 1999, 175: 23–7.

Farnell S, Maxwell L, Tan S, Rhodes A, Philips B. Temperature measurement: comparison of non-invasive methods used in adult critical care. *Journal of Clinical Nursing* 2005, 14: 632–9.

Feeney M, Clegg A, Winwood P, Snook J, for the East Dorset Gastroenterology Group. A case-control study of measles vaccination and inflammatory bowel disease. *Lancet* 1997, 350: 764–6.

Field A. *Discovering Statistics Using SPSS for Windows*. London: Sage, 2009.

Foley K, Vasey J, Markson LE. Development and validation of the hyperlipidemia attitudes & beliefs in treatment (HABIT) survey for physicians. *Journal of General Internal Medicine* 2003, 18(12): 984–90.

Freedland SJ, Humphreys EB, Mangold LA, Eisenberger M, Dorey FJ, Walsh PC, Partin AW. Death in patients with recurrent prostate cancer after radical prostatectomy: prostate-specific antigen doubling time subgroups and their associated contributions to all-cause mortality. *Journal of Clinical Oncology* 2007, 25: 1765–71.

Gaist F, Vaeth M, Tsiropoulos I, Christensen K, Corder E, Olsen J, *et al*. Risk of subarachnoid haemorrhage in first degree relatives of patients with subarachnoid haemorrhage: follow up study based on national registries in Denmark. *BMJ* 2000, 320: 141–5.

Gebre T, Ayele B, Zerihun M, Genet A, Stoller NE, Zhou Z, *et al*. Comparison of annual versus twice-yearly mass azithromycin treatment for hyperendemic trachoma in Ethiopia: a cluster-randomised trial. *Lancet* 2012, 379: 143–51.

Gibbs S, Harvey I, Sterling JC, Stark R. Local treatments for cutaneous warts. *Cochrane Database of Systematic Reviews* 2005, 3: CD001781.

Goldhaber SZ, Visani L, De Rosa M. Acute pulmonary embolism: clinical outcomes in the International Cooperative Pulmonary Embolism Registry (ICOPER). *Lancet* 1999, 353: 1386–9.

Graham W, Smith P, Kamal A, Fitzmaurice A, Smith N, Hamilton N. Randomised controlled trial comparing effectiveness of touch screen with leaflet for providing women with information on prenatal tests. *BMJ* 2000, 320: 155–60.

Grandjean P, Bjerve KS, Weihe P, Steuerwald U. Birthweight in a fishing community: significance of essential fatty acids and marine food contaminants. *International Journal of Epidemiology* 2000, 30: 1272–7.

Grant C, Goodenough T, Harvey I, Hine C. A randomised controlled trial and economic evaluation of a referrals facilitator between primary care and the voluntary sector. *BMJ* 2000, 320: 419–23.

Griffin S. Diabetes care in general practice: meta-analysis of randomised control trials. *BMJ* 1998, 317: 390–6.

Haelterman E, Bréart G, Paris-Llado J, Dramaix M, Tchobroutsky C. Effect of uncomplicated chronic hypertension on the risk of small-for-gestational age birth. *American Journal of Epidemiology* 1997, 145: 689–95.

Hagen S, Bugge C, Alexander H. Psychometric properties of the SF-36 in the early post-stroke phase. *Journal of Advanced Nursing* 2003, 44: 461–8.

Hammerlid E, Taft C. Health-related quality of life in long-term head and neck cancer survivors: a comparison with general population norms. *British Journal of Cancer* 2001, 84: 149–56.

Hawton K, Bergen H, Casey D, Simkin S, Palmer B, Cooper J, *et al*. Self-harm in England: a tale of three cities. Multicentre study of self-harm. *Social Psychiatry and Psychiatric Epidemiology* 2007, 42: 513–21.

He Y, Lam TH, Li LS, Du RY, Jia GL, Huang JY, *et al*. Passive smoking at work as a risk factor for coronary heart disease in Chinese women who have never smoked. *BMJ* 1994, 308: 380–4.

Hearn J, Higginson IJ, on behalf of the Palliative Care Core Audit Project Advisory Group. Development and validation of a core outcome measure for palliative care: the palliative care outcome scale. *Quality in Health Care* 1999, 8: 219–27.

Heart Protection Study Collaborative Group. C-reactive protein concentration and the vascular benefits of statin therapy: an analysis of 20 536 patients in the Heart Protection Study. *Lancet* 2011, 377: 469–76.

Heianza Y, Hara S, Arase Y, Saito K, Fujiwara K, Tsuji H, *et al*. HbA$_{1c}$ 5.7–6.4% and impaired fasting plasma glucose for diagnosis of prediabetes and risk of progression to diabetes in Japan (TOPICS 3): a longitudinal cohort study. *Lancet* 2011, 378(9786): 147–55.

Henderson RD, Wliasziw M, Fox AJ, Rothwell PM, Barnett HJM, for the North American Symptomatic Carotid Endarterectomy Trial Group. Angiographically defined collateral circulation and risk of stroke in patients with severe carotid artery stenosis. *Stroke* 2000, 31: 128–32.

Hesse-Biber SN, Leavy P. *The Practice of Qualitative Research*, 2nd edn. London: Sage, 2011.

Hesselgard K, Larsson S, Romner B, Strömblad L-G, Reinstrup P. Validity and reliability of the Behavioural Observational Pain Scale for postoperative pain measurement in children 1–7 years of age. *Pediatric Critical Care Medicine* 2007, 8: 102–8.

Higgins JPT, Thompson SG. Quantifying heterogeneity in a meta-analysis. *Statistics in Medicine* 2002, 21: 1539–58.

Ho Cheung W, Lopez V. Children's emotional manifestation scale: development and testing. *Journal of Clinical Nursing* 2003, 14: 223–9.

Hosmer DW, Lemeshow S. *Applied Logistic Regression*, 2nd edn. Chichester: Wiley, 2013.

Hosmer DW, Lemeshow S. *Applied Survival Analysis*. Chichester: Wiley, 1999.

Houwelling TAJ, Prasanta T, Nirmala N, Shibanand R, Suchitra R, Rajkumar G, *et al*. The equity impact of participatory women's groups to reduce neonatal mortality in India: secondary analysis of a cluster-randomised trial. *International Journal of Epidemiology* 2013, 42: 520–32.

Hundley V, Milne J, Leighton-Beck L, Graham W, Fitzmaurice A. Raising research awareness among midwives and nurses: does it work? *Journal of Advanced Nursing* 2000, 31: 78–88.

Jernström H, Olsson H. Breast size in relation to endogenous hormone levels, body constitution, and oral contraceptive use in healthy nulligravid women aged 19–25 years. *American Journal of Epidemiology* 1997, 45: 571–80.

Jones IR, Ahmed N, Catty J, McLaren S, Rose D, Wykes T, *et al*. Illness careers and continuity of care in mental health services: a qualitative study of users and carers. *Social Science & Medicine* 2009, 69: 632–9.

Jozwiak M, Oude Rengerink K, Benthem M, van Beek E, Dijksterhuis MGK, de Graaf IM, *et al*. Foley catheter versus vaginal prostaglandin E$_2$ gel for induction of labour at term (PROBAAT trial): an open-label, randomised controlled trial for the PROBAAT Study Group. *Lancet* 2011, 378: 2095–103.

Kobayashi T, Saji T, Otani T, Takeuchi K, Nakamura T, Arakawa H, *et al*., on behalf of the RAISE Study Group Investigators. Efficacy of immunoglobulin plus prednisolone for prevention of coronary artery abnormalities in severe Kawasaki disease (RAISE study): a randomised, open-label, blinded-endpoints trial. *Lancet* 2012, 379: 1613–20.

Kokkinos PF, Faselis C, Myers J, Panagiotakos D, Doumas M. Interactive effects of fitness and statin treatment on mortality risk in veterans with dyslipidaemia: a cohort study. *Lancet* 2013, 381: 394–9.

Kong S. Day treatment programme for patients with eating disorders: randomized controlled trial. *Journal of Advanced Nursing* 2005, 51: 5–14.

Kremer C, Duffy S, Moroney M. Patient satisfaction with outpatient hysteroscopy versus day case hysteroscopy: randomised controlled trial. *BMJ* 2000, 320: 279–82.

Kroman N, Jensen M-B, Wohlfahrt J, Mouridsen HT, Andersen PK, Melbye M. Factors influencing the effect of age on prognosis in breast cancer: population based study. *BMJ* 2000, 320: 474–9.

Kwakkel G, Wagenaar RC, Twisk JWR, Lankhorst GJ, Koetsier JC. Intensity of leg and arm training after primary middle-cerebral-artery stroke: a randomised trial. *Lancet* 1999, 354: 191–6.

Lachal J, Speranza M, Taieb O, Falissard B, Lefevre H, Moro M-R, *et al*. Qualitative research using photo-elicitation to explore the role of food in family relationships among obese adolescents. *Appetite* 2012, 58: 1099–105.

Lacy AM, Garcia-Valdecasas JC, Delgado S, Castells A, Taura P, Pique JM, *et al*. Laparoscopy-assisted colectomy versus open colectomy for treatment of non-metastatic colon cancer: a randomised trial. *Lancet* 2002, 359: 2224–9.

Ledergerber B, Egger M, Opravil M, Telenti A, Hirschel B, Battegay M, *et al*. Clinical progression and virological failure on highly active antiretroviral therapy in HIV-1 patients: a prospective cohort study. *Lancet* 1999, 353: 863–8.

Leon DA, Smith GD. Infant mortality, stomach cancer, stroke, and coronary heart disease: ecological analysis. *BMJ* 2000, 320: 1705–6.

Levene S. More injuries from "bouncy castles". *BMJ* 1992, 304: 1311–2.

Lin L-C, Wang TG, Chen MY, Wu SC, Portwood MJ. Depressive symptoms in long-term care residents in Taiwan. *Journal of Advanced Nursing* 2005, 51: 30–7.

Little P. GP documentation of obesity: what does it achieve? *British Journal of General Practice* 1998, 48: 890–4.

Lobbana F, Barrowclough C, Jeffery S, Bucci S, Taylor K, Mallinson S, *et al*. Understanding factors influencing substance use in people with recent onset psychosis: a qualitative study. *Social Science & Medicine* 2010, 70: 1141–7.

Long EM, Martin HL, Kriess JK, Rainwater SMJ, Lavreys L, Jackson DJ, *et al*. Gender differences in HIV-1 diversity at time of infection. *Nature Medicine* 2000, 6: 71–5.

Lowe AJ, Carlin JB, Bennett CM, Hosking CS, Allen KJ, Robertson CF, *et al*. Paracetamol use in early life and asthma: prospective birth cohort study. *BMJ* 2010, 341: c4616.

Macarthur A, Macarthur C, Weeks S. Epidural anaesthesia and low back pain after delivery: a prospective cohort study. *BMJ* 1995, 311: 1336–9.

Mahmood A, Chaudhury H, Michael YL, Campo M, Hay K, Sarte A. A photovoice documentation of the role of neighbourhood physical and social environments in older adults' physical activity in two metropolitan areas in North America. *Social Science and Medicine* 2012, 74: 1180–92.

Marshall M, Lockwood A, Gath D. Social services case-management for long-term mental disorders: a randomised controlled trial. *Lancet* 1995, 345: 409–12.

McKee M, Hunter D. Mortality league tables: do they inform or mislead? *Quality in Health Care* 1995, 4: 5–12.

McKeown-Eyssen GE, Sokoloff ER, Jazmaji V, Marshall LM, Baines CJ. Reproducibility of the University of Toronto self-administered questionnaire used to assess environmental sensitivity. *American Journal of Epidemiology* 2000, 151: 1216–22.

Mejdahl MK, Andersen KG, Gärtner R, Kroman N, Kehlet H. Persistent pain and sensory disturbances after treatment for breast cancer: six year nationwide follow-up study. *BMJ* 2013, 346: f1865.

MERIT-HF Study Group. Effect of metoprolol CR/XL in chronic heart failure: Metoprolol CR/XL Randomised Intervention Trial in Congestive Heart Failure (MERIT-HF). *Lancet* 1999, 353: 2001–7.

Middleton S, McElduff P, Ward J, Grimshaw JM, Dale S, D'Este C, *et al*., on behalf of the QASC Trialists Group. Implementation of evidence-based treatment protocols to manage fever, hyperglycaemia, and swallowing dysfunction in acute stroke (QASC): a cluster randomised controlled trial. *Lancet* 2011, 378: 1699–706.

Miles K, Penny N, Power R, Mercy D. Comparing doctor- and nurse-led care in sexual health clinics: patient satisfaction questionnaire. *Journal of Advanced Nursing* 2002, 42: 64–72.

Mosack KE, Abbott M, Singer M, Weeks MR, Rohena L. If I didn't have HIV, I'd be dead now: illness narratives of drug users living with HIV/AIDS. *Qualitative Health Research* 2005, 15: 586–605.

Moore RA, Tramèr MR, Carroll D, Wiffen PJ, McQuay HJ. Quantitative systematic review of topically applied non-steroidal anti-inflammatory drugs. *BMJ* 1998, 316: 333–8.

Morris CR, Kato GJ, Poljakovic M, Wang X, Blackwelder WC, Sachdev V, *et al*. Dysregulated arginine metabolism, hemolysis-associated pulmonary hypertension, and mortality in sickle cell disease. *Journal of the American Medical Association* 2005, 294: 81–90.

Möttönen T, Hannonen P, Leirisalo-Repo M, Nissilä M, Kautiainen H, Korpela M, *et al*. Comparison of combination therapy with single-drug therapy in early rheumatoid arthritis: a randomised trial. *Lancet* 1999, 353: 1568–73.

Naumburg E, Bellocco R, Cnattingius S, Hall P, Ekbom A. Prenatal ultrasound examinations and risk of childhood leukaemia: case-control study. *BMJ* 2000, 320: 282–3.

Nikolajsen L, Ilkjaer S, Christensen JH, Krøner K, Jensen TS. Randomised trial of epidural bupivacaine and morphine in prevention of stump and phantom pain in lower-limb amputation. *Lancet* 1998, 350: 1353–7.

Peabody JW, Gertler PJ. Are clinical criteria just proxies for socioeconomic status? A study of low birthweight in Jamaica. *Journal of Epidemiology and Community Health* 1997, 51: 90–5.

Pinnock H, Bawden R, Proctor S, Wolfe S, Scullion J, Price D, *et al*. Accessibility, acceptability, and effectiveness in primary care of routine telephone review of asthma: pragmatic, randomised controlled trial. *BMJ* 2003, 326: 477–9.

Pisacane A, Sansone R, Impagliazzo N, Coppola A, Rolando P, D'Apuzzo A, *et al*. Iron deficiency anaemia and febrile convulsions: case-control study in children under 2 years. *BMJ* 1996, 313: 343.

Platt S, Tannahill A, Watson J, Fraser E. Effectiveness of antismoking telephone helpline: follow up survey. *BMJ* 1997, 314: 1371–5.

Plugge E, Douglas N, Fitzpatrick R. Patients, prisoners, or people? Women prisoners' experiences of primary care in prison: a qualitative study. *British Journal of General Practice* 2008, 58(554): e1–8.

Poulter NR, Chang CL, MacGregor AJ, Snieder H, Spector TD. Association between birthweight and adult blood pressure in twins: historical cohort study. *BMJ* 1999, 319: 1330–3.

Powell P, Murphy VE, Taylor DR, Hensley MJ, McCaffery K, Giles W, *et al*. Management of asthma in pregnancy guided by measurement of fraction of exhaled nitric oxide: a double-blind, randomised controlled trial. *Lancet* 2011, 378: 983–90.

Premawardhena AP, de Silva CE, Fonseka MMD, Gunatilake SB, de Silva HJ. Low dose subcutaneous adrenaline to prevent acute adverse reactions to antivenom serum in people bitten by snakes: randomised, placebo controlled trial. *BMJ* 1999, 318: 1041–3.

Reidy A, Minassian DC, Vafidis G, Joseph J, Farrow S, Wu J, *et al*. Prevalence of serious eye disease and visual impairment in a north London population: population based, cross sectional study. *BMJ* 1998, 316: 1643–6.

Rini BI, Escudier B, Tomczak P, Kaprin A, Szczylik C, Hutson TE, *et al*. Comparative effectiveness of axitinib versus sorafenib in advanced renal cell carcinoma (AXIS): a randomised phase 3 trial. *Lancet* 2011, 378: 1931–9.

Rodgers M, Miller JE. Adequacy of hormone replacement therapy for osteoporosis prevention assessed by serum oestradiol measurement, and the degree of association with menopausal symptoms. *British Journal of General Practice* 1997, 47: 161–6.

Rogers SL, Farlow MR, Doody RS, Mohs R, Friedhoff LT, for the Donepezil Study Group. A 24-week, double-blind, placebo-controlled trial of donepezil in patients with Alzheimer's disease. *Neurology* 1998, 50: 136–45.

Ros-Bullón MR, Sánchez-Pedreño P, Martínez-Liarte JH. Serum tyrosine hydroxylase activity is increased in melanoma patients. An ROC curve analysis. *Cancer Letters* 1998, 129: 151–5.

Roscigno CI, Swanson KM. Parents' experiences following children's moderate to severe traumatic brain injury: a clash of cultures. *Qualitative Health Research* 2011, 21: 1413–26.

Rubinstein F, Micone P, Bonotti A, Wainer V, Schwarcz A, Augustovski F, *et al*., on behalf of 'EVA' Study Research Group (Estudio 'Embarazo y Vacuna Antigripal'). Influenza A/H1N1 MF59 adjuvanted vaccine in pregnant women and adverse perinatal outcomes: multicentre study. *BMJ* 2013, 346: f393 [correction: f990].

Salmon G, James A, Smith DM. Bullying in schools: self reported anxiety, depression, and self esteem in secondary school children. *BMJ* 1998, 317: 924–5.

Selman L, Higginson IJ, Godfrey A, Dinat N, Downing J, Gwyther L, *et al*. Meeting information needs of patients with incurable progressive disease and their families in South Africa and Uganda: multicentre qualitative study. *BMJ* 2009, 338: b1326.

Singer G, Freedman LS. Injuries sustained on "bouncy castles". *BMJ* 1992, 304: 912.

Singh A, Crockard HA. Quantitative assessment of cervical spondylotic myelopathy by a simple walking test. *Lancet* 1999, 354: 370–3.

Singh-Manoux A, Kivimaki M, Glymour MM, Elbaz A, Berr C, Ebmeier KP, *et al*. Timing of onset of cognitive decline: results from Whitehall II prospective cohort study. *BMJ* 2012, 344: 1–8.

Søyseth V, Kongerud J, Haarr D, Strand O, Bolle R, Boe J. Relation of exposure to airway irritants in infancy to prevalence of bronchial hyper-responsiveness in schoolchildren. *Lancet* 1995, 345: 217–20.

Stephens C, Budge C, Carryer J. What is this thing called hormone replacement therapy? Discursive construction of medication in situation practice. *Qualitative Health Research*, 2002, 12: 347–59.

Subramanian P, Kantharuban S, Subramanian V, Willis-Owen SAG, Willis-Owen CA. Orthopaedic surgeons: as strong as an ox and almost twice as clever? Multicentre prospective comparative study. *BMJ* 2011, 343: d7506.

Tang JL, Armitage JM, Lancaster T, Silagy CA, Fowler GH, Neil HAW. Systematic review of dietary intervention trials to lower blood total cholesterol in free-living subjects. *BMJ* 1998, 316: 1213–9.

Taylor DW, Barnett HJM, Haynes RB, Ferguson GG, Sackett DL, Thorpe KE, *et al*. Low-dose and high-dose acetylsalicyclic acid for patients undergoing carotid endarterectomy: a randomised controlled trial. *Lancet* 1999, 353: 2179–84.

Tebartz van Elst L, Woermann FG, Lemieux L, Thompson PJ, Trimble MR. Affective aggression in patients with temporal lobe epilepsy: a quantitative MRI study of the amygdala. *Brain* 2000, 123: 234–43.

Thompson C, Kinmonth AL, Stevens L, Peveler RC, Stevens A, Ostler KJ, *et al*. Effects of a clinical-practice guideline and practice-based education on detection and outcome of depression in primary care: Hampshire Depression Project randomised controlled trial. *Lancet* 2000, 355: 185–9.

Turnbull D, Holmes A, Shields N, Cheyne H, Twaddle S, Gilmour WH, *et al*. Randomised, controlled trial of efficacy of midwife-managed care. *Lancet* 1996, 348: 213–8.

Unwin C, Blatchley N, Coker W, Fery S, Hotopf M, Hull L, *et al*. Health of UK servicemen who served in the Persian Gulf War. *Lancet* 1999, 353: 169–78.

Veseth M, Binder PE, Borg M, Davidson L. Toward caring for oneself in a life of intense ups and downs: a reflexive-collaborative exploration of recovery in bipolar disorder. *Qualitative Health Research* 2012, 22: 119–133.

Wald NJ, Law MR, Morris JK, Bagnall AM. *Helicobacter pylori* infection and mortality from ischaemic heart disease: negative result from a large, prospective study. *BMJ* 1997, 315: 1199–201.

Watson JM, Kang'ombe AR, Soares MO, Chuang L-H, Worthy G, Bland JM, *et al.*, on behalf of the VenUS III Team. Use of weekly, low dose, high frequency ultrasound for hard to heal venous leg ulcers: the VenUS III randomised controlled trial. *BMJ* 2011, 342: d1092.

Wilson HS, Hutchinson SA, Holzemer WL. Reconciling incompatibilities: a grounded theory of HIV medication adherence and symptom management. *Qualitative Health Research* 2002, 12: 1309.

Wolfe CDA, Rudd AG, Howard R, Coshall C, Stewart J, Hajat C, *et al.* Incidence and case fatality rates of stroke subtypes in a multiethnic population: the South London Stroke Register. *Journal of Neurology, Neurosurgery & Psychiatry* 2002, 72: 211–6.

Zinkstok SM, Roos YB, on behalf of the ARTIS Investigators. Early administration of aspirin in patients treated with alteplase for acute ischaemic stroke: a randomised controlled trial. *Lancet* 2012, 380: 731–7.

Zoltie N, de Dombal FT. The hit and miss of ISS and TRISS. Yorkshire Trauma Audit Group. *BMJ* 1993, 307: 906.

Index

Understanding Clinical Papers, Third Edition. David Bowers, Allan House, David Owens and Bridgette Bewick.
© 2014 John Wiley & Sons, Ltd. Published 2014 by John Wiley & Sons, Ltd.